Head and Neck Cutaneous Cancer

Editors

CECELIA E. SCHMALBACH
KELLY M. MALLOY

OTOLARYNGOLOGIC CLINICS OF NORTH AMERICA

www.oto.theclinics.com

Consulting Editor
SUJANA S. CHANDRASEKHAR

April 2021 • Volume 54 • Number 2

ELSEVIER

1600 John F. Kennedy Boulevard • Suite 1800 • Philadelphia, Pennsylvania, 19103-2899

http://www.oto.theclinics.com

OTOLARYNGOLOGIC CLINICS OF NORTH AMERICA Volume 54, Number 2
April 2021 ISSN 0030-6665, ISBN-13: 978-0-323-81317-4

Editor: Stacy Eastman
Developmental Editor: Diana Ang

Otolaryngologic Clinics of North America (ISSN 0030-6665) is published bimonthly by Elsevier, Inc., 360 Park Avenue South, New York, NY 10010-1710. Months of issue are February, April, June, August, October, and December. Business and Editorial Offices: 1600 John F. Kennedy Blvd., Suite 1800, Philadelphia, PA 19103-2899. Customer Service Office: 6277 Sea Harbor Drive, Orlando, FL 32887-4800. Periodicals postage paid at New York, NY and additional mailing offices. Subscription prices are $437.00 per year (US individuals), $1278.00 per year (US institutions), $100.00 per year (US & Canadian student/resident), $559.00 per year (Canadian individuals), $1348.00 per year (Canadian institutions), $610.00 per year (international individuals), $1348.00 per year (international institutions), $270.00 per year (international student/resident). Foreign air speed delivery is included in all *Clinics'* subscription prices. All prices are subject to change without notice. **POSTMASTER:** Send address changes to *Otolaryngologic Clinics of North America*, Elsevier Health Sciences Division, Subscription Customer Service, 3251 Riverport Lane, Maryland Heights, MO 63043. **Telephone: 1-800-654-2452 (U.S. and Canada); 314-447-8871 (outside U.S. and Canada). Fax: 314-447-8029. E-mail: journalscustomerservice-usa@elsevier.com (for print support); journalsonlinesupport-usa@elsevier.com (for online support).**

Reprints. For copies of 100 or more of articles in this publication, please contact the Commercial Reprints Department, Elsevier Inc., 360 Park Avenue South, New York, NY 10010-1710. Tel.: 212-633-3874; Fax: 212-633-3820; E-mail: reprints@elsevier.com.

Otolaryngologic Clinics of North America is also published in Spanish by McGraw-Hill Interamericana Editores S.A., P.O. Box 5-237, 06500 Mexico D.F., Mexico.

Otolaryngologic Clinics of North America is covered in *MEDLINE/PubMed (Index Medicus), Current Contents/Clinical Medicine, Excerpta Medica, BIOSIS, Science Citation Index,* and *ISI/BIOMED.*

Contributors

CONSULTING EDITOR

SUJANA S. CHANDRASEKHAR, MD, FACS, FAAOHNS
Consulting Editor, *Otolaryngologic Clinics of North America*, Past President, American Academy of Otolaryngology–Head and Neck Surgery, Secretary-Treasurer, American Otological Society, Partner, ENT & Allergy Associates LLP, Clinical Associate Professor, Department of Otolaryngology–Head and Neck Surgery, Icahn School of Medicine at Mount Sinai, New York, New York; Clinical Professor, Department of Otolaryngology–Head and Neck Surgery, Donald and Barbara Zucker School of Medicine at Hofstra-Northwell, Hempstead, New York

EDITORS

CECELIA E. SCHMALBACH, MD, MSc, FACS
David Myers, MD Professor and Chair, Department of Otolaryngology–Head and Neck Surgery, Lewis Katz School of Medicine, Temple University, Director, Head and Neck Institute, Temple University Health System, Philadelphia, Pennsylvania

KELLY M. MALLOY, MD, FACS
Associate Professor of Otolaryngology–Head and Neck Surgery, University of Michigan Medical School, University of Michigan, Program Director, Head and Neck Surgical Oncology and Mircrovascular Reconstruction Fellowship, Associate Chief Clinical Officer of Surgical and Rehabilitation Services, University Hospital, Michigan Medicine, Ann Arbor, Michigan

JENNIFER A. VILLWOCK, MD, FAAOA
Department of Otolaryngology–Head and Neck Surgery, University of Kansas Medical Center, Kansas City, Kansas

AUTHORS

NISHANT AGRAWAL, MD
Department of Surgery, Section of Otolaryngology–Head and Neck Surgery, University of Chicago Medicine, Chicago, Illinois

ONEIDA A. AROSARENA, MD, FACS
Professor, Department of Otolaryngology–Head and Neck Surgery, Office of Health Equity, Associate Dean, Diversity and Inclusion, Lewis Katz School of Medicine, Temple University, Philadelphia, Pennsylvania

SEMIRRA L. BAYAN, MD
Assistant Professor, Department of Otorhinolaryngology, Mayo Clinic, Rochester, Minnesota

CRISTINA CABRERA-MUFFLY, MD
Associate Professor, Department of Otolaryngology–Head and Neck Surgery, University of Colorado School of Medicine, Aurora, Colorado

KAREN Y. CHOI, MD
Assistant Professor, Department of Otolaryngology–Head and Neck Surgery, The Pennsylvania State University, College of Medicine, Hershey, Pennsylvania

DONTRE' M. DOUSE, MD
Department of Otorhinolaryngology, Mayo Clinic, Rochester, Minnesota

KRISTEN A. ECHANIQUE, MD
Department of Head and Neck Surgery, University of California, Los Angeles Medical Center, Los Angeles, California

ISSAM N. EID, MD, FACS
Assistant Professor, Department of Otolaryngology–Head and Neck Surgery, Lewis Katz School of Medicine, Temple University, Philadelphia, Pennsylvania

KEVIN EMERICK, MD
Associate Professor of Otolaryngology Head and Neck Surgery, Harvard Medical School, Massachusetts Eye and Ear Infirmary, Boston, Massachusetts

LESLIE A. FECHER, MD
Clinical Associate Professor of Medicine and Dermatology, University of Michigan, Rogel Cancer Center, Clinical Associate Professor of Medicine and Dermatology, Ann Arbor, Michigan

BRIAN B. HUGHLEY, MD, FACS
Department of Otolaryngology–Head and Neck Surgery, University of Florida, Gainesville, Florida

GINA D. JEFFERSON, MD, MPH, FACS
Professor, Division Chief, Head and Neck Oncologic and Microvascular Surgery, Department of Otolaryngology–Head and Neck Surgery, University of Mississippi Medical Center, Jackson, Mississippi

ADITYA JULOORI, MD
Department of Radiation and Cellular Oncology, Duchossois Center for Advanced Medicine, Chicago, Illinois

KIRAN KAKARALA, MD, FACS
Associate Professor, Head and Neck Surgery and Microvascular Reconstruction, Patient Safety and Quality Improvement Officer, Co-Director, Head and Neck Fellowship, Departments of Otolaryngology–Head and Neck Surgery and Health Policy and Management, University of Kansas School of Medicine, Kansas City, Kansas

ROHAN KATIPALLY, MD
Department of Radiation and Cellular Oncology, Duchossois Center for Advanced Medicine, Chicago, Illinois

ALOK R. KHANDELWAL, PhD
Department of Otolaryngology–Head and Neck Surgery, LSU Health Sciences Center, Shreveport, Louisiana

MIRIAM LANGO, MD
Professor, Department of Head and Neck Surgery, The University of Texas MD Anderson Cancer Center, Houston, Texas

JEFFREY C. LIU, MD
Department of Otolaryngology–Head and Neck Surgery, Lewis Katz School of Medicine, Temple University, Division of Head and Neck Oncology, Fox Chase Cancer Center, Philadelphia, Pennsylvania

SUSAN McCAMMON, MFA, MD, FACS
John W. Poynor Professor in Otolaryngology, Professor, Department of Otolaryngology–Head and Neck Surgery, Department of Internal Medicine, Division of Gerontology, Geriatrics and Palliative Care, The University of Alabama at Birmingham, Birmingham, Alabama

CAITLIN P. McMULLEN, MD
Assistant Professor, Department of Head and Neck – Endocrine Oncology Program, Moffit Cancer Center, Tampa, Florida, USA

KELLY M. MALLOY, MD, FACS
Associate Professor of Otolaryngology–Head and Neck Surgery, University of Michigan Medical School, University of Michigan, Program Director, Head and Neck Surgical Oncology and Mircrovascular Reconstruction Fellowship, Associate Chief Clinical Officer of Surgical and Rehabilitation Services, University Hospital, Michigan Medicine, Ann Arbor, Michigan

LAWRENCE MARK, MD, PhD
Department of Dermatology, Indiana University School of Medicine, Indianapolis, Indiana

MARCUS MONROE, MD, FACS
Associate Professor, Head and Neck Surgery, Physician Lead, Head and Neck Clinical Trials Program, Co-Lead, Head and Neck Disease-Oriented Team, Huntsman Cancer Institute, University of Utah School of Medicine, Salt Lake City, Utah

CHERIE ANN NATHAN, MD, PhD
Department of Head and Neck Surgery, University of California, Los Angeles Medical Center, Los Angeles, California; Jack Pou Endowed Professor and Chairman, Department of Otolaryngology–Head and Neck Surgery, LSU Health-SHV, Director of Head and Neck Surgical Oncology, Feist-Weiller Cancer Center, Shreveport, Louisiana

ERIN K. O'BRIEN, MD
Associate Professor, Department of Otorhinolaryngology, Mayo Clinic, Rochester, Minnesota

MIRIAM A. O'LEARY, MD
Assistant Professor, Chief, Division of Head & Neck Surgery, Department of Otolaryngology–Head and Neck Surgery, Tufts Medical Center, Boston, Massachusetts

ALYSSA K. OVAITT, MD
Department of Otolaryngology–Head and Neck Surgery, The University of Alabama at Birmingham, Birmingham, Alabama

THOMAS J. OW, MD, MS
Associate Professor, Departments of Otorhinolaryngology–Head and Neck Surgery, and Pathology, Montefiore Medical Center/Albert Einstein College of Medicine, Bronx, New York

BRAD RUMANCIK, PharmD
Department of Dermatology, Indiana University School of Medicine, Indianapolis, Indiana

CECELIA E. SCHMALBACH, MD, MSc, FACS
David Myers, MD Professor and Chair, Department of Otolaryngology–Head and Neck Surgery, Lewis Katz School of Medicine, Temple University, Director, Head and Neck Institute, Temple University Health System, Philadelphia, Pennsylvania

ROSH SETHI, MD, MPH
Instructor in Otolaryngology-Head and Neck Surgery, Harvard Medical School, Brigham and Women's Hospital, Boston, Massachusetts

YELIZAVETA SHNAYDER, MD
Professor, Department of Otolaryngology–Head and Neck Surgery, University of Kansas School of Medicine, Kansas City, Kansas

MAIE ST. JOHN, MD, PhD
Department of Head and Neck Surgery, University of California, Los Angeles Medical Center, Department of Head and Neck Surgery, UCLA Head and Neck Cancer Program, David Geffen School of Medicine, UCLA, Los Angeles, California

JANALEE K. STOKKEN, MD
Associate Professor, Department of Otorhinolaryngology, Mayo Clinic, Rochester, Minnesota

BRITTNY N. TILLMAN, MD
Department of Otolaryngology–Head and Neck Surgery, University of Texas Southwestern Medical School, Dallas, Texas

KATHRYN M. VAN ABEL, MD
Associate Professor, Department of Otorhinolaryngology, Mayo Clinic, Rochester, Minnesota

STEVEN J. WANG, MD
Professor, Chair, Department of Otolaryngology–Head and Neck Surgery, University of Arizona College of Medicine, Tucson, Arizona

MELISSA A. WILSON, MD, PhD
Associate Professor of Medical Oncology, Sidney Kimmel Cancer Center, Thomas Jefferson University, Associate Professor of Medical Oncology, Philadelphia, Pennsylvania

VIVIAN F. WU, MD, MPH
Senior Staff Surgeon, Department of Otolaryngology–Head and Neck Surgery, Henry Ford Health System, Clinical Assistant Professor, Wayne State University, School of Medicine

Contents

Cutaneous malignancy is becoming an increasing public health burden in terms of morbidity and cost, associated with changing environmental exposures and increased longevity of the general and the immunosuppressed population. Yet the understanding of the scope of this problem is hindered by lack of robust registries for nonmelanoma skin cancer. The risk factor responsible for most of these cancers, exposure to ultraviolet radiation, can be mitigated. However, greater consensus is necessary to enact effective prevention and screening programs. New developments, including identification of biomarkers and use of artificial intelligence, show promise for targeting screening efforts.

There has been a drastic increase in the incidence of nonmelanoma (NMSC), including squamous, basal cell, and melanoma skin cancers worldwide. Most cases of skin cancer can be treated effectively with surgery; fewer than 10% of cases are advanced and may require additional therapies. A better understanding of the biology of skin cancer will help contribute to better prognostic information and identification of possible new therapeutic targets. Herein, the authors review the biology and pathogenesis of both NMSC and melanoma, focusing on critical cell signaling pathways mediating the disease and current therapeutic strategies targeted to underlying genetic pathways.

Basal cell carcinoma is the most common skin malignancy worldwide. While early basal cell carcinomas can be treated with simple excision, advanced basal cell cancers require a multidisciplinary management approach. The mainstay of treatment remains surgical excision with appropriate reconstruction. Some advanced tumors may require radical resections; however, extensive, high-risk surgery may be justified by the indolent biology of the disease and the likelihood of cure. Other options, such as radiation or systemic targeted therapy, may be considered in selected patients who either refuse or are not candidates for surgery. The focus of this article is primarily on management of these high-risk cases.

Sentinel lymph node biopsy is the most precise and accurate staging technique for malignant melanoma. This resulted from international collaborations and technical innovations across subspecialties and systematic and methodical study of real-time clinical problems. This article describes sentinel node biopsy from conception to current techniques. Indications for the procedure and evidence of its prognostic value are discussed. Controversies surrounding results of Multicenter Selective Lymphadenectomy Trial I and II and German Dermatologic Cooperative Oncology Group Selective Lymphadenectomy trial are reviewed. Head and neck melanoma is presented as a unique subsite for performing sentinel node biopsy and when considering completion cervical lymphadenectomy.

Sentinel lymph node biopsy has the potential to impact regional control and survival for high-risk cutaneous malignancy. The outcome of sentinel lymph node biopsy is a potential guide for treatment and surveillance. The population of high-risk nonmelanoma patients that will benefit from sentinel lymph node biopsy remains to be determined. Any cutaneous malignancy with a greater than 10% risk of occult metastasis should be considered for sentinel lymph node biopsy or active surveillance. Localized cutaneous squamous cell carcinoma lesions with multiple high-risk features and nearly all patients with localized Merkel cell carcinoma should be considered for sentinel lymph node biopsy.

Radiation therapy plays an integral role in the management of cutaneous malignancies of the head and neck. This article highlights the use of radiation therapy in the definitive and adjuvant setting for basal cell carcinoma, cutaneous squamous cell carcinoma, melanoma, and Merkel cell carcinoma. Themes that emerge include the overall efficacy of radiation therapy as a local therapy, the relevance of cosmesis, functional outcomes, late toxicities as secondary end points, and the multitude of treatment modalities that are used.

The treatment of advanced melanoma has changed dramatically over the last decade. With the discovery of activating BRAF mutations and the development of targeted therapies and checkpoint inhibitors, the overall survival of patients with advanced melanoma has improved. This article provides an overview of systemic therapies, including the pivotal agents that have led to these advances.

Caitlin P. McMullen and Thomas J. Ow

Systemic therapy for patients with head and neck cutaneous squamous cell carcinoma (HNCSCC) generally is used for patients with advanced disease and most often employed for patients in the palliative setting when disease is unresectable and/or widely metastatic. Cytotoxic agents and epidermal growth factor receptor pathway targeted therapy have been utilized most commonly, with few clinical data to support their efficacy. Adjuvant postoperative chemoradiation with platinum has been called into question based on recent data. Programmed cell death protein 1 receptor immune checkpoint inhibitors have demonstrated profound activity in HNCSCC, and cemiplimab and pembrolizumab now are approved for use for unresectable/metastatic disease.

Miriam Lango and Yelizaveta Shnayder

The incidence of Merkel cell carcinoma (MCC) continues to increase. Understanding of MCC biology has advanced rapidly, with current staging providing valuable prognostic information. MCC treatment often is multidisciplinary. Surgery remains an important component in the staging and treatment, most commonly involving wide excision of the cancer and sentinel lymph node biopsy. Lymphadenectomy is used to treat nodal disease. Radiotherapy enhances locoregional control and possibly survival. Systemic therapies, in particular novel immunotherapies, may be promising in the treatment of advanced or recurrent and metastatic disease.

Brittny N. Tillman and Jeffrey C. Liu

Cutaneous sarcomas represent a rare group of tumors presenting in the head and neck. In this article, we discuss specific sarcoma tumor types and their presentation, pathogenesis, histologic findings, and management recommendations. Tumors to be reviewed include dermatofibrosarcoma protuberans, atypical fibroxanthoma, pleomorphic dermal sarcoma, cutaneous leiomyosarcoma, and angiosarcoma.

Issam N. Eid and Oneida A. Arosarena

The goals of cutaneous malignancy reconstruction are to restore the best functional and aesthetic outcome. Reconstruction should aim to restore all defects layers. While local flaps are the mainstay of head and neck Mohs reconstruction, the range of reconstructive options varies from healing by secondary intention to microvascular free tissue transfer.

The immunosuppressed (IS) population encompasses a diverse cohort of patients to include iatrogenically immunocompromised organ transplant recipients as well as patients with chronic lymphoid malignancies, human immunodeficiency virus/acquired immunodeficiency syndrome, and autoimmune disorders. Cutaneous cancers in this high-risk patient group are clinically distinct from the general immunocompetent population, showing aggressive behavior with associated poor outcomes. This article reviews the pathogenesis, epidemiology, incidence, prognosis, and special considerations required in managing cutaneous cancers in the IS patient population.

Discussions of ethics in surgery generally focus on the principles of beneficence, nonmalfeasance, autonomy, and justice. Caring for elderly patients with advanced cutaneous malignancies often requires the added consideration of narrative ethics to account for the expanded circle of care, complex medical conditions, and different goals of treatment often seen in this population. By focusing on the patient's illness narrative and relying on the collective experiences of the patient and surgeon, compassionate and appropriate care can be provided for these often-devastating disease processes.

Head and neck cutaneous melanomas pose many treatment challenges. Intratumoral injectables offer local and possibly systemic therapy in unresectable lesions. Talimogene laherparepvec, an injectable oncolytic type 1 herpes simplex virus, can improve durable response rates compared with systemic granulocyte-macrophage colony-stimulating factor therapy in patients with stage IIIB to IVM1a unresectable melanoma. These benefits were most noticed in lower-stage subsets and treatment naive patients. Efficacy of talimogene laherparepvec was maintained in patients with head and neck melanoma. Talimogene laherparepvec plus systemic immunotherapies is being studied, with promising preliminary data. Numerous ongoing clinical trials are investigating other viral and nonviral injectables.

Mohs micrographic surgery (MMS) represents an excellent means to address basal cell carcinoma and some squamous cell carcinomas (cSCCs) of the head and neck region, achieving excellent outcomes with respect to local recurrence rates and disease-specific survival. MMS by virtue of its technique maximally preserves uninvolved tissues of the head and neck, thereby maintaining form, cosmesis, and function to the greatest extent as dictated by the disease. However, the application of

MMS for managing high-risk cSCC and melanoma requires additional investigation. MMS may also prove beneficial in treating rare cutaneous diseases such as Merkel cell carcinoma and dermatofibrosarcoma protuberans.

Mentorship and sponsorship are critically important for otolaryngologists at all levels of their career. Mentorship is typically found within a long-term professional relationship and provides career advice and support. Sponsorship is a more transactional relationship that promotes the mentee for specific career advancement opportunities. Both help mentees achieve more in their careers and have higher career satisfaction. This article defines mentorship and sponsorship and the current state of these within otolaryngology. Strategies for being an effective mentor and mentee are listed. Mentorship needs among women and underrepresented minorities within otolaryngology are discussed.

Otolaryngology continues to have one of the lowest percentages of Black physicians of any surgical specialty, a number than has not improved in recent years. The history of exclusion of Black students in medical education as well as ongoing bias affecting examination scores, clerkship grades and evaluations, and honors society acceptance of Black students may factor into the disproportionately low number of Black otolaryngology residents. In order to increase the number of Black physicians in otolaryngology, intentional steps must be taken to actively recruit, mentor, and train Black physicians specializing in otolaryngology.

OTOLARYNGOLOGIC CLINICS
OF NORTH AMERICA

SERIES OF RELATED INTEREST

Facial Plastic Surgery Clinics
Available at: https://www.facialplastic.theclinics.com/

THE CLINICS ARE AVAILABLE ONLINE!
Access your subscription at:
www.theclinics.com

Foreword

As Plain as The Nose on Your Face?

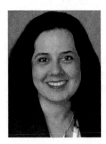

Sujana S. Chandrasekhar, MD, FACS, FAAOHNS
Consulting Editor

When I was a senior resident, a patient came into the Veterans Administration hospital with a huge fungating squamous cell tumor that had essentially replaced three-fourths of his nose. He was homeless, an alcohol abuser, malnourished and had unfortunately allowed this to grow over time. Resection resulted in significant cosmetic compromise, and reconstructive planning had to take into account the tumor, the defect, and the attendant socioeconomic and nutritional aspects pertaining to this patient. I had cared for an elderly man, a church leader, with a similar defect in the private hospital, who had undergone Mohs surgery under ketamine anesthesia in the dermatologist's office. Eight hours later, he was admitted to our service for bleeding control from what was essentially a rhinectomy, which then required reconstruction.

Cutaneous cancer of the head and neck poses particular challenges for the patient and their health care team. As the Guest Editors of this issue of *Otolaryngologic Clinics of North America*, Drs Cecelia Schmalbach and Kelly Malloy, point out, skin cancers are the most common cancers in the United States, and the majority of them occur on the sun-exposed regions of the head and neck. As with other otolaryngologic cancers, the goal is maximal tumor control while maintaining as normal a cosmetic appearance as possible. With cutaneous cancer defects, this can be particularly taxing.

Even though the risks of sun exposure and tanning have been known for some time, there was a staggering 26% increase in skin squamous cell carcinoma between the 1980s and 2010. As a result, the cost of care has increased dramatically, and it is 5 times as high as for other cancer sites. But this increased experience has a silver lining; it has resulted in significant improvements in treatments and outcomes. Key thought-leaders in this space, Drs Schmalbach and Malloy have compiled a comprehensive issue on Cutaneous Head and Neck Cancer, with articles by experts in the field.

To tackle a problem, one must know whom it affects and how to teach the public about prevention. Without understanding tumor biology, a given surgeon's one hammer

Otolaryngol Clin N Am 54 (2021) xiii–xiv
https://doi.org/10.1016/j.otc.2021.01.002
0030-6665/21/© 2021 Published by Elsevier Inc.

oto.theclinics.com

will be the wrong implement in many cases. Basal cell carcinoma (BCCa) is considered "easy," that is, early BCCa is treated locally by our dermatology colleagues alone or along with otolaryngology if a larger resection or flap reconstruction is needed, and incorporating, say, oculoplastics involvement if the eyelids are affected. However, advanced BCCa behaves differently and is more challenging. Understanding the predictive nature and importance of sentinel node biopsy is important, as we consider degree of resection, radiation therapy, and systemic therapy for various tumor types. This issue includes an article on reconstruction, which is vital for the diagnostic and extirpative physician and surgeon to understand. The patient examples I gave above highlight the need for the articles on special care for individuals who are immunocompromised and elderly, on when to consider offering injectables, on what Mohs surgery is and does, and where we, as otolaryngologists, interface with other specialty colleagues.

Again, I compliment Drs Schmalbach and Malloy on curating this comprehensive reference issue on cutaneous cancer of the head and neck. Although the tumor may be as plain as the nose on your face, the treatments are often varied. The otolaryngologist who takes the time and energy to read this cover to cover will find themselves better able to care for these patients in a comprehensive manner.

Sujana S. Chandrasekhar, MD, FACS, FAAOHNS
Consulting Editor
Otolaryngologic Clinics of North America
Past President
American Academy of Otolaryngology–
Head and Neck SurgerySecretary-Treasurer
American Otological Society
Partner, ENT & Allergy Associates LLP
18 East 48th Street, 2nd Floor
New York, NY 10017, USA

Clinical Professor
Department of Otolaryngology–
Head and Neck Surgery
Zucker School of Medicine at Hofstra-Northwell
Hempstead, NY, USA

Clinical Associate Professor
Department of Otolaryngology–
Head and Neck Surgery
Icahn School of Medicine at Mount Sinai
New York, NY, USA

E-mail address:
ssc@nyotology.com

Website:
http://www.ears.nyc

Preface

Head and Neck Cutaneous Cancer

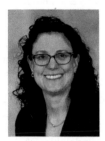   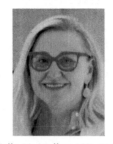

Cecelia E. Schmalbach, MD, MSc, FACS   Kelly M. Malloy, MD, FACS

Editors

Cutaneous cancer is the most commonly diagnosed malignancy in the United States with an estimated 3.5 million cases of nonmelanoma skin cancer diagnosed annually, in addition to 60,000 invasive melanoma cases.[1,2] The incidence is growing at epidemic proportions: there has been a 263% increase in cutaneous squamous cell carcinoma (cSCC) between the time periods of 1976 to 1984 and 2000 to 2010.[1] This exponential growth is attributed to our aging patient population, outdoor lifestyle changes, increased use of tanning beds, sun-worshipping tendencies, advances in solid organ transplantation, and changes to the ozone.[3]

The cost to diagnose and treat this growing patient population of cutaneous cancer patients continues to skyrocket as well. Within the United States, the total annual national cost increased from $3.6 billion to $8.1 billion between the time periods of 2002 to 2006 and 2007 to 2011.[1] This 125.2% increase is exorbitant when compared with the 25.1% cost increase reported for all other cancer sites. Consequently, cutaneous cancer is a public health priority with a significant associated economic burden.

The majority of cutaneous cancers occur on the sun-exposed regions of the head and neck. For this reason, we dedicated an entire issue of *Otolaryngologic Clinics of North America* to this important topic. In the following pages, we present a contemporary and comprehensive overview of the most common cancers, such as melanoma, cSCC, basal cell carcinoma (BCC), as well as the rarer tumors that head and neck surgeons may encounter in practice (Merkel cell carcinoma, sarcoma). All treatment modalities are discussed, from surgical therapies and innovations, to radiation therapy, systemic treatment options, and injectables. Challenges faced in treating both the immunosuppressed and the geriatric patient population are also highlighted.

The field of cutaneous cancer has experienced exciting changes over the past decade. From the diagnostic standpoint, sentinel node biopsy has become standard of care for localized melanoma[4,5] and Merkel cell carcinoma.[4,5] Impactful modifications have been made to the American Joint Committee on Cancer staging for both

Otolaryngol Clin N Am 54 (2021) xv–xvi
https://doi.org/10.1016/j.otc.2021.01.001
0030-6665/21/© 2021 Published by Elsevier Inc.

melanoma[2] and cSCC,[6] allowing for better risk stratification and counseling of our patients. Alternative treatment options are finally available for patients with recalcitrant and often unresectable skin cancers, from hedgehog inhibitors for advanced BCC and programmed cell death inhibitors-1 in advanced cSCC,[7] to biologic therapies in melanoma.[4] We have witnessed the first significant impact in melanoma survival rates since 1968, thanks to these developments in targeted therapy and immunotherapies.[8]

Building a comprehensive issue on a diverse and rapidly changing field would not be possible without a cadre of talented and dedicated surgical, medical, and radiation oncologists. We would like to thank our authors for sharing their time, passion, and expertise in their respective areas of head and neck cutaneous malignancy. They are truly the leading experts in the field.

Cecelia E. Schmalbach, MD, MSc, FACS
3440 North Broad Street
Kresge West, 3rd Floor, 309
Philadelphia, PA 19140, USA

Kelly M. Malloy, MD, FACS
1500 East Medical Center Drive
#1904 TC Spc 5312
Ann Arbor, MI 48109, USA

E-mail addresses:
Cecelia.Schmalbach@tuhs.temple.edu (C.E. Schmalbach)
kellymal@med.umich.edu (K.M. Malloy)

REFERENCES

1. Guy GP Jr, Machlin SR, Ekwueme DU, et al. Prevalence and costs of skin cancer treatment in the U.S., 2002-2006 and 2007-2011. Am J Prev Med 2015;48(2):183–7.
2. Gershenwald JE, Scolyer RA, Hess KR, et al. Melanoma of the skin. In: Amin MB, et al, editors. AJCC Cancer Staging Manual. Eighth Edition. Chicago: Springer; 2017.
3. Stang A, Khil L, Kajüter H, et al. Incidence and mortality for cutaneous squamous cell carcinoma: comparison across three continents. J Eur Acad Dermatol Venereol 2019;33(Suppl 8):6–10.
4. National Comprehensive Cancer Network (NCCN). NCCN Clinical Practice Guidelines in Oncology. Cutaneous melanoma. Version 4.2020. Available at: https://www.nccn.org/professionals/physician_gls/pdf/cutaneous_melanoma.pdf. Accessed September 3, 2020.
5. National Comprehensive Cancer Network (NCCN). NCCN Clinical Practice Guidelines in Oncology. Merkel cell carcinoma. Version 1.2020. Available at: https://www.nccn.org/professionals/physician_gls/pdf/mcc_blocks.pdf. Accessed September 3, 2020.
6. Califano JA, Lydiatt WM, Nehal KS, et al. Cutaneous squamous cell carcinoma of the head and neck. In: Amin MB, et al, editors. AJCC Cancer Staging Manual. Eighth Edition. Chicago: Springer; 2017.
7. National Comprehensive Cancer Network (NCCN). NCCN Clinical Practice Guidelines in Oncology. Squamous cell skin cancer. Version 2.2020. Available at: http://NCCN.org/professionals/physician_gls/pdf/squamous.pdf. Accessed August 1, 2020.
8. Siegel RL, Miller KD, Jemal A. Cancer statistics, 2019. CA Cancer J Clin 2019;69:7–34.

Epidemiology and Prevention of Cutaneous Cancer

Miriam A. O'Leary, MD[a],*, Steven J. Wang, MD[b]

KEYWORDS

- Nonmelanoma skin cancer • Melanoma • Epidemiology • UV radiation
- Indoor tanning • Screening • Prevention

KEY POINTS

- Nonmelanoma skin cancer is the most common malignancy in the United States; melanoma is the fifth most common cancer in the United States but is the leading cause of death among skin cancers.
- Lack of mandated reporting for nonmelanoma skin cancers hinders the ability to accurately study their incidence, outcomes, and cost.
- Incidence of cutaneous malignancies is rapidly increasing, in association with increased longevity, a growing immunosuppressed population, and changes in patterns of ultraviolet radiation exposure.
- The United States does not have a national skin cancer prevention program, because of lack of consensus regarding the efficacy and evidence of beneficial outcomes.
- Universal skin-cancer screening may not be cost-effective, but targeted screening of high-risk populations is generally accepted by experts as worthwhile.

INCIDENCE

Cutaneous malignancy is the most common human cancer, in the United States and worldwide. The incidence of skin cancer is higher than all other cancers combined. In the United States alone, more than 9500 people are diagnosed with skin cancer every day, and more than two people die of the disease every hour.[1] One in five Americans develop skin cancer by the age of 70.[2] Incidence is difficult to assess accurately because the most common types, basal cell carcinoma (BCC) and squamous cell carcinoma (SCC), are not required to be reported to cancer registries.[3] A 2015 study

[a] Department of Otolaryngology–Head and Neck Surgery, Tufts Medical Center, Box #850, 800 Washington Street, Boston, MA 02111, USA; [b] Department of Otolaryngology–Head and Neck Surgery, University of Arizona College of Medicine, 1501 North Campbell Avenue, Room 5401, Tucson, AZ 85724, USA
* Corresponding author.
E-mail address: moleary@tuftsmedicalcenter.org

Otolaryngol Clin N Am 54 (2021) 247–257
https://doi.org/10.1016/j.otc.2020.11.001
oto.theclinics.com

using Medicare databases and national survey data found that 5.4 million cases of nonmelanoma skin cancer (NMSC) were treated in 3.3 million patients in 2012.[4] BCC is the most common cutaneous malignancy, accounting for roughly 80% of NMSC, with approximately 4.3 million cases diagnosed in the United States each year, whereas more than 1 million cases of SCC are diagnosed annually.[5]

Invasive melanoma is mandated by law to be reported to cancer registries. Therefore, we better understand the numbers for this disease, although there is evidence that melanomas are underreported. Proposed reasons include the outpatient treatment of many melanomas, which may lead them to go undetected by automated surveillance systems.[6] Despite potential reporting inaccuracies, it is clear that invasive melanoma constitutes a small proportion of all cutaneous malignancies (1% according to the Surveillance, Epidemiology, and End Results database) but is responsible for the preponderance of skin cancer mortality. This year, new melanoma diagnoses will number around 100,350 in the United States, and 6850 people will die of the disease.[7] Although it is orders of magnitude less common than NMSC, melanoma is the fifth most common reported cancer in the United States, trailing only breast, lung, prostate, and colorectal malignancies. Melanoma currently accounts for 5.6% of all reported new cancer diagnoses in this country.[7] Most cutaneous malignancies occur in Whites, which, in combination with climate, dictates the geographic distribution around the globe. According to research cited by Bradford,[8] skin cancer accounts for approximately 35% to 45% of all cancers in Whites, 4% to 5% in Hispanics, 2% to 4% in Asians, and 1% to 2% in Blacks. Sixty percent to 75% of melanomas in Blacks, Asians, and native Hawaiians occur on the palms, soles, mucous membranes, and nail regions, which contain less melanin.[9]

Among Whites, skin cancer risk is highest in those with light skin pigmentation, light hair and eye color, and skin that burns easily.[10,11] Risk of melanoma and NMSC is more common in men and in older people. BCC incidence is 30% higher in men than women. Fifty-five to 75 year olds have a 100-fold higher rate of BCC compared with those younger than 20 years of age.[12] For SCC, incidence is 50 to 300 times higher in those older than 75 years versus those younger than 45 years old.[13] Melanoma is more common in women than men in people younger than 50 years of age, but rates in men far outpace those in women with increasing age, with a 2:1 ratio by age 65 and a 3:1 ratio by age 80. Several factors may explain these differences, including gender and age variations in occupational and recreational exposure to ultraviolet radiation (UVR), and divergences in health care use.[14] Aside from the commonly acknowledged at-risk population of older White patients, cutaneous malignancy is an underappreciated disease in other distinct populations, namely young women, patients of Hispanic ethnicity, and homosexual men.[15] A concerning development is the increase in NMSC diagnoses among American younger than 45 years of age, especially women.[16] Christenson and Borrowman[16] hypothesize that this trend is associated with increased use of tanning beds and increased sun exposure, and greater public awareness of cutaneous malignancy, leading to improved surveillance.

Most NMSCs are curable, especially if the cancer is detected and treated early. Mortality from BCC and SCC is known to be uncommon, but again difficult to track because reporting is not mandated for these cancers. However, given the prevalence of these diseases, the mortality burden is substantial. It is estimated that more than 15,000 people die of SCC in the United States each year, more than twice the number of mortalities from melanoma.[17] Worldwide, more than 5400 people die of NMSC skin cancer every month.[18] Death from NMSC occurs mostly in the elderly, those who present at an advanced stage, and the immunosuppressed. Although melanoma is also frequently curable when detected in its earliest stages, its propensity for regional and distant metastasis far exceeds NMSC. The overall 5-year relative survival rate for melanoma is 92%.[3] Fortunately, 84% of cases are diagnosed at a localized stage, for which the 5-year survival rate is 99%. Survival drops substantially with regional metastases (65%) and distant metastases (25%). Recent breakthroughs in systemic treatment have led to one noteworthy improvement: more than half of patients diagnosed with distant-stage disease now survive at least 1 year. Black patients have significantly poorer outcomes, with an estimated 5-year overall melanoma survival rate of only 70%.[3] Hispanic and Black patients are typically diagnosed at a more advanced stage than are non-Hispanic White patients; 52% of Black patients and 26% of Hispanic patients are diagnosed with melanoma at an advanced stage, compared with 16% of non-Hispanic White patients.[19]

Already the most commonly diagnosed human cancer, cutaneous malignancy is rapidly growing in incidence. Diagnosis of NMSC in the United States increased by 77% between 1994 and 2014. Between 2010 and 2020, the number of melanoma diagnoses has increased by 47%.[3] Multiple factors seem to contribute to this trend. Developments in outdoor activities over the past five decades, evolution of clothing styles, lengthened lifespan, particularly for patients with immunocompromised immune systems, ozone depletion, and advances in skin cancer detection all seem to play a role.[2]

RISK FACTORS

Ninety percent of NMSC and 86% of melanomas are caused by exposure to UVR,[20,21] a type of electromagnetic radiation that is located between X-radiation and light on the electromagnetic spectrum. UVR is released by the sun and by devices, such as tanning beds, which can emit UVR in amounts 10 to 15 times higher than the sun at its peak intensity.[22] UVR causes cutaneous malignancy through a combination of mechanisms: DNA damage, suppression of the immune system, tumor promotion, and mutations in the *p53* tumor suppressor gene. DNA absorbs UVR, causing base modifications, strand breaks, cross-links, and DNA-protein cross-links. These DNA "photoproducts" lead to gene mutations, triggering cellular responses, such as cytokine release that stimulate tumor promotion, tumor progression, and immunosuppression. One of the most common gene mutations is in the *p53* tumor suppressor gene, found in more than 90% of cutaneous SCC. In fact, specific *p53* mutations caused by C to T or C:C to T:T transitions at pyrimidine-pyrimidine sequences are frequent enough to be considered a trademark of UVR carcinogenesis. These mutations have been found in 74% of sun-exposed normal human skin samples and only 5% of unexposed skin samples. UVR exposure has been shown in multiple studies, in humans and experimental animals, to diminish immune function.[23] Greater epidermal melanin in people with darker skin filters twice as much UVR as does the epidermis in Whites, explaining the demographic differences in skin cancer incidence.[24] Multiple studies have shown variations in the patterns of sun exposure that correlate with different cutaneous malignancies. Total cumulative sun exposure correlates with development of BCC and SCC, whereas intense intermittent exposure, including sunburns and childhood exposure, is more strongly associated with the development of melanoma, including areas of the body only intermittently exposed to the sun, such as the back in men and the legs in women.[25] Several studies have linked occupational sun exposure to SCC, including a case-control study by Schmitt and colleagues,[26] which found an almost two-fold risk of SCC in patients with high levels of sun exposure through their work.

UV-emitting tanning beds are categorized as a group 1 carcinogen by the International Agency for Research on Cancer, an affiliate of the World Health Organization, placing them in the same class as tobacco and asbestos.[27] More people now develop skin cancer because of indoor tanning than develop lung cancer caused by smoking. Indoor tanning is responsible for more than 450,000 new skin cancers annually, including more than 10,000 melanomas, 245,000 BCCs, and 168,000 SCCs.[28] Any history of indoor tanning increases one's lifetime risk of BCC by 29% and risk of SCC by 83%.[29] More specifically, it increases one's risk of developing BCC before the of age 40 by 69%.[30] A large cohort study of women in Norway over more than two decades demonstrated a dose-response association between tanning bed use and risk of cutaneous SCC.[29] Women with highest cumulative exposure to indoor tanning had a hazard ratio of 1.83 compared with never users for the development of cutaneous SCC. This correlation between cumulative indoor tanning exposure and cancer risk was not impacted by duration of use or age at initiation.[29]

A similar study by the same authors found that risk of developing melanoma also showed a dose-response association with tanning bed use, with highest cumulative exposure to tanning beds having an adjusted relative risk of 1.32. This study showed that age at initiation of use of less than 30 years carried a higher risk of developing melanoma, and at a slightly younger age (2.2 years earlier).[31] A 2012 meta-analysis demonstrated that any use of tanning beds was associated with a summary relative risk of melanoma of 1.20, and a 1.8% increase in risk of melanoma with each tanning bed exposure per year. Age of initiation of use less than 35 years of age increased the summary relative risk to 1.87.[32] Compounding this risk of malignancy is the correlation of tanning booth use with behaviors such as reduced use of protective clothing and shade when outdoors.[33] Even "sunless tanning" can lead people to increase their risk by neglecting to wear sunscreen and otherwise limit their sun exposure. Misguided beliefs about the benefits of tanning beds for seasonal depressive disorder and perceived vitamin D deficiency thwart educational efforts about the risks of UVR exposure.[34]

Family history of NMSC and melanoma has been shown to increase the risk of developing these diseases.[25] Genetic factors are suggested by multiple studies to play a role but is challenging to separate from the influence of shared cutaneous phenotypes and similar environmental exposures among families. There are several rare inherited disorders that markedly increase risk of cutaneous malignancy. Xeroderma pigmentosum and oculocutaneous albinism are associated with heightened risk of BCC and SCC. Nevoid BCC syndrome (Gorlin syndrome) and Bazex-Dupre-Christol syndrome increase risk of BCC, whereas epidermolysis bullosa and epidermodysplasia verruciformis increase risk of SCC. Familial atypical multiple mole and melanoma syndrome and atypical mole syndrome (also known as dysplastic nevus syndrome) increase risk of melanoma.[25]

IMMUNE SYSTEM FACTORS

A variety of immunocompromising conditions have a notable impact on the immune system's capacity to recognize and eliminate cutaneous malignancies. The most striking example of this is organ transplantation. More than half of White transplant recipients (solid organ transplant recipients [SOTRs]) develop cutaneous malignancy, on average 3 to 8 years after transplantation. Most of these are NMSC, with a predominance of SCC over BCC, versus the preponderance of BCC in the general population. SCC has a 65- to 250-fold increased incidence in SOTRs, whereas BCC has a 10-fold increased incidence.[35] Melanoma has a two- to five-fold increased incidence, and work by Fattouh and colleagues[36] demonstrates a steadily increasing incidence over the past two decades. Frequent routine skin cancer surveillance for transplant patients may be a contributing factor. Risk of cutaneous malignancy correlates with exposure to immunosuppressive medications, because incidence of NMSC increases with higher doses, longer duration, and increased numbers of these drugs. This helps explain why heart and lung transplants have the highest risk of skin cancers, because they require the highest levels of immunosuppression, compared with kidney and liver transplants. SOTRs are characteristically afflicted with many skin cancers, and with more aggressive skin cancers than those in the general population.[34] SCCs in transplant patients often grow rapidly. These patients have a 13.4% local recurrence rate, usually within the first 6 months after resection, and a 5% to 8% rate of metastasis, typically in the second year after resection.[37]

Patients with chronic lymphocytic leukemia, the most common adult leukemia in the United States, have an increased risk of cutaneous malignancy, with an eight-fold increased risk of NMSC and a two- to four-fold increased incidence of melanoma.[35] As in SOTRs, disease recurrence and mortality are more common than in the general population. Patients with human immunodeficiency virus overall have a two-fold increase in risk of BCC and five-fold increase in risk of SCC, and risk increases in those with poorly controlled disease, with lower CD4 counts and higher viral loads.[38] Patients treated with biologic agents for autoimmune diseases (including psoriatic arthritis, rheumatoid arthritis, and inflammatory bowel disease) have an increased risk of NMSC, mostly SCC, but not melanoma. These biologic agents include inhibitors of tumor necrosis factor and the interleukin-17 pathway.[39] Finally, immunosenescence, the gradual deterioration of the immune system that occurs with advancing age, has been linked to increasing risk of cancer, likely associated with deterioration in T-cell function that diminishes tumor immunosurveillance.[40,41]

PREVENTION

NMSC is the most common malignancy in the United States.[1] Melanoma is the fifth most common cancer in the United States but is the leading cause of death among skin cancers.[3] The average annual cost of skin cancer treatment in the United States more than doubled between 2002 and 2011 to $8.1 billion, whereas the costs of all other cancer treatment only increased by 25%.[42] The increasing incidence of NMSC and melanomas, and the increasing health care and economic costs related to the treatment and management of cutaneous cancers, suggests potential benefit of prevention and screening to decrease severity of this disease burden. However, there remains controversy and conflicting evidence regarding many prevention and screening methods including the efficacy of public health campaigns, benefits of sunscreen use, and cost-effectiveness of skin cancer screening.

Some of the best data regarding skin cancer prevention comes from Australia. In the 1980s, Australia implemented a national skin cancer prevention program focused on clothing, sunscreen, wearing hats, and seeking shade.[43] Between 1988 and 2011, the campaign is estimated to have prevented 50,000 cancers and 1400 deaths and produced a net savings of $92 million.[44] In another Australian study, 25- to 75-year-old people who applied sunscreen regularly for 5 years were found to have reduced melanoma incidence 10 years later.[45]

Although there are various programs focused on education and sun safety that have been reported in the United States, there has never been a national skin cancer prevention program.[15,43] A lack of consensus regarding the efficacy and evidence of beneficial outcomes of skin cancer prevention programs is likely responsible for the current state.

There is no consensus regarding recommendations for sunscreen use. This controversy exists because of some studies showing no decrease and other studies actually showing an increase in skin cancer incidence with sunscreen use.[46–48] The reasons for these conflicting data may be caused by individuals using lower than recommended SPF or insufficient amounts of sunscreen may be applied to their skin.[49] The use of sunscreen may create a false sense of security leading individuals to possibly have longer sun exposure.[50] Some studies may not have followed study participants long enough, because it may take decades to see the beneficial impact of sunscreen use.[51] The annual cost of sunscreen is $200 to $400 for the average adult, which may be a socioeconomic barrier to use.[52] Free sunscreen dispensers have been suggested and exist in many countries.

Children are an especially vulnerable population because their skin is thinner, has finer hair follicles, and allows greater percutaneous absorption of UVR.[53] Children also tend to spend more time outdoors. Thus, approximately 50% of the estimated total lifetime exposure to radiation occurs before the age of 18.[54] Therefore, public health prevention efforts in children are especially important.

Indoor tanning, despite its obvious risks, remains a popular activity among young people, especially White women.[28] UVR from tanning booths is a known carcinogen and efforts to inform and persuade against this destructive practice is important.[55] Yet evidence points to need to use nontraditional platforms of outreach to more effectively convey this public health message to the target population.

SCREENING

In 2016, the US Preventative Services Task Force found insufficient evidence to recommend skin cancer screening for early detection.[56] A recent Cochrane review found similarly no evidence of benefit from universal screening programs for preventing melanoma.[57] Skin cancer screening for the general public might lead to overdiagnosis and a potential surge in treatment costs without significant mortality benefit.[58] It has been suggested that targeted screening of high-risk populations for cutaneous malignancies may be more worthwhile. By focusing on high-risk populations, it may be possible to prevent delayed diagnosis of melanomas or other skin cancers, which could mean avoiding costlier treatment, more invasive surgery, and the need for systemic treatment as opposed to simple excision.

Supporting the benefits of public skin cancer screening is the German experience of its SCREEN campaign, conducted in 2003 to 2004.[59] As part of a population-based skin cancer awareness campaign, the program included clinician and patient education and training and screening of nearly 20% of eligible adults aged 20 or older with a single annual clinical visual skin examination. On average, identified melanomas were 50% thinner, and there was an 8% relative reduction in melanoma mortality by 2009, suggesting earlier diagnosis and a benefit to the screening campaign. Unfortunately, the mortality benefit could not be sustained with further implementation of the German public health campaign.[60]

Although universal screening may not be cost-effective, targeted screening of high-risk populations is generally accepted by experts as worthwhile. Dermatologic societies have typically considered high-risk population groups to recommend for skin cancer screening to include patients with history of skin cancer or melanoma, organ-transplant patients, Fitzpatrick skin type I to III, family history of melanoma, severely sun-damaged skin, or history of indoor tanning.[56] Individuals from high-risk populations may have up to a 60-fold higher risk for developing skin cancer.[46] For example, people with a history of multiple skin cancers have a probability of developing another skin cancer of 50% within 1 year and 70% within 3 years of their last skin cancer diagnosis.[46]

The goal of screening of high-risk populations is earlier skin cancer diagnosis to allow for less radical surgery and eliminate need for systemic therapy. Ultimately, improved survival is the goal. However, the method of screening even for high-risk populations remains unclear. Increased public awareness and skin self-examination practices have been promoted for the general population by the American Cancer Society.[61] However, the prevalence of doing skin self-examinations in even high-risk groups remains low.[62] Full-body skin cancer screenings by health providers is possible but is fraught with different challenges. Given the higher regularity of visits to primary care providers, these providers would seem well positioned to lead in screenings; however, studies have shown primary care providers may lack sufficient preparation and training to identify early skin cancers.[63] Dermatologists, however, may lack sufficient numbers of providers and adequate time during visits to be able to meet the screening needs of even those at most risk.[59,64] But considering the significant cost savings that could be derived by reducing the burden of advanced skin cancer treatment, a concerted effort to improve quality and the resources available to provide comprehensive skin cancer screening for a defined at-risk population seems an important goal.

New research may provide additional tools to facilitate identification and screening of high-risk populations. UVR is a known risk factor for skin cancer; however, there may be decades between sunburn events and visible skin lesions. Studies have identified biomarkers, including p53, E-cadherin, Snail, Slug, and Twist, that are associated with UV-related progression to SCC and their precursor lesions, actinic kerotoses.[65–67] Multiple heritable mutations are known to be associated with risk for NMSC and melanoma, such as xeroderma pigmentosum and basal cell nevus syndrome.[68,69] Use of biomarkers may facilitate better risk-stratification of populations that would most benefit from skin cancer screening.

Artificial intelligence and machine learning may also provide additional tools to improve the accuracy and availability of skin cancer screenings. A recent promising study using artificial intelligence systems and a neural network trained on 129,450 clinical images found similar performance compared with 21 experienced clinical dermatologists.[70] Implementation of such a tool could potentially allow for tele-remote skin cancer screening location by nondermatologic health care providers.

In summary, cutaneous malignancy is becoming an increasing public health burden in terms of morbidity and cost, associated with changing environmental exposures and increased longevity of the general and the immunosuppressed population. Yet the understanding of the scope of this problem is hindered by lack of robust registries for NMSC. The risk factor responsible for most of these cancers (exposure to UVR) can be mitigated. However, greater consensus is necessary to enact effective prevention and screening programs. New developments, including identification of biomarkers and use of artificial intelligence, show promise for targeting screening efforts.

CLINICS CARE POINTS

- Cutaneous malignancy is becoming an increasing public health burden in terms of morbidity and cost, associated with changing environmental exposures and increased longevity of the general and the immunosuppressed population.
- Exposure to ultraviolet radiation is the risk factor responsible for most of these cancers, and tanning booth use substantially contributes to the incidence of cutaneous malignancies, particularly in younger people.
- Screening programs targeted at high risk populations could significantly reduce the morbidity and cost associated with advanced skin cancer treatment.

DISCLOSURE

M.A. O'Leary has no commercial or financial conflicts of interest to disclose. S.J. Wang has no commercial or financial conflicts of interest to disclose.

REFERENCES

1. Available at: https://www.skincancer.org/skin-cancer-information/skin-cancer-facts/ Accessed August 20, 2020.
2. Stern RS. Prevalence of a history of skin cancer in 2007: results of an incidence-based model. Arch Dermatol 2010;146(3):279–82.
3. Cancer Facts and Figures 2020. American Cancer Society. Available at: https://www.cancer.org/content/dam/cancer-org/research/cancer-facts-and-statistics/annual-cancer-facts-and-figures/2020/cancer-facts-and-figures-2020.pdf. Accessed August 26, 2020.
4. Rogers HW, Weinstock MA, Feldman SR, et al. Incidence estimate of nonmelanoma skin cancer (keratinocyte carcinomas) in the US population, 2012. JAMA Dermatol 2015;151(10):1081–6.
5. What are basal and squamous cell skin cancers? American Cancer Society. Available at: http://www.cancer.org/cancer/skincancer-basalandsquamouscell/detailedguide/skin-cancer-basal-and-squamous-cell-what-is-basal-and-squamous-cell. Accessed August 26, 2020.
6. Cockburn M, Swetter SM, Peng D, et al. Melanoma under-reporting: why does it happen, how big is the problem, and how do we fix it? J Am Acad Dermatol 2008; 59(6):1081.
7. Surveillance, Epidemiology, and End Results Program, National Cancer Institute. SEER stat fact sheets: melanoma of the skin. Available at: http://seer.cancer.gov/statfacts/html/melan.html. Accessed August 26, 2020.
8. Bradford PT. Skin cancer in skin of color. Dermatol Nurs 2009;21(4):170–8.
9. Gloster HM, Neal K. Skin cancer in skin of color. J Am Acad Dermatol 2006;55: 741–60.
10. Khalesi M, Whiteman DC, Tran B, et al. A meta-analysis of pigmentary characteristics, sun sensitivity, freckling and melanocytic nevi and risk of basal cell carcinoma of the skin. Cancer Epidemiol 2013;37:534.
11. Zanetti R, Rosso S, Martinez C, et al. The multicentre South European study 'Helios'. I: skin characteristics and sunburns in basal cell and squamous cell carcinomas of the skin. Br J Cancer 1996;73:1440.
12. Scotto J, Fears TR, Fraumeni JF Jr, et al. Incidence of nonmelanoma skin cancer in the United States in collaboration with Fred Hutchinson Cancer Research Center. NIH publication No. 83-2433. Bethesda (MD): U.S. Dept. of Health and Human Services, Public Health Service, National Institutes of Health, National Cancer Institute; 1983. p. 113, xv.
13. Gray DT, Suman VJ, Su WP, et al. Trends in the population-based incidence of squamous cell carcinoma of the skin first diagnosed between 1984 and 1992. Arch Dermatol 1997;133:735.
14. Skin Cancer Facts and Statistics. Available at: https://www.cancer.org/content/dam/cancer-org/research/cancer-facts-and-statistics/annual-cancer-facts-and-figures/2020/cancer-facts-and-figures-2020.pdf. Accessed August 26, 2020.
15. Linos E, Katz K, Colditz G. Skin cancer—the importance of prevention. JAMA Intern Med 2016;176(10):1435–6.
16. Christenson LJ, Borrowman TA. Incidence of basal cell and squamous cell carcinomas in a population younger than 40 years. JAMA 2005;294(6):681.

17. Mansouri B, Housewright C. The treatment of actinic keratoses—the rule rather than the exception. J Am Acad Dermatol 2017;153(11):1200.
18. Global Burden of Disease Cancer Collaboration. Global, regional and national cancer incidence, mortality, years of life lost, years lived with disability, and disability-adjusted life-years for 29 cancer groups, 1990 to 2017. JAMA Oncol 2019;5(12):1749–68.
19. Hu S, Soza-Vento RM, Parker DF, et al. Comparison of stage at diagnosis of melanoma among Hispanic, black, and white patients in Miami-Dade County, Florida. Arch Dermatol 2006;142(6):704–8.
20. Koh HK, Geller AC, Miller DR, et al. Prevention and early detection strategies for melanoma and skin cancer: Current status. Arch Dermatol 1996;132(4):436–42.
21. Parkin DM, Mesher D, Sasieni P. Cancers attributable to solar (ultraviolet) radiation exposure in the UK in 2010. Br J Cancer 2011;105:S66–9.
22. Le Clair MZ, Cockburn MG. Tanning bed use and melanoma: establishing risk and improving prevention interventions. Prev Med Rep 2016;3:139–44.
23. Ultraviolet-radiation-related exposures. Broad-spectrum UVR, pp. 1-5. NTP (National Toxicology Program). 2014. Report on Carcinogens, Thirteenth Edition. Research Triangle Park, NC: U.S. Department of Health and Human Services, Public Health Service. Available at: http://ntp.niehs.nih.gov/ntp/roc/content/profiles/ultravioletradiationrelatedexposures.pdf. Accessed August 26, 2020.
24. Montagna W. The architecture of black and white skin. J Am Acad Dermatol 1991;24:29–37.
25. Wu PA. Epidemiology, pathogenesis, and clinical features of basal cell carcinoma. Available at: https://www.uptodate.com/contents/epidemiology-pathogenesis-and-clinical-features-of-basal-cell-carcinoma. Accessed August 26, 2020.
26. Schmitt J, Haufe E, Trautmann F, et al. Is ultraviolet exposure acquired at work the most important risk factor for cutaneous squamous cell carcinoma? Results of the population-based case-control study FB-181. Br J Dermatol 2018;178(2):462.
27. El Ghissassi F, Baan R, Straif K, et al. Special report: policy. A review of human carcinogens—part D: radiation. Lancet 2009;10(8):751–2.
28. Wehner MR, Chren MM, Nameth D, et al. International prevalence of indoor tanning: a systematic review and meta-analysis. JAMA Dermatol 2014;150(4):390–400.
29. Lergenmuller S, Ghiasvand R, Robsahm TE, et al. Association of lifetime indoor tanning and subsequent risk of cutaneous squamous cell carcinoma. JAMA Dermatol 2019;155(12):1350–7.
30. Ferrucci LM, Cartmel B, Molinaro AM, et al. Indoor tanning and risk of early-onset basal cell carcinoma. J Am Acad Dermatol 2012;67(4):552–62.
31. Ghiasvand R, Rueegg CS, Weiderpass E, et al. Indoor tanning and melanoma risk: long-term evidence from a prospective population-based cohort study. Am J Epidemiol 2017;185(3):147–56.
32. Boniol M, Autier P, Boyle P, et al. Cutaneous melanoma attributable to sunbed use: systematic review and meta-analysis. BMJ 2012;345:4757.
33. Fischer AH, Wang TS, Yenokyan G, et al. Association of indoor tanning frequency with risky sun protection practices and skin cancer screening. JAMA Dermatol 2016;153(2):168–74.
34. Julian A, Thorburn S, Geldhof GJ. Health beliefs about UV and skin cancer risk behaviors. Cancer Control 2020;27:1–6.
35. Euvrard S, Kanitakis J, Claudy A. Skin cancers after organ transplantation. N Engl J Med 2003;348(17):1681–91.

36. Fattouh K, Ducroux E, Decullier E, et al. Increasing incidence of melanoma after solid organ transplantation:a retrospective epidemiological study. Transpl Int 2017;30(11):1172–80.

37. Howard MD, Su JC, Chong AH. Skin cancer following solid organ transplantation: a review of risk factors and models of care. Am J Clin Dermatol 2018;19(4): 585–97.

38. Collins L, Quinn A, Stasko T. Skin cancer and immunosuppression. Dermatol Clin 2019;37:83–94.

39. Chen Y, Friedman M, Liu G, et al. Do tumor necrosis factor inhibitors increase cancer risk in patients with chronic immune-mediated inflammatory disorders? Cytokine 2018;101:78–88.

40. Foster AD, Sivarapatna A, Gress RE. The aging immune system and its relationship with cancer. Aging Health 2011;7(5):707–18.

41. Mohan SV, Chang AL. Advanced basal cell carcinoma: epidemiology and therapeutic innovations. Curr Dermatol Rep 2014;3(1):40–5.

42. Guy GP Jr, Machlin SR, Ekwueme DU, et al. Prevalence and costs of skin cancer treatment in the US, 2002-2006 and 2007-2011. Am J Prev Med 2015;48(2): 183–7.

43. Trager MH, Queen D, Samie FH, et al. Advances in prevention and surveillance of cutaneous malignancies. Am J Med 2020;133(4):417–23.

44. Shih STF, Carter R, Heward S, et al. Skin cancer has a large impact on our public hospitals but prevention programs continue to demonstrate strong economic credentials. Aust N Z J Public Health 2017;41(4):371–6.

45. Green AC, Williams Gm, Logan V, et al. Reduced melanoma after regular sunscreen use: randomized trial follow-up. J Clin Oncol 2011;29(3):257–63.

46. Westerdahl J, Ingvar C, Masback A, et al. Sunscreen use and malignant melanoma. Int J Cancer 2000;87(1):145–50.

47. Wolf P, Quehenberger F, Mullegger R, et al. Phenotypic markers, sunlight-related factors and sunscreen use in patients with cutaneous melanoma: an Austrian case-control study. Melanoma Res 1998;8(4):370–8.

48. Green A, Williams G, Neale R, et al. Daily sunscreen application and betacarotene supplementation in prevention of basal-cell and squamous cell carcinomas of the skin: a randomized controlled trial. Lancet 1999;354(9180):723–9.

49. Kim SM, Oh BH, Lee YW, et al. The relation between the amount of sunscreen applied and the sun protection factor in Asian skin. J Am Acad Dermatol 2010; 62(2):218–22.

50. Autier P, Boniol M, Dore JF. Sunscreen use and increased duration of intentional sun exposure: still a burning issue. Int J Cancer 2007;121(1):1–5.

51. van der Pols JC, Williams GM, Pandeya N, et al. Prolonged prevention of squamous cell carcinoma of the skin by regular sunscreen use. Cancer Epidemiol Biomarkers Prev 2006;15(12):2546–8.

52. Johal R, Leo MS, Ma B, et al. The economic burden of sunscreen usage. Dermatol Online J 2014;20(6). 13030/qt6v0352fw.

53. Green AC, Wallingford SC, McBride P. Childhood exposure to ultraviolet radiation and harmful skin effects: epidemiological evidence. Prog Biophys Mole Biol 2011; 107(3):349–55.

54. Stern RS, Weinstein MC, Baker SG. Risk reduction for nonmelanoma skin cancer with childhood sunscreen use. JAMA Dermatol 1986;122(5):537–45.

55. Falzone AE, Brindis CD, Chren MM, et al. Teens, tweets, and tanning beds: rethinking the use of social media for skin cancer prevention. Am J Prev Med 2017;53(3S1):S86–94.

56. Johnson MM, Leachman SA, Aspinwall LG, et al. Skin cancer screening: recommendations for data-driven screening guidelines and a review of the US Preventive Services Task Force controversy. Melanoma Manag 2017;(1):13–37.

57. Johansson M, Brodersen J, Gøtzsche PC, et al. Screening for reducing morbidity and mortality in malignant melanoma. Cochrane Database Syst Rev 2019;6(6): CD012352.

58. Curiel-Lewandrowski C, Chen SC, Swetter SM, Melanoma Prevention Working Group-Pigmented Skin Lesion Sub-Committee. Screening and prevention measures for melanoma: is there a survival advantage? Curr Oncol Rep 2012;14(5): 458–67.

59. Breitbart EW, Waldmann A, Nolte S, et al. Systematic skin cancer screening in Northern Germany. J Am Acad Dermatol 2012;66(2):201–11.

60. Stang A, Jockel KH. Does skin cancer screening save lives? A detailed analysis of mortality time trends in Schleswig-Holstein and Germany. Cancer 2016;122(3): 432–7.

61. Be Safe in the Sun. American Cancer Society website. Available at: https://www.cancer.org/healthy/be-safe-in-sun/skin-exams.html. Accessed August 22, 2020.

62. Aitken JF, Janda M, Lowe JB, et al. Prevalence of whole-body skin self-examination in a population at high risk for skin cancer (Australia). Cancer Causes Control 2004;15:453–63.

63. Moore MM, Geller AC, Zhang Z, et al. Skin cancer examination teaching in US medical education. Ach Dermatol 2006;143:439–44.

64. Oliveria SA, Heneghan MK, Cushman LF, et al. Skin cancer screening by dermatologists, family practitioners, and internists: barriers and facilitating factors. Arch Dermatol 2011;147:39–44.

65. Trager MH, Geskin LJ, Samie FH, et al. Biomarkers in melanoma and non-melanoma skin cancer prevention and risk stratification. Exp Dermatol 2020. https://doi.org/10.1111/exd.14114.

66. Criscione VD, Weinstock MA, Naylor MF, et al. Actinic keratoses: natural history and risk of malignant transformation in the Veterans Affairs Topical Tretinoin Chemoprevention Trial. Cancer 2009;115(11):2523–30.

67. Bakshi A, Shafi R, Nelson J, et al. The clinical course of actinic keratosis correlates with underlying molecular mechanisms. Br J Dermatol 2019;182(4): 995–1002.

68. Kraemer KH, Patronas NJ, Schiffmann R, et al. Xeroderma pigmentosum, trichothiodystrophy and Cockayne syndrome: a complex genotype-phenotype relationship. Neuroscience 2007;145(4):1388–96.

69. Hahn H, Wicking C, Zaphiropoulous PG, et al. Mutations of the human homolog of Drosophila patched in the nevoid basal cell carcinoma syndrome. Cell 1996; 85(6):841–51.

70. Esteva A, Kuprel B, Novoa RA, et al. Dermatologist-level classification of skin cancer with deep neural networks. Nature 2017;342(7639):115–8.

Cutaneous Cancer Biology

Alok R. Khandelwal, PhD[a,1], Kristen A. Echanique, MD[b,1],
Maie St. John, MD, PhD[b,c,d], Cherie Ann Nathan, MD, PhD[e,*]

KEYWORDS

- Head and neck cancer • Cutaneous skin cancer • Squamous cell carcinoma
- Basal cell carcinoma • Melanoma • Merkel cell carcinoma

KEY POINTS

- Most cases of skin cancer can be treated effectively with surgery; fewer than 10% of cases are advanced and may require additional therapies.
- There has been a drastic increase in the incidence of nonmelanoma, skin cancers, including squamous and basal cell, and melanoma skin cancers worldwide.
- A better understanding of the biology of skin cancer will help contribute to better prognostic information and identification of possible new therapeutic targets.

CUTANEOUS SQUAMOUS CELL CARCINOMA

The incidence of cutaneous squamous cell carcinoma (cSCC) has now surpassed the combined incidence of breast, prostate, lung, and colon cancers combined.[1–3] The primary cause for cutaneous cancers is exposure to UV radiation. In response to UV radiation, skin keratinocytes mount a physiologic response and prevent the replication of UV-induced DNA damaged cells. Keratinocytes repair UV-B–induced DNA damage, become senescent, or after extreme UV-B exposure, undergo apoptosis. The pathogenesis of cSCC involves multiple steps, including formation of precancerous lesions characterized by actinic keratosis, followed by conversion to carcinoma in situ, and finally progressing into invasive cSCC. Subsequent steps include

[a] Department of Otolaryngology, Head and Neck Surgery, LSU Health Sciences Center, Shreveport, LA 71130, USA; [b] Department of Head and Neck Surgery, University of California, Los Angeles Medical Center, 10833 Le Conte Avenue, CHS 62-132, Los Angeles, CA 90095, USA; [c] Department of Head and Neck Surgery, David Geffen School of Medicine at University of California, Los Angeles (UCLA), Los Angeles, CA, USA; [d] UCLA Head and Neck Cancer Program, David Geffen School of Medicine at UCLA, Los Angeles, CA, USA; [e] Department of Otolaryngology/HNS, LSU Health-SHV, Feist-Weiller Cancer Center, 1501 Kings Highway, Shreveport, LA 71130, USA
[1] Equal contribution.
* Corresponding author. Department of Otolaryngology/HNS, LSU Health-SHV, Feist-Weiller Cancer Center, 1501 Kings Highway, Shreveport, LA 71130.
E-mail address: cnatha@lsuhsc.edu

Otolaryngol Clin N Am 54 (2021) 259–269
https://doi.org/10.1016/j.otc.2020.11.002
0030-6665/21/Published by Elsevier Inc.

oto.theclinics.com

neoangiogenesis, invasion into surrounding tissues, and formation of distant organ metastasis.[4]

In preclinical studies, the multistage model of skin carcinogenesis is composed of three stages: initiation, promotion, and progression.[5] In response to UV radiation or a genotoxic carcinogen, such as 7,12-dimethyl benz(a)-anthracene, irreversible genetic mutations in *H-ras* are induced that do not lead to any immediate morphologic changes. However, with subsequent exposure, these mutated epidermal cells undergo clonal expansion leading to hyperproliferation, hyperplasia, and development of premalignant papillomas.[5] Several key growth factor signaling mechanisms are activated, including epidermal growth factor receptor (EGFR), fibroblast growth factor receptor (FGFR), ERB2, STAT3, c-SRC, and AKT, that induce autonomous cell growth and invasion.[5]

Initiated cells can also undergo epithelial to mesenchymal transition (EMT) leading to metastatic and invasive carcinomas that are associated with inflammation and adaptive immunity. In the UV-B–induced model of cSCC, high-risk papillomas share a gene expression pattern with those at high risk for malignant conversion. The normal human epidermis is composed of the stratum corneum, lucidum, granulosum, spinosum, and basale. In response to UV or environmental stimuli, keratinocytes can become atypical and enlarged and undergo activation, overexpression, and amplification of tumor promoter genes, such as *RAS* and *BCL2*.[4] Additional alterations can occur, including a decrease in tumor suppressor genes, such as *p53*, leading to genomic instability and chromosome alterations. With subsequent induction, these enlarged and atypical keratinocytes may invade the dermis. Similar to the response to UV-B in preclinical studies, several cell-signaling pathways, such as ERB1 (EGFR), AKT, STAT3, and extracellular regulated kinase (ERK)/mitogen activated protein kinase (MAPK), are induced in human cSCC.[6] There is a subsequent increase in angiogenetic mediators, such as VEGF, MMPs, and the induction of EMT markers that promote metastasis.[6]

One well-recognized mutation present in nearly 90% of cSCC is a loss of function of *TP53*. Known as the guardian of the genome, loss of heterozygosity in *TP53* is associated with a significant increase in mutation burden.[7,8] UV light has been shown to produce pyrimidine dimers that promote uncontrolled proliferation of keratinocytes.[8] In a recent study by Zilberg and colleagues,[7] 90% of cSCC exhibited loss-of-function mutations in TP53. In oral SCC, mutations within the TP53 binding domain have been noted to be independent predictors of poor disease-specific survival.[9] Although this is yet to be validated in the cSCC literature, pilot data support that this may be predictive of prognosis in these patients as well.

Genetic Predisposition to Cutaneous Squamous Cell Carcinoma

Several hereditary syndromes exist that lead to the development of cSCC, including xeroderma pigmentosum, Ferguson-Smith syndrome, oculocutaneous albinism, and epidermodysplasia verruciformis (EV). Recent candidate gene studies have identified genes such as melanocortin 1 receptor (MC1R), tyrosinase (TYR), and interferon regulating factor (IRF4) to increase susceptibility to cSCC. In addition, specific populations have been studied recently through genome-wide association studies with loci identified that lead to pigmentary changes.[10] A rare autosomal recessive disorder, xeroderma pigmentosum, is caused by defects in the nucleotide excision repair mechanism that is essential for correcting and removing DNA damage caused by Ultraviolet Radiation (UVR).[11] Oculocutaneous albinism represents an autosomal recessive inherited group of disorders with defects in the biosynthesis of melanin leading to skin, hair, and eye hypopigmentation and increased susceptible to vision deficits and cSCC. Among the most common genetic mutations are mutations in the tyrosinase (*TYR*) gene as well as mutations in the *SLC452A* gene.[12] Also known as multiple self-healing squamous epitheliomas, Ferguson-Smith syndrome is a rare autosomal dominant disease marked by multiple tumors of the nose, ears, and mouth that have the ability to spontaneously regress. Although histologically indistinguishable from well-differentiated SCC, it is distinct in its ability for the tumor to involute. While healing, the ulcer displays dermal fibrosis, loss of elastic fibers, and keratin absorption. This syndrome is incredibly rare, with less than 100 reports described in the literature. It is marked by loss of heterozygosity in the *TGFBR1*. EV is an exceedingly rare autosomal recessive disease with a prevalence of less than 1 in 1,000,000. EV is unique because of its concurrent genetic predisposition for susceptibility to specific human papillomaviruses (HPVs). This genetic predisposition is due to gene mutations in the transmembrane channel *TMC6/EVER1* or *TMC8/EVER2* genes. Although the pathogenesis of disease is still poorly understood, cutaneous malignancy is thought to result from concurrent HPV infection in the setting of the aforementioned genetic mutations.[13]

BASAL CELL CARCINOMA

Basal cell carcinomas (BCCs) classically appear as slow-growing, translucent, elevated lesions on sun-exposed skin.[3] Locally invasive, BCCs are indolent epithelial neoplasms that arise from the basilar layer of the epidermis. These lesions tend to develop gradually, with the neoplastic cells spreading in a three-dimensional manner throughout the papillary and reticular dermis. Unlike cSCC wherein several signaling pathways can be involved, BCC is mainly associated with the Sonic Hedgehog (SHH) signaling axis.[14] The SHH signaling pathway is named after the family of extracellular hedgehog (HH) ligands, of which there are three in mammals: SHH, Indian hedgehog, and desert hedgehog.[15] Patched 1 (PTCH1) is the receptor to which the HH ligands bind and leads to disinhibition of the pathway induced by unbound PTCH1. A cascade of interacting proteins, including suppressor of fused, is then triggered that culminates in the activation of the downstream Gli family of transcription factors.[16] The stability of these molecules is controlled by phosphorylation and ubiquitination-proteolytic destruction.[17] In studies of mice engineered to conditionally express GLI-2, BCC regression is seen when GLI-2 expression is inactivated.[18] The absence of precursor lesions in BCC supports further research into biomolecular mechanisms underlying the initiation and histologic differentiation of BCC to allow for screening and early detection.

Genetic Predisposition to Basal Cell Carcinoma

Although far less common than primary BCC, nevoid basal cell carcinoma syndrome (NBCCS) is characterized by multiple BCCs. NBCCS is an autosomal dominant disorder with complete penetrance and variable expressivity. NBCCS is primarily caused by mutations in PTCH1 leading to constitutive activation of the HH pathway.[19] In addition to the development of BCCs at an early age, patients are also prone to developing other tumors, such as medulloblastoma.[20]

MELANOMA

The development and progression of melanoma is complex. Melanocytic nevi arise that go on to develop hyperplasia and dysplasia and finally lead to the radial growth phase of primary melanoma. Melanoma is characterized by a vertical growth phase, which unchecked leads to metastatic melanoma.[21] UVR is the primary cause of cutaneous melanoma and culminates into stereotypical nucleotide adducts known as cyclobutane pyrimidine dimers that support formation of pyrimidine dimer mutations, in which a cytosine located in a dipyrimidine sequence becomes mutated to thymidine. Exomic deep sequencing of human melanomas confirms the role of UVR in melanoma development, demonstrating an abundance of UV-derived genomic mutations within melanomas.[22] Exposure to UVR can also trigger the loss of cellular adhesion molecules, such as E-cadherin, P-cadherin, desmoglein, and connexins.[23]

Microphthalmia-associated transcription factor (MITF), a melanocytic lineage-specific transcription factor, is identified as a master regulator for melanocyte function and pigmentation. MITF is also recognized as a lineage survival factor for melanocytes. In addition, MITF regulates antiapoptotic genes, such as *BCL2*, *BCL2A1*, and cell-cycle regulatory genes, such as *CDK2*, thus playing an important role in melanocyte proliferation, survival, and melanoma progression. In melanoma, MITF is phosphorylated by MAPK leading to subsequent ubiquitin-dependent proteolysis.[24]

Genetic Predisposition to Melanoma

It is estimated that nearly 5% to 10% of all cases of cutaneous melanoma occur in families and are inherited in an autosomal dominant fashion with incomplete penetrance. Of these cases, 20% to 40% are noted to harbor germline mutations in CDKN2A. Other predisposing genes have been identified but are rare and collectively contribute to only 10% of additional familial cases. These genes include CDK4, BAP1, TERT, POT1, ACD, TERF2IP, and MITF.[25] It is recommended that suspected cases of familial melanoma should be offered genetic testing to screen for CDKN2A and CDK4.[25]

MERKEL CELL CARCINOMA

Merkel cell carcinoma (MCC) is a rare and aggressive neuroendocrine dermal neoplasm mainly associated with immunosuppression and aging. MCC is characterized by a solitary red to violaceous nodule usually less than 2 cm in size. The pathophysiology of MCC is often driven by infection with Merkel cell polyomavirus (MCPyV). Although most frequently found in the dermis, MCC can arise from any layer of the skin, ranging from intraepidermal to subcutaneous.[26]

Of significant clinical interest, the cell type responsible for MCC formation remains controversial. Several cell populations of, including but not limited to fibroblasts, pro-B cells or pre-B cells, dermal mesenchymal stem cells, and epidermal progenitor cell populations may potentially be involved in MCC.[27] In cases of virus-positive MCC, MCPyV binds to skin cells via heat shock proteins. The virus then integrates into the host cell and directly interacts with the retinoblastoma-associated protein (RB) binding motif. Responsible for direct inhibition of RB, MCPyV enables cell-cycle progression to S phase. Interestingly, 2 viral oncoproteins, truncated large T antigen (LT-t) and small T antigen (ST), are expressed in MCC host cells. MCPyV ST is hypothesized as the main driver of cellular transformation via an increase in LT protein levels through the activity of its large-T stabilization domain (LSD). The LSD of the virus inhibits E3 ubiquitin ligase activity via interactions with F-box/WD repeat-containing protein 7 and cell division cycle protein 20 homologue, resulting in increased oncoprotein stability and cap-dependent messenger RNA (mRNA) translation, respectively.[28] The ST antigen associates with protein phosphatase complex PP4 to inhibit nuclear factor-kappa B (NF-κB) signaling, eukaryotic translation initiation factor 4E-binding protein 1 (4E-BP1), CR1, conserved region 1, NEMO (NF-κB essential modulator), and the nuclear localization signal.

Other types of skin cancer that constitute less than 1% of all skin malignancies include dermatofibrosarcoma protuberans, atypical fibroxanthoma, adnexal carcinoma, and sebaceous carcinoma, but they are beyond the scope of this review.

MOLECULAR SIGNALING IN SKIN CANCER

The molecular signaling mechanisms involved in BCC and melanoma are complex and well understood. However, those affecting cSCC are less well defined. In response to external stimuli, growth factor receptors (GFRs) activate downstream signaling pathways, including MAPK, PI3/AKT, STAT3, and c-SRC.[29] Chronic exposure to stimuli can further lead to constitutive activation of these signaling pathways, thus leading to cutaneous carcinoma. Several preclinical studies have established growth factor receptors to modulate multiple events in pathogenesis of cSCC, including but not limited to proliferation, apoptosis, angiogenesis, cell adhesion, and migration.[30] Therefore, targeting GFR signaling and subsequent downstream signaling pathways could potentially prevent and treat epithelial cancers, including skin cancer. For the purpose of this review, the authors focus on EGFR and FGFR system, two major growth factor signaling pathways in the pathogenesis of skin cancer.[31]

EPIDERMAL GROWTH FACTOR RECEPTOR

EGFR is the first identified member of the ERB family and has been implicated in a variety of cancers, including but not limited to, pancreatic, colon, lung, and ovarian.[32–35] Located on the chromosomal region 7p12, EGFR encodes a 170-kDa transmembrane tyrosine kinase receptor. In response to ligand binding, EGFR dimerizes and triggers auto-phosphorylation of tyrosine kinases, thus leading to activation of various intracellular downstream pathways, including the PI3K/AKT, RAF/MEK/ERK, and STAT3.[36]

The binding of EGFR ligands to EGFR leads to activation of multiple events in the pathogenesis of cSCC, including cellular proliferation, apoptosis, invasion, angiogenesis, and metastasis. In addition, EGFR is responsible for including migrating keratinocytes and the promotion of cell survival and resistance to apoptosis. EGFR overexpression is detectable in well-differentiated human cSCC. Furthermore, several skin tumor promoter agents, such as okadaic acid, 12-O-tetradecanoylphorbol-13-acetate (TPA), and chrysarobin, induce EGFR expression in mouse epidermis. Topical treatment with EFGR inhibitor GW2974 and transgenic mice expressing dominant-negative EGFR have further established a cause and effect for the role of EGFR in epithelial carcinogenesis.[37] Recent studies have identified EGFR overexpression as an independent prognostic factor in cSCC. In cSCC of the head and neck, overexpression of EGFR is associated with lymphatic progression and increased disease severity. Furthermore, increased expression of EGFR is also observed in advanced or metastatic cSCC tumor tissue.[38–40] Therefore, targeting EGFR in cSCC is a valid rationale that demands further exploration.

EGFR signaling is also implicated in BCC; however, the role is controversial. EGFR is identified as a prognostic marker for BCC, with EGFR significantly higher in the recurrent tumors when compared with primary tumors.[41] Interestingly, both genetic and pharmacologic inhibition of EGFR signaling was associated with a reduction in tumor growth in mouse models of HH/GLI driven BCC.[42] Moreover, positive regulatory interactions between EGFR and FGF19, CXCR4, JUN, and SOX9 were determined to selectively amplify the expression of HH-EGFR regulated genes by maintaining high-level expression of HH-EGFR response genes required for sustained tumor growth.[42] Brunner and colleagues[43] demonstrated lack of EGFR staining in MCC. Similar findings were obtained by Maubec and colleagues.[44] Veija and colleagues[45,46] analyzed the expression of EGFR at an mRNA level, observing underexpression in MCC tumors as compared with normal skin. However, EGFR mutations were observed in 22% of 27 MCC tumors.[45] Because the low number of EGFR-positive cases poses a challenge in analyzing correlations to clinical data, further evaluation in larger sample size is needed.

As relevant mutations exist within the EGFR pathway, drugs targeting these mutations are of interest and include gefitinib and cetuximab.[47]

The role of EGFR in melanoma is controversial.[48] Interestingly, although EGFR is not expressed in normal melanocytes, it is expressed in melanoma. In human uveal melanoma, EGFR overexpression correlates with an increased capacity to metastasize to the liver, an increased resistance to Tumor Necrosis Factor-Alpha (TNF-alpha)–mediated lysis, and decreased survival.[49] In a cohort of 114 patients with primary cutaneous melanoma, Boone and colleagues[50] determined expression of EGFR proteins to be associated with a positive sentinel lymph node but not with survival. Furthermore, using in vitro studies of melanoma cell lines, cetuximab attenuated invasion with no effect on cell growth and viability; this suggests a role for EGFR in progression of melanoma with potential benefit in patients with advanced disease.[50] In melanoma, activation of EGFR leads to subsequent activation of the RAS/RAF/MEK/ERK pathway and may lead to metastases.[51] In addition, in samples of BRAF V600-mutant melanomas, the expression of EGFR has been associated with acquired resistance to BRAF inhibitors. Therefore, combination therapies that include an EGFR inhibitor are suggested to address this resistance.

FIBROBLAST GROWTH FACTOR RECEPTOR

FGFRs are transmembrane receptor tyrosine kinases (RTKs) of the immunoglobulin superfamily. In humans, the FGFR family consists of four genes encoding closely related transmembrane RTKs.[52] Upon binding of fibroblast growth factors (FGFs) to FGFRs, receptor dimerization is induced and results in a conformational change that enables transphosphorylation of tyrosines in the intracellular domain, including the kinase domain and the C-terminus. FGFs and their receptors convey multiple biological activities, including proliferation, differentiation, and motility.[53] Phosphorylation of FGFR activates multiple intracellular signaling cascades, including RAS-RAF–MAPK-ERK, PI3/AKT, and Stat3/NFKB pathway.[54,55] The FGFR transcript then undergoes alternative splicing, resulting in Fgrf2 IIIb and Fgrf2 IIIc isoforms; these isoforms are predominantly expressed in the epithelial and mesenchymal cells, respectively.[56] Ligands for epithelium-expressed FGFR2b are mainly produced by mesenchymal cells during normal skin development, resulting in paracrine signaling.[57] Compared with cell lines, whole tumors express high levels of FGFR2b ligands, including FGF1, FGF2, FGF7, and FGF10.[58]

Although FGFR2 is required for the normal growth and development of the epidermis, studies in mice with constitutive genetic deletion of Fgfr2 (K5-R2) using K5-Cre/Lox system demonstrated impaired skin barrier function, abnormal appendages, hair follicle growth, and cutaneous homeostasis.[59] In addition, epidermal deletion of FGFR2 (Fgfr2b^flox/flox; K5-Cre positive) sensitized animals to chemical-induced skin papillomas and cSCC.[59] However, it is important to note that increased keratinocyte proliferation was observed in these mice because of progressive inflammation and not because of cell-autonomous effects, as K5-R2 keratinocytes exhibited a normal rate of proliferation in vitro.

Deletion of FGFR2 leads to upregulation of FGFR1, which suggests a protective role of FGFR2 in cancer development. Despite this, FGFR2 signaling initiates keratinocyte proliferation and promotes skin papilloma formation that can be reversed by genetic ablation of *Ffgr2* in PTEN-deficient epidermal mice.[60] UV-B exposure induced FGF-2 expression in epidermal keratinocytes in vitro and in vivo in mice epidermis, and inhibition of FGFR using a pharmacologic inhibitor significantly decreased UV-B–induced epidermal hyperproliferation.[61]

Melanocytes are anchored to the basement membrane and are under constant paracrine control from the skin keratinocytes. In response to UV-B, FGF2 from keratinocytes and fibroblasts stimulates pigmentation and melanocyte proliferation and induces a phenotypic change via melanocyte receptors.[62] Furthermore, a higher level of FGF2 in the microenvironment of dermal nevus-derived melanocytes could potentially allow melanocytes to adapt to grow in the dermis, which is hypothesized as important for the development of melanoma. Melanoma progression was shown to be accompanied by increased FGF2 expression in the nevi by Giehl and colleagues.[63] Interestingly, FGF2 was detected in 72% of nondysplastic nevi and only in 18% of dysplastic nevi.

Because FGF2 is overexpressed in BCC, use of an FGF inhibitor, dobesilate, inhibits infiltrative BCC via the STAT-3 pathway, as well as inhibits angiogenesis and cell survival. Use of an FGFR inhibitor significantly increased apoptosis and attenuates cell proliferation and angiogenesis.[64] Interestingly, in a study of high-risk cSCC, somatic missense mutations in the tyrosine kinase FGFR2 were only identified in patients with perineural invasion.[7]

Nguyen and colleagues[65] evaluated FGFR2 signaling in an MCC mouse model and determined SOX9(+) cells located within the developing hair placodes to give rise to Merkel cells through FGFR2-mediated signaling. Other preclinical studies include mapping the MCC genomic landscape, determined polyomavirus-positive and polyomavirus-negative MCC to display independent patterns of genomic alterations. Interestingly, virus-negative tumors exhibit increased genomic instability with a higher mutation burden and a more characteristic UV signature.[66] In addition, potentially targetable gene alterations involving the FGFR2 pathway have been identified in the virus-negative disease. Despite this, available data on its response to tyrosine kinase inhibitors are scarce. To date, there are only 2 studies that report the effect of Pazopanib in MCC patients. A clinical trial evaluating the effect of Pazopanib in metastatic MCC determined only 3 out of 16 patients with a partial response. Similar findings have also been described in a single case report.[67]

SUMMARY

Numerous advancements in the understanding of the causes underlying cutaneous malignancies have been discovered in recent years. These findings have led to an increased understanding of skin cancer biology as well as exciting and promising targeted treatments. Further research into the basis of cutaneous malignancies is needed to address resistance to current therapeutics as well as to identify additional gene candidates that can serve as targets for precision therapy.

CLINICS CARE POINTS

- Nearly 90% of cutaneous SCCs exhibit a loss of function in TP53 which is associated with significant increase in mutation burden. Additionally, early data supports TP53 mutations as independent predictors of poor disease-specific survival in patients with cutaneous SCC.

- Recent candidate gene studies have identified melanocortin 1 receptor, tyrosinase, and interferon regulating factor to be involved in the pathogenesis of cSCC.

- In numerous cases of melanoma, microphthalmia-associated transcription factor (MITF) is constitutively activated, leading to upregulation of antiapoptotic genes such as BCL2, BCL2A1,and cell-cycle regulatory genes, such as CDK2.
- Some cases of melanoma are inherited in an autosomal dominant fashion with incomplete penetrance; as such, the authors recommend that suspected cases of familial melanoma undergo genetic testing to screen for CDKN2A and CDK4 mutations.
- Growth factor receptors have been identified in preclinical studies to module multiple events in the pathogenesis of cSCC. As such, these pathways may represent potential treatment pathways that may be targeted to both prevent and treat epithelial cancers.
- EGFR has been identified as a prognostic marker for BCC, found significantly upregulated in recurrent tumors when compared to primary tumors. Drugs that target the EGFR pathway, such as gefitinib and cetuximab may hold promise in the treatment of cutaneous SCC.
- FGF2 is overexpressed in BCC and the use of dobesilate, an FGF inhibitor, has been shown to increase apoptosis and attenuate cell proliferation and angiogenesis.
- In a cohort of patients with high-risk cSCC, somatic missense mutations in the tyrosine kinase FGFR2 were identified in patients with perineural invasion.

DISCLOSURE

The authors have no commercial or financial conflicts of interest pertaining to this article.

REFERENCES

1. Erb P, Ji J, Kump E, et al. Apoptosis and pathogenesis of melanoma and nonmelanoma skin cancer. Adv Exp Med Biol 2008;624:283–95.
2. Ahmed SR, Petersen E, Patel R, et al. Cemiplimab-rwlc as first and only treatment for advanced cutaneous squamous cell carcinoma. Expert Rev Clin Pharmacol 2019;12(10):947–51.
3. Castanheira A, Boaventura P, Pais Clemente M, et al. Head and neck cutaneous basal cell carcinoma: what should the otorhinolaryngology head and neck surgeon care about? Acta Otorhinolaryngol Ital 2020;40(1):5–18.
4. Ratushny V, Gober MD, Hick R, et al. From keratinocyte to cancer: the pathogenesis and modeling of cutaneous squamous cell carcinoma. J Clin Invest 2012; 122(2):464–72.
5. Abel EL, Angel JM, Kiguchi K, et al. Multi-stage chemical carcinogenesis in mouse skin: fundamentals and applications. Nat Protoc 2009;4(9):1350–62.
6. Zhang X, Wu L, Xiao T, et al. TRAF6 regulates EGF-induced cell transformation and cSCC malignant phenotype through CD147/EGFR. Oncogenesis 2018; 7(2):17.
7. Zilberg C, Lee MW, Yu B, et al. Analysis of clinically relevant somatic mutations in high-risk head and neck cutaneous squamous cell carcinoma. Mod Pathol 2018; 31(2):275–87.
8. Uribe P, Gonzalez S. Epidermal growth factor receptor (EGFR) and squamous cell carcinoma of the skin: molecular bases for EGFR-targeted therapy. Pathol Res Pract 2011;207(6):337–42.
9. Li L, Fukumoto M, Liu D. Prognostic significance of p53 immunoexpression in the survival of oral squamous cell carcinoma patients treated with surgery and neoadjuvant chemotherapy. Oncol Lett 2013;6(6):1611–5.

10. Green AC, Olsen CM. Cutaneous squamous cell carcinoma: an epidemiological review. Br J Dermatol 2017;177(2):373–81.
11. Moriwaki S, Kanda F, Hayashi M, et al. Xeroderma pigmentosum clinical practice guidelines. J Dermatol 2017;44(10):1087–96.
12. Schidlowski L, Liebert F, Iankilevich PG, et al. Non-syndromic oculocutaneous albinism: novel genetic variants and clinical follow up of a brazilian pediatric cohort. Front Genet 2020;11:397.
13. Burger B, Itin PH. Epidermodysplasia verruciformis. Curr Probl Dermatol 2014; 45:123–31.
14. Athar M, Li C, Kim AL, et al. Sonic hedgehog signaling in basal cell nevus syndrome. Cancer Res 2014;74(18):4967–75.
15. Kakanj P, Reuter K, Sequaris G, et al. Indian hedgehog controls proliferation and differentiation in skin tumorigenesis and protects against malignant progression. Cell Rep 2013;4(2):340–51.
16. Niewiadomski P, Niedziolka SM, Markiewicz L, et al. Gli proteins: regulation in development and cancer. Cells 2019;8(2):147.
17. Cohen M, Kicheva A, Ribeiro A, et al. Ptch1 and Gli regulate Shh signalling dynamics via multiple mechanisms. Nat Commun 2015;6:6709.
18. Hutchin ME, Kariapper MS, Grachtchouk M, et al. Sustained Hedgehog signaling is required for basal cell carcinoma proliferation and survival: conditional skin tumorigenesis recapitulates the hair growth cycle. Genes Dev 2005;19(2): 214–23.
19. Martinez MF, Romano MV, Martinez AP, et al. Nevoid basal cell carcinoma syndrome: PTCH1 mutation profile and expression of genes involved in the hedgehog pathway in argentinian patients. Cells 2019;8(2):144.
20. Pellegrini C, Maturo MG, Di Nardo L, et al. Understanding the molecular genetics of basal cell carcinoma. Int J Mol Sci 2017;18(11):2485.
21. Clark WH Jr, Elder DE, Guerry Dt, et al. A study of tumor progression: the precursor lesions of superficial spreading and nodular melanoma. Hum Pathol 1984; 15(12):1147–65.
22. Hodis E, Watson IR, Kryukov GV, et al. A landscape of driver mutations in melanoma. Cell 2012;150(2):251–63.
23. Li G, Schaider H, Satyamoorthy K, et al. Downregulation of E-cadherin and Desmoglein 1 by autocrine hepatocyte growth factor during melanoma development. Oncogene 2001;20(56):8125–35.
24. Wu M, Hemesath TJ, Takemoto CM, et al. c-Kit triggers dual phosphorylations, which couple activation and degradation of the essential melanocyte factor Mi. Genes Dev 2000;14(3):301–12.
25. Rossi M, Pellegrini C, Cardelli L, et al. Familial melanoma: diagnostic and management implications. Dermatol Pract Concept 2019;9(1):10–6.
26. Harms PW. Update on Merkel cell carcinoma. Clin Lab Med 2017;37(3):485–501.
27. Zur Hausen A, Rennspiess D, Winnepenninckx V, et al. Early B-cell differentiation in Merkel cell carcinomas: clues to cellular ancestry. Cancer Res 2013;73(16): 4982–7.
28. Nwogu N, Ortiz LE, Kwun HJ. Surface charge of Merkel cell polyomavirus small T antigen determines cell transformation through allosteric FBW7 WD40 domain targeting. Oncogenesis 2020;9(5):53.
29. Chan KS, Carbajal S, Kiguchi K, et al. Epidermal growth factor receptor-mediated activation of Stat3 during multistage skin carcinogenesis. Cancer Res 2004;64(7): 2382–9.

30. Rho O, Kim DJ, Kiguchi K, et al. Growth factor signaling pathways as targets for prevention of epithelial carcinogenesis. Mol Carcinog 2011;50(4):264–79.

31. Khandelwal AR, Kent B, Hillary S, et al. Fibroblast growth factor receptor promotes progression of cutaneous squamous cell carcinoma. Mol Carcinog 2019; 58(10):1715–25.

32. Bian Y, Yu Y, Wang S, et al. Up-regulation of fatty acid synthase induced by EGFR/ERK activation promotes tumor growth in pancreatic cancer. Biochem Biophys Res Commun 2015;463(4):612–7.

33. Milagre CS, Gopinathan G, Everitt G, et al. Adaptive upregulation of EGFR limits attenuation of tumor growth by neutralizing IL6 antibodies, with implications for combined therapy in ovarian cancer. Cancer Res 2015;75(7):1255–64.

34. Suda K, Mitsudomi T. Role of EGFR mutations in lung cancers: prognosis and tumor chemosensitivity. Arch Toxicol 2015;89(8):1227–40.

35. Vene R, Tosetti F, Minghelli S, et al. Celecoxib increases EGF signaling in colon tumor associated fibroblasts, modulating EGFR expression and degradation. Oncotarget 2015;6(14):12310–25.

36. Roberts PJ, Der CJ. Targeting the Raf-MEK-ERK mitogen-activated protein kinase cascade for the treatment of cancer. Oncogene 2007;26(22):3291–310.

37. El-Abaseri TB, Putta S, Hansen LA. Ultraviolet irradiation induces keratinocyte proliferation and epidermal hyperplasia through the activation of the epidermal growth factor receptor. Carcinogenesis 2006;27(2):225–31.

38. Bumpous J. Metastatic cutaneous squamous cell carcinoma to the parotid and cervical lymph nodes: treatment and outcomes. Curr Opin Otolaryngol Head Neck Surg 2009;17(2):122–5.

39. Canueto J, Cardenoso E, Garcia JL, et al. Epidermal growth factor receptor expression is associated with poor outcome in cutaneous squamous cell carcinoma. Br J Dermatol 2017;176(5):1279–87.

40. Sweeny L, Dean NR, Magnuson JS, et al. EGFR expression in advanced head and neck cutaneous squamous cell carcinoma. Head Neck 2012;34(5):681–6.

41. Yerebakan O, Ciftcioglu MA, Akkaya BK, et al. Prognostic value of Ki-67, CD31 and epidermal growth factor receptor expression in basal cell carcinoma. J Dermatol 2003;30(1):33–41.

42. Eberl M, Klingler S, Mangelberger D, et al. Hedgehog-EGFR cooperation response genes determine the oncogenic phenotype of basal cell carcinoma and tumour-initiating pancreatic cancer cells. EMBO Mol Med 2012;4(3):218–33.

43. Brunner M, Thurnher D, Pammer J, et al. Expression of VEGF-A/C, VEGF-R2, PDGF-alpha/beta, c-kit, EGFR, Her-2/Neu, Mcl-1 and Bmi-1 in Merkel cell carcinoma. Mod Pathol 2008;21(7):876–84.

44. Maubec E, Duvillard P, Velasco V, et al. Immunohistochemical analysis of EGFR and HER-2 in patients with metastasizing melanoma, Merkel carcinoma and squamous cell carcinoma of the skin. Ann Dermatol Venereol 2006;133(3):274–6.

45. Veija T, Koljonen V, Bohling T, et al. Aberrant expression of ALK and EZH2 in Merkel cell carcinoma. BMC Cancer 2017;17(1):236.

46. Veija T, Sarhadi VK, Koljonen V, et al. Hotspot mutations in polyomavirus positive and negative Merkel cell carcinomas. Cancer Genet 2016;209(1–2):30–5.

47. Lewis CM, Glisson BS, Feng L, et al. A phase II study of gefitinib for aggressive cutaneous squamous cell carcinoma of the head and neck. Clin Cancer Res 2012;18(5):1435–46.

48. Real FX, Rettig WJ, Chesa PG, et al. Expression of epidermal growth factor receptor in human cultured cells and tissues: relationship to cell lineage and stage of differentiation. Cancer Res 1986;46(9):4726–31.

49. Ma D, Niederkorn JY. Role of epidermal growth factor receptor in the metastasis of intraocular melanomas. Invest Ophthalmol Vis Sci 1998;39(7):1067–75.
50. Boone B, Jacobs K, Ferdinande L, et al. EGFR in melanoma: clinical significance and potential therapeutic target. J Cutan Pathol 2011;38(6):492–502.
51. Mirmohammadsadegh A, Mota R, Gustrau A, et al. ERK1/2 is highly phosphorylated in melanoma metastases and protects melanoma cells from cisplatin-mediated apoptosis. J Invest Dermatol 2007;127(9):2207–15.
52. Johnson DE, Williams LT. Structural and functional diversity in the FGF receptor multigene family. Adv Cancer Res 1993;60:1–41.
53. Grose R, Dickson C. Fibroblast growth factor signaling in tumorigenesis. Cytokine Growth Factor Rev 2005;16(2):179–86.
54. Ahmad I, Iwata T, Leung HY. Mechanisms of FGFR-mediated carcinogenesis. Biochim Biophys Acta 2012;1823(4):850–60.
55. Ornitz DM, Itoh N. The fibroblast growth factor signaling pathway. Wiley Interdiscip Rev Dev Biol 2015;4(3):215–66.
56. Ranieri D, Rosato B, Nanni M, et al. Expression of the FGFR2 mesenchymal splicing variant in epithelial cells drives epithelial-mesenchymal transition. Oncotarget 2016;7(5):5440–60.
57. Ornitz DM, Xu J, Colvin JS, et al. Receptor specificity of the fibroblast growth factor family. J Biol Chem 1996;271(25):15292–7.
58. Ramsey MR, Wilson C, Ory B, et al. FGFR2 signaling underlies p63 oncogenic function in squamous cell carcinoma. J Clin Invest 2013;123(8):3525–38.
59. Grose R, Fantl V, Werner S, et al. The role of fibroblast growth factor receptor 2b in skin homeostasis and cancer development. EMBO J 2007;26(5):1268–78.
60. Hertzler-Schaefer K, Mathew G, Somani AK, et al. Pten loss induces autocrine FGF signaling to promote skin tumorigenesis. Cell Rep 2014;6(5):818–26.
61. Khandelwal AR, Rong X, Moore-Medlin T, et al. Photopreventive effect and mechanism of AZD4547 and curcumin C3 complex on UVB-induced epidermal hyperplasia. Cancer Prev Res (Phila) 2016;9(4):296–304.
62. Teixeira BL, Amarante-Silva D, Visoni SB, et al. FGF2 stimulates the growth and improves the melanocytic commitment of trunk neural crest cells. Cell Mol Neurobiol 2020;40(3):383–93.
63. Giehl KA, Nagele U, Volkenandt M, et al. Protein expression of melanocyte growth factors (bFGF, SCF) and their receptors (FGFR-1, c-kit) in nevi and melanoma. J Cutan Pathol 2007;34(1):7–14.
64. Jee SH, Chu CY, Chiu HC, et al. Interleukin-6 induced basic fibroblast growth factor-dependent angiogenesis in basal cell carcinoma cell line via JAK/STAT3 and PI3-kinase/Akt pathways. J Invest Dermatol 2004;123(6):1169–75.
65. Nguyen MB, Cohen I, Kumar V, et al. FGF signalling controls the specification of hair placode-derived SOX9 positive progenitors to Merkel cells. Nat Commun 2018;9(1):2333.
66. Goh G, Walradt T, Markarov V, et al. Mutational landscape of MCPyV-positive and MCPyV-negative Merkel cell carcinomas with implications for immunotherapy. Oncotarget 2016;7(3):3403–15.
67. Davids MS, Charlton A, Ng SS, et al. Response to a novel multitargeted tyrosine kinase inhibitor pazopanib in metastatic Merkel cell carcinoma. J Clin Oncol 2009;27(26):e97–100.

Management of Advanced Basal Cell Carcinoma of the Head and Neck

Marcus Monroe, MD[a],*, Kiran Kakarala, MD[b,c]

KEYWORDS

- Basal cell carcinoma • Management • Surgery • Radiation • Neoadjuvant • PD-1
- Immunotherapy

KEY POINTS

- Management of advanced basal cell carcinoma often requires a multidisciplinary team approach.
- Surgery remains the current standard of care for locally advanced basal cell carcinoma.
- Radiation or systemic therapy may be considered in patients who refuse or are not candidates for surgery.
- Hedgehog inhibitors are targeted agents against BCC, but have less efficacy than surgery or radiation, and should be reserved for patients who are not candidates for these treatments.

INTRODUCTION

Basal cell carcinoma (BCC) is the most common human malignancy. While the exact incidence is unknown, BCC likely affects more than 2 million people in the United States each year.[1] The incidence is increasing despite efforts to mitigate risk factors. Patients with lighter skin tones (Fitzpatrick types I and II) who have significant sun exposures (ultraviolet radiation) account for most BCC cases, and these tumors tend to occur on sun-exposed areas of the head and neck.[2] Other risk factors include exposure to ionizing radiation; immunosuppression; and rarely, genetic syndromes (basal cell nevus syndrome, xeroderma pigmentosum).

Mortality from BCC is rare because most lesions are easily managed with surgical or nonsurgical treatments. However, the cost to patients and society to manage these

[a] Head and Neck Surgery, Head and Neck Clinical Trials Program, Head and Neck Disease-Oriented Team, Huntsman Cancer Institute, University of Utah School of Medicine, 2000 Circle of Hope Drive, Salt Lake City, UT 84132, USA; [b] Head and Neck Surgery and Microvascular Reconstruction, Head and Neck Fellowship, Department of Otolaryngology-Head and Neck Surgery, University of Kansas School of Medicine, 3901 Rainbow Boulevard, Kansas City, KS 66160, USA; [c] Department of Health Policy and Management, University of Kansas School of Medicine, 3901 Rainbow Boulevard, Kansas City, KS 66160, USA
* Corresponding author.
E-mail address: marcus.monroe@hsc.utah.edu

Otolaryngol Clin N Am 54 (2021) 271–280
https://doi.org/10.1016/j.otc.2020.11.003
0030-6665/21/Published by Elsevier Inc.

cancers is substantial, given the high incidence.[3] A small subset of patients with BCC develop advanced tumors of the head and neck region that present unique management challenges and often merit a multidisciplinary approach. The focus of this article primarily is on the management of these high-risk cases, reviewing surgical and nonsurgical options to achieve cure wherever possible while minimizing morbidity and maximizing quality of life.

DISCUSSION
Management of Low-Risk Basal Cell Carcinoma

Most BCC are amenable to management with surgical techniques. Curettage with electrodessication is a destructive technique to remove low-risk BCC without assessment of margins. It is highly effective in experienced hands, but should be avoided for deeper lesions approaching subcutaneous fat, and lesions in areas with terminal hair growth (eg, scalp, beard, axilla, groin).[4] Simple excision with primary closure, secondary intention healing, or skin graft is also highly effective. Rotational flaps should be avoided unless frozen section margin clearance is achieved. A clinical margin of 4 mm is recommended to minimize risk of recurrence, and achieves negative margins in more than 95% of low-risk cases, obviating frozen section margin control or Mohs micrographic surgery (MMS) in appropriate cases.[5]

For patients who are not candidates for curettage with electrodessication or excision, a variety of nonsurgical treatments are available. Radiation is usually reserved for those patients older than 60 because of long-term sequalae, but achieves high rates of cure in low-risk cases. Topical therapies, such as imiquimod and 5-FU, although not as effective as surgical treatments, may have superior cosmetic outcomes in selected cases. Other options that may be considered are cryosurgery and photodynamic therapy.[6]

Management of High-Risk Basal Cell Carcinoma

Although most BCCs are considered low-risk and treated with simple excision or other local destructive measures as described previously, high-risk lesions are more likely to require a multidisciplinary approach. Any regionally or distantly metastatic tumor is considered high risk by default. For locally advanced tumors, several clinical and pathologic features are known to increase the risk of morbidity and/or recurrence and have been included in the definition for high-risk BCC contained in the National Comprehensive Cancer Network guidelines.[5] Within this definition, high-risk BCCs are those that include any of the following features: (1) recurrent; (2) poorly defined borders; (3) patient immunosuppression; (4) occurrence in site of prior radiotherapy; (5) demonstration of aggressive growth pattern (infiltrative micronodular, morpheaform, sclerosing, carcinosarcomatous, or basosquamous differentiation in any part of the tumor); (6) perineural invasion; and (7) size greater than or equal to 10 mm on the cheek, forehead, scalp and/or neck, or any in the H areas of the face (central face, eyelids, eyebrows, periorbital, nose, lips, chin, mandible, preauricular, postauricular, temple, ear).

SURGICAL THERAPY

Surgery is the preferred curative treatment of locally advanced BCC.[5] Achieving negative margins is critical to preventing recurrence and associated morbidity and possible mortality. Two main strategies for intraoperative margin assessment are available: MMS and wide excision with intraoperative frozen section of circumferential skin and deep soft tissue margins. MMS is performed by a dermatologist with surgical and dermatopathology training. The lesion is excised with small margins, in multiple layers if necessary. After each layer of excision, the entire margin of excision is examined in full by the Mohs surgeon to determine the need for further resection. This procedure is most often done in an office setting with local anesthesia. In contrast, in wide local excision the lesion is removed with a margin of normal-appearing tissue, and then the circumferential skin and deep margins are sampled by the surgeon and sent for intraoperative assessment by a pathologist using frozen sections. MMS was compared with wide local excision in a prospective randomized trial in the Netherlands.[7] After 10-year follow-up, the rate of recurrence in patients with high-risk facial BCC was lower in those treated with MMS compared with standard surgical excision, although this finding was only statistically significant for those patient with recurrent high-risk BCC.

Locally advanced BCC of the head and neck often presents unique challenges for surgical resection and reconstruction. Critical structures for function and cosmesis, such as cartilage, bone, cranial nerves, and sensory organs (eye, ear, nose), may be involved with cancer or need to be removed to achieve negative margins. Although MMS is most often used in an outpatient clinic setting under local anesthesia, there have been reports describing the successful use of MMS in the operating room setting under general anesthesia to remove larger/deeper tumors.[8]

Locally advanced tumors involving the skull base often require a multidisciplinary surgical approach. For example, advanced lateral skull base tumors might require a neurotologist to complete a temporal bone resection, a neurosurgeon if there is intracranial involvement, and a head and neck surgeon with capability to complete the reconstruction (**Fig. 1**). If cranial nerves (eg, facial, spinal accessory) are functional preoperatively, then they should be preserved unless gross disease will be left as a result. Similarly, tumors involving the anterior skull base might benefit from the involvement of an oculoplastic surgeon if there is orbital invasion but the eye is functional preoperatively and the goal is orbit preservation. In resections involving dura or brain, a reliable reconstruction, often using free tissue transfer, is important to minimizing postoperative morbidity (eg, meningitis, cerebrospinal fluid leak).[9] In tumors with high-risk features where adjuvant radiation is planned, using well-vascularized tissues for coverage of critical structures (eg, free tissue transfer or pedicled local/regional flaps), is important to prevent wound complications. These resections entail high risk of morbidity to the patient despite maximal reconstructive efforts; however, they may be justified given the likelihood of cure given the relative indolence of the pathology. Radical resections that would not be considered for other cancers because of the low likelihood of survival benefit, might be appropriate for BCC.[10]

Although surgery is the gold standard for the management of high-risk BCC, certain cases may benefit from alternative management strategies discussed later. Morbidity from surgery may be unacceptable to certain patients with locally advanced tumors. Patient preferences for quality and quantity of life must be elicited and respected. Other patients may not be good surgical candidates because of medical comorbidity. Surgery for locally advanced tumors requiring multidisciplinary surgical resection and reconstruction may take many hours with risk of significant blood loss, which may represent unacceptable perioperative risk of morbidity and mortality in some patients. Advanced age alone should not be a contraindication for proceeding with an aggressive surgery and reconstruction; rather careful risk stratification using assessments, such as frailty, should guide decision-making.[11] Thus, management of locally advanced head and neck BCC must be tailored to the individual patient. If surgery is not feasible or acceptable, then radiation or systemic therapy should be considered.

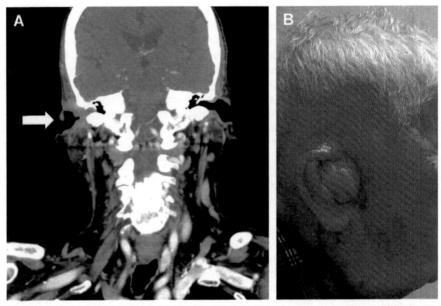

Fig. 1. An 86-year-old man presented with a basal cell cancer of the right ear, involving the conchal bowl and ear canal. He had undergone two previous surgical resections with positive margins at another institution, and subsequently underwent radiation therapy for local recurrence. Three months following the completion of radiation therapy he was noted to have persistent disease involving the ear canal. Imaging was obtained, showing tumor abutting but not invading the temporal bone and no evidence of perineural spread (*A, arrow*). Partial auriculectomy with lateral temporal bone resection was recommended, but the patient opted for therapy with vismodegib. There was no response to treatment, and he agreed to proceed with surgery 5 months later because of worsening ear pain. Surgical resection with submental artery island flap reconstruction was performed and negative frozen section skin and deep soft tissue margins were achieved (B). Final pathology revealed basal cell cancer, morpheaform type, with squamous differentiation. After being lost to follow-up, he returned 3 years later, age 89, with right otalgia and facial paresis. Imaging revealed likely recurrence along the skull base. He declined any further treatments and was alive with disease at last follow-up at age 91.

RADIATION
Primary Radiotherapy

Radiation therapy for advanced BCC of the head and neck is primarily considered when surgical resection is deemed unlikely to be curative, carries unacceptable surgery-related morbidity, or is deemed unsafe because of patient comorbidities and/or advanced age.

In the only randomized controlled trial to date comparing surgery with radiation therapy, surgical therapy demonstrated superior oncologic and cosmetic outcomes.[12] Avril and colleagues[12] compared surgical excision with frozen section margin clearance versus radiation therapy for BCCs of the head and neck less than 4 cm in size. Three radiation techniques were allowed, including interstitial brachytherapy to 65 to 70 Gy; superficial contact therapy with two, 18 to 20 Gy treatments; or conventional radiotherapy to 60 Gy. The primary end point of the study, cure rate at 4 years, was superior in the surgical treatment arm with 0.7% failure compared with 7.5% with radiotherapy. Cosmetic outcome as assessed by a panel of five judges was also deemed superior with 87% of the surgically treated patients compared with 69% of the radiation-treated patients having a cosmetic outcome rated as good.

Data on radiation therapy control rates for more advanced BCCs are limited to case series. As might be expected, with increasing high-risk features, the effectiveness of primary radiotherapy decreases. In a study of 108 aggressive BCCs of the head and neck (defined as primary lesion >10 mm, >2 recurrences, or extracutaneous extension), primary radiation achieved a locoregional control rate of 87% and a recurrence-free survival rate of 82%.[13] Aggressive histologic subtypes and those in which delineation of the tumor margins is difficult, such as morpheaform BCC, are associated with lower rates of cure. In a series of 127 patients with morpheaform BCC, the 5-year cure rate was 81%.[14]

Adjuvant Radiotherapy

The use of adjuvant radiation therapy following surgical excision has been recommended when significant perineural invasion is noted or when surgical margins are positive and not amenable to further excision.[5,15] Recurrent disease with prior negative margins and invasion of muscle and/or bone have also been recommended as criteria for when adjuvant radiation therapy should be considered.[15] However, robust evidence to support these recommendations remains limited. No randomized trials have been conducted and evidence remains limited to small uncontrolled case series.[13,16]

SYSTEMIC THERAPY FOR BASAL CELL CARCINOMA
Cytotoxic Chemotherapy

Cytotoxic chemotherapy regimens reported in the literature typically involve a backbone of a platinum agent. Although these regimens are less frequently used today given the development of better-performing and better-tolerated targeted and immune-based therapies, they remain options in refractory disease or when a rapid response for symptom control is needed. In the largest reported series combining BCC and squamous cell carcinomas of the skin, Guthrie and colleagues[17] documented an overall response rate of 68% to the combination of cisplatin and doxorubicin. Rapid symptomatic response has been noted with the combination of cisplatin and paclitaxel or cisplatin and doxorubicin.[17–19]

Hedgehog Pathway Inhibitors: Vismodegib and Sonidegib

Initially discovered as the genetic cause of basal cell nevus syndrome, mutations in the hedgehog pathway have also been demonstrated to occur frequently in sporadic BCC. In a study of 42 BCCs, mutations in the sonic hedgehog pathway genes *PTCH*, *SMOH*, and *SUFUH* occurred in 67%, 10%, and 5%, respectively.[20] Mutations in PTCH and SMO, key receptor proteins in the hedgehog pathway, result in activation of GLI and downstream initiation of basal cell growth and proliferation. The two available hedgehog pathway inhibitors, vismodegib (Erivedge) and sonidegib (Odomzo), are small-molecule inhibitors that bind to SMO and inhibit downstream activation of these target genes.

In 2012 the Food and Drug Administration approved vismodegib for locoregionally advanced or metastatic BCC on the results of the ERIVANCE study.[21] This phase 2 trial evaluated vismodegib, 150 mg daily, in patients with metastatic or locally advanced BCC. For patients with locally advanced disease, inclusion criteria included a size of 1 cm or more that was considered either inoperable or surgery was not advised because of a history of two or more recurrences or anticipated substantial morbidity. Patients were required to have had prior radiation therapy unless contraindicated. The primary end point of the study was an objective response of 30% reduction in visible or radiographic dimensions. In the initial report, of 33 patients with metastatic BCC, a response rate of 30% was noted. Of the 63 patients with locally advanced disease, 54% responded with a 21% complete response rate. The median duration of response was 7.6 months in both cohorts. In the final reported update, the investigator-assessed response rate was 48.5% in the metastatic cohort and 60.3% in the locally advanced. Twenty patients achieved a complete response. The median duration of response was 14.8 months.[22] Adverse events (AE) were common with more than 30% experiencing muscle spasms, alopecia, dysgeusia, weight loss, and/or fatigue. Approximately 25% experienced serious AE with seven reported deaths.

These results were replicated in the Safety Events In Vismodegib (STEVIE) trial,[23] an international open label study of vismodegib for patients with locally advanced or metastatic BCC. In the study of 1215 patients, investigator-assessed response rates of 69% for locally advanced and 37% for patients with metastasis were reported. Complete responses were reported in 34% of patients with locally advanced disease and 7% in the metastatic cohort. AE occurred in most patients (98%), with 24% experiencing serious AEs.

In 2015, sonidegib was approved for locally advanced BCC based on the results of the BOLT trial.[24] This trial was a multicenter randomized controlled trial comparing 200 mg and 800 mg of daily sonidegib. Inclusion criteria included a diagnosis of locally advanced BCC where surgery or radiation therapy was not indicated or metastatic. In all, 230 patients were randomized. With a 13.9-month median follow-up, an objective response was achieved in 43% of locally advanced patients and 15% of patients with metastasis in the 200-mg cohort. Only 5% of patients were noted to have a complete response. No improvement in response was noted in the 800-mg group (38% locally advanced, 17% metastatic, no complete responses) at the cost of a higher rate of AE. The most common AE included muscle spasms, alopecia, dysgeusia, nausea, and elevations of creatine kinase. Serious AE occurred in 14% of the 200-mg cohort and 30% of the 800-mg group.

Differences in outcome measures between the Erivance and BOLT studies complicate comparisons with regards to efficacy. A similar profile of adverse effects is present, although serious AEs were reported to be lower with sonidegib compared with vismodegib. For patients who initially fail vismodegib, significant response rates have not been noted with sonidegib,[25] suggesting that an agent with a different mechanism of action should be tried once patients fail to respond to one of the currently available hedgehog pathway inhibitors.

A significant criticism of both of these studies include ambiguity in the criteria used to define surgically unresectable disease. For these studies the decision was left up to the patient's surgeon, a group including Mohs, plastic, and head and neck surgical specialists. Given the significant differences in surgical extirpative training and experience among these surgical disciplines, it is reasonable to assume that the definition of surgically resectable might vary considerably. In both studies objective response rates were less than 50% for locally advanced disease and 30% or less for metastatic disease. Although higher rates of response were reported for follow-up studies,[22,23] these data are subject to potential bias given that they were determined by individual investigators and not centrally reviewed. Given that these response rates remain significantly less than what has been reported for surgery and radiation therapy, these medications should not be viewed as equivalent treatment options in patients who are candidates for surgery and/or radiation.

The role of these therapies in a neoadjuvant setting remain exploratory. In a single-institution open label trial, 15 patients with BCC were given 3 to 6 months of neoadjuvant vismodegib at 150 mg daily before Mohs excision.[26] Eleven of the 15 patients completed the trial. Twenty-nine percent of patients were unable to complete more than 3 months of therapy because of treatment-related side effects. Vismodegib did reduce the surgical defect area by 27% from baseline. With a short-term mean follow-up of 11.5 months (range, 4–21), one patient recurred. Of seven patients with complete clinical response, only four demonstrated no residual tumor histologically following excision, underscoring the concept that complete clinical response does not equate to cure. Of concern, four patients in this trial did not complete standard of care surgical therapy because of either being lost to follow-up or experiencing side effects from vismodegib and withdrawing from the study. Although they might have received care subsequently, the potential for neoadjuvant vismodegib to hinder the delivery of curative therapy remains concerning and deserves further exploration.

Taken together, these data support the role of hedgehog pathway inhibitors as the current first-line treatment option in patients that are not deemed surgical or radiation candidates. Neoadjuvant hedgehog pathway inhibition should only be administered in the context of a clinical trial given the lack of long-term control data and concern regarding potential interference with curative therapy.

Immunotherapy

Based on the high mutational burden present in BCC,[27] and success with other cutaneous malignancies, immunotherapeutic strategies targeting the PD-1/PD-L1 pathway are currently being explored. In an investigator-initiated nonrandomized study of 16 patients, pembrolizumab was given with or without concurrent vismodegib.[28] In the nine patients receiving pembrolizumab monotherapy, four (44%) achieved a response, with a median duration of 67 weeks. This small series and other case reports demonstrating response to PD-1/PD-L1 inhibition[29,30] suggest that immunotherapy may become a viable treatment option. An ongoing multi-institutional phase II study of cemiplimab in advanced BCC has shown an objective response rate of 29% with locally advanced (n = 84) and 21% with metastatic (n = 29) BCC and 21% in an early press release of the data.[31] The final data from this study are anticipated to provide the most definitive picture regarding the usefulness of immunotherapy in this patient population.

SUMMARY

Locally advanced BCC requires a multidisciplinary treatment strategy. For most patients, surgery remains standard of care based on evidence demonstrating improved disease control. For patients in whom surgery is not possible because of patient comorbidities or unacceptable morbidity, radiation therapy remains a viable option with long-term disease control capabilities. Systemic treatments are available but are associated with inferior response rates to traditional therapies, such as surgery and radiation, and should be considered only for patients whom are not good candidates for these therapies.

CLINICS CARE POINTS

- Management of advanced BCC often requires a multidisciplinary team approach.
- Surgery with or without adjuvant radiation remains the current standard of care for locally advanced BCC.
- Radiation therapy has demonstrated long-term disease control potential that, although inferior to surgery, surpasses what is reported for systemic therapy and remains the second-line treatment of choice in patients with locally advanced BCC that are not surgical candidates.
- Hedgehog pathway inhibitors (vismodegib and sonidegib) are Food and Drug Administration approved systemic therapies with response rates ranging from 43% to 67% in locally advanced and 15% to 49% with metastatic disease. Complete responses to treatment occur in a minority of 20% to 30% with locally advanced and 7% with metastatic BCC. Complete clinical response correlates with histologic response in 57% of patients.
- PD-1/PD-L1 targeted immunotherapy approaches show promise in preliminary published evidence. Results of ongoing studies will clarify the role of these medications in the BCC treatment paradigm.

DISCLOSURE

M. Monroe has served on cutaneous squamous cell carcinoma advisory boards for Merck, Sanofi-Adventis, and Regeneron. He has research funding from the NIH (NIDCR), American Head and Neck Society, and Huntsman Cancer Institute. K. Kakarala has no disclosures.

REFERENCES

1. Rogers HW, Weinstock MA, Harris AR, et al. Incidence estimate of nonmelanoma skin cancer in the United States, 2006. Arch Dermatol 2010;146(3):283–7.
2. Gallagher RP, Hill GB, Bajdik CD, et al. Sunlight exposure, pigmentary factors, and risk of nonmelanocytic skin cancer. I. Basal cell carcinoma. Arch Dermatol 1995;131(2):157–63.
3. Chen JG, Fleischer AB Jr, Smith ED, et al. Cost of nonmelanoma skin cancer treatment in the United States. Dermatol Surg 2001;27(12):1035–8.
4. Thissen MR, Neumann MH, Schouten LJ. A systematic review of treatment modalities for primary basal cell carcinomas. Arch Dermatol 1999;135(10):1177–83.
5. National Comprehensive Cancer Network. Basal Cell Skin Cancer (Version 1.2021). Available at: https://www.nccn.org/professionals/physician_gls/pdf/nmsc.pdf. Accessed February 23, 2021.
6. Roozeboom MH, Arits AH, Nelemans PJ, et al. Overall treatment success after treatment of primary superficial basal cell carcinoma: a systematic review and meta-analysis of randomized and nonrandomized trials. Br J Dermatol 2012;167(4):733–56.
7. van Loo E, Mosterd K, Krekels GA, et al. Surgical excision versus Mohs' micrographic surgery for basal cell carcinoma of the face: a randomised clinical trial with 10 year follow-up. Eur J Cancer 2014;50(17):3011–20.
8. Seth R, Revenaugh PC, Vidimos AT, et al. Simultaneous intraoperative Mohs clearance and reconstruction for advanced cutaneous malignancies. Arch Facial Plast Surg 2011;13(6):404–10.

9. Kwon D, Iloreta A, Miles B, et al. Open anterior skull base reconstruction: a contemporary review. Semin Plast Surg 2017;31(4):189–96.

10. Backous DD, DeMonte F, El-Naggar A, et al. Craniofacial resection for nonmelanoma skin cancer of the head and neck. Laryngoscope 2005;115(6):931–7.

11. Ørum M, Gregersen M, Jensen K, et al. Frailty status but not age predicts complications in elderly cancer patients: a follow-up study. Acta Oncol 2018;57(11):1458–66.

12. Avril MF, Auperin A, Margulis A, et al. Basal cell carcinoma of the face: surgery or radiotherapy? Results of a randomized study. Br J Cancer 1997;76(1):100–6.

13. Rishi A, Hui Huang S, O'Sullivan B, et al. Outcome following radiotherapy for head and neck basal cell carcinoma with 'aggressive' features. Oral Oncol 2017;72:157–64.

14. Caccialanza M, Piccinno R, Cuka E, et al. Radiotherapy of morphea-type basal cell carcinoma: results in 127 cases. J Eur Acad Dermatol Venereol 2014;28(12):1751–5.

15. Likhacheva A, Awan M, Barker CA, et al. Definitive and postoperative radiation therapy for basal and squamous cell cancers of the skin: an ASTRO clinical practice guideline. Pract Radiat Oncol 2020;10(1):8–20.

16. Duinkerken CW, Lohuis PJFM, Crijns MB, et al. Orthovoltage X-rays for postoperative treatment of resected basal cell carcinoma in the head and neck area. J Cutan Med Surg 2017;21(3):243–9.

17. Guthrie TH Jr1, Porubsky ES, Luxenberg MN, et al. Cisplatin-based chemotherapy in advanced basal and squamous cell carcinomas of the skin: results in 28 patients including 13 patients receiving multimodality therapy. J Clin Oncol 1990;8(2):342–6.

18. Jefford M, Kiffer JD, Somers G, et al. Metastatic basal cell carcinoma: rapid symptomatic response to cisplatin and paclitaxel. ANZ J Surg 2004;74(8):704–5.

19. Jaal J, Putnik K. Induction cisplatin-based chemotherapy and following radiotherapy in locally advanced basal cell carcinoma of the skin. Acta Oncol 2012;51(7):952–4.

20. Reifenberger 1 J, Wolter M, Knobbe CB, et al. Reifenberger Somatic mutations in the PTCH, SMOH, SUFUH and TP53 genes in sporadic basal cell carcinomas. Br J Dermatol 2005;152(1):43–51.

21. Sekulic A, Migden MR, Oro AE, et al. Efficacy and safety of vismodegib in advanced basal-cell carcinoma. N Engl J Med 2012;366(23):2171–9.

22. Sekulic A, Migden MR, Basset-Seguin N, et al, ERIVANCE BCC Investigators. Long-term safety and efficacy of vismodegib in patients with advanced basal cell carcinoma: final update of the pivotal ERIVANCE BCC study. BMC Cancer 2017;17(1):332.

23. Basset-Séguin N, Hauschild A, Kunstfeld R, et al. Vismodegib in patients with advanced basal cell carcinoma: primary analysis of STEVIE, an international, open-label trial. Eur J Cancer 2017;86:334–48.

24. Migden MR, Guminski A, Gutzmer R, et al. Treatment with two different doses of sonidegib in patients with locally advanced or metastatic basal cell carcinoma (BOLT): a multicentre, randomised, double-blind phase 2 trial. Lancet Oncol 2015;16(6):716–28.

25. Danial C, Sarin KY, Oro AE, et al. An investigator-initiated open-label trial of sonidegib in advanced basal cell carcinoma patients resistant to vismodegib. Clin Cancer Res 2016;22(6):1325–9.

26. Ally MS, Aasi S, Wysong A, et al. An investigator-initiated open-label clinical trial of vismodegib as a neoadjuvant to surgery for high-risk basal cell carcinoma. J Am Acad Dermatol 2014;71(5):904–11.

27. Jayaraman SS, Rayhan DJ, Hazany S, et al. Mutational landscape of basal cell carcinomas by whole-exome sequencing. J Invest Dermatol 2014;134(1):213–22.

28. Chang ALS, Tran DC, Cannon JGD, et al. Pembrolizumab for advanced basal cell carcinoma: an investigator-initiated, proof-of-concept study. J Am Acad Dermatol 2019;80(2):564–6.

29. Cannon JGD, Russell JS, Kim J, et al. A case of metastatic basal cell carcinoma treated with continuous PD-1 inhibitor exposure even after subsequent initiation of radiotherapy and surgery. JAAD Case Rep 2018;4(3):248–50.

30. Fischer S, Hasan Ali O, Jochum W, et al. Anti-PD-1 therapy leads to near-complete remission in a patient with metastatic basal cell carcinoma. Oncol Res Treat 2018;41(6):391–4.

31. Libtayo (cemiplimab) shows clinically meaningful and durable responses in second-line advanced basal cell carcinoma [news release]. Paris and Tarrytown, NY. Published May 5, 2020. Available at: sanofi.com/en/media-room/press-releases/2020/2020-05-05-07-00-00. Accessed August 1, 2020.

Sentinel Node Biopsy for Head and Neck Cutaneous Melanoma

Vivian F. Wu, MD, MPH[a], Kelly M. Malloy, MD[b],*

KEYWORDS

• Melanoma • Sentinel node biopsy • MSLT • Head and neck • Lymphadenectomy

KEY POINTS

- Sentinel node biopsy provides the most precise staging information for patients with any thickness melanoma allowing for accurate prognostication and guidance toward adjuvant care.
- Completion nodal dissection for sentinel node–positive patients with low disease burden demonstrates no additional survival benefit as long as the patient undergoes close and frequent clinical observation, including serial ultrasound, for at least 2 years.
- Sentinel node biopsy is safe and accurate for head and neck melanoma. Despite lack of data indicating survival benefit, completion neck dissection reduces regional recurrence. Surgeons must walk patients through this lengthy risk/benefit discussion to ensure shared decision making.
- Low enrollment of patients with head and neck melanoma in large clinical trials renders the conclusions less generalizable to this patient population.

INTRODUCTION

The most important prognostic factors as reflected in the current staging of melanoma include:

- Primary tumor depth of invasion.
- Ulceration at the primary site.
- Regional lymph node involvement.

This article explores the birth and evolution of sentinel node biopsy for melanoma and the controversies surrounding its application in the head and neck (HN). The story provides fascinating study into how new technology is often fraught with opposition

[a] Department of Otolaryngology-HNS, Henry Ford Health System, 2799 West Grand Boulevard, Detroit, MI 48202, USA; [b] Department of Otolaryngology-HNS, University of Michigan Medical School, 1904 Taubman Center, 1500 East Medical Center Drive, Ann Arbor, MI 48109-5321, USA
* Corresponding author.
E-mail address: kellymal@med.umich.edu

Otolaryngol Clin N Am 54 (2021) 281–294
https://doi.org/10.1016/j.otc.2020.11.004
oto.theclinics.com

and what it takes to foster the collaborations necessary to provide evidence of its benefits. The progression of data from Multicenter Selective Lymphadenectomy Trial I (MSLT-I) to the designing and resulting of Multicenter Selective Lymphadenectomy Trial II (MSLT-II) affirms that evidence-based medicine is the key component in advancing practice change.

SENTINEL LYMPH NODE BIOPSY: A BRIEF HISTORY

Gould and coworkers[1] published the first case series of sentinel lymph node biopsy (SLNB) in 1960. During a parotidectomy, his team astutely observed "a normal-appearing node at the junction of the anterior and posterior facial vein" and sent this for frozen section. The node was reported as "metastatic tumor" and the surgeons proceeded with radical neck dissection. Twenty-eight additional cases were similarly performed and results are seen in **Box 1**.[1] It was from this work that the term "sentinel node" was coined.

Sixteen years later, Cabanas[2] presented his series of penile cancer cases using lymphangiograms to locate sentinel lymph nodes. His study of 100 patients concluded that (1) lymphangiograms identify the sentinel node; (2) the sentinel node is the first site of metastasis; and (3) positive SLNB should be followed by lymphadenectomy, whereas negative SLNB can be observed.[2]

In the 1980s, Morton[3] and his team began to use these concepts and mapping techniques toward the management of melanoma. Early adopters were spurred by concerns regarding significant lymphedema associated with routine elective lymphadenectomy for melanoma, particularly because only 20% patients who underwent elective lymph node dissection demonstrated positive nodes[3]; knowing which patients would truly benefit from comprehensive lymphadenectomy would spare those with N0 disease the morbidity of a full lymph node dissection.[3] As such, SLNB is considered one of the first forms of targeted therapy.

EARLY TECHNIQUE

SLNB aims to identify the primary echelon of nodal drainage from a specific anatomic region. Initial work in melanoma used vital blue dye alone to identify cutaneous drainage.[4] Morton's early work was performed in cats where blue dye injection reliably identified the lymphatic watershed. Subsequent clinical study examined 223 consecutive patients and successfully identified 194 sentinel nodes in 237 lymphatic basins.[4] This "open and see approach"[5] posed a challenge because early surgeries were burdensome given the requirement to lift large areas of skin flaps and thoroughly trace lymphatic drainage pathways down to nodes of interest.

Box 1

The follow-up, 6–8 years, on the group of patients with neck dissection and parotidectomy shows all patients living and well except one who died of encephalomalacia 8 years after surgery. The four patients who had malignant parotid tumors but negative lymph nodes, and who therefore did not have a radical neck dissection, have been observed for 2–8 years, and none shows evidence of either recurrence or metastasis.

From Gould ED, Winship T, Philbin PH, Kerr HH. Observations on a "sentinel node" in cancer of the parotid. *Cancer.* 1960 Jan-Feb; 13:77-8, with permission.

Lymphoscintigraphy for cutaneous lesions was first described in 1953 when the authors found this technique could reliably predict lymphatic flow.[6] Because of the complex lymphatic patterns in HN, it is no surprise that an otolaryngologist was part of the first team[7] to apply this technique intraoperatively for malignant melanoma, building on Morton's work. Because blue dye alone is not visible on the skin surface, lymphoscintigraphy with gamma probe use in the operating room allowed for localizing radiocolloid tracer in the preoperative and intraoperative setting (**Box 2**). Lymphoscintigraphy planar images helped to better localize lymphatic drainage patterns and paved the way for more innovative "see and open approaches."[5] Despite this advancement, planar images were not precise for deep nodes, could not distinguish nodes near the injection site, had less sensitivity with doublet nodes, and were challenging to use with complex lymphatic drainage.[5] Single-photon emission computed tomography (SPECT) uses three-dimensional functional imaging fused with anatomic computed tomography (CT) correlates to improve localization of sentinel nodes. SPECT/CT can distinguish a sentinel node from a lymphangioma, lymphatic lake, or skin contamination.[5] Using blue dye in addition to SPECT/CT technology, the surgeon can "see, open, hear and see" to improve chances of accurately identifying sentinel nodes and minimizing false negatives.

SLNB needs to be gracefully orchestrated among the surgeon, nuclear medicine team, and pathologist. There is a learning curve for each specialty involved. The surgeon requires comfort with minimally invasive approaches and reliance on sight and sound to identify nodes. The nuclear medicine team must learn the timing in which to capture and map lymphatic drainage. The pathology workflow includes the need for additional processing and evaluation of nodal tissue to identify micrometastasis. With so many moving parts, validation of this new technique required a multicenter clinical trial.

MULTICENTER SELECTIVE LYMPHADENECTOMY TRIAL

MSLT-I was initiated to study whether SLNB can identify patients with clinically occult nodal metastases.[8] Its goal was to confirm the accuracy of nodal staging based on SLNB and determine whether immediate completion lymphadenopathy (CLND) in patients with tumor-positive sentinel nodes can improve outcome. **Fig. 1** describes the schema of the trial.[8]

Box 2
Gamma-probe localization has several advantages

- Aids in the precise location of the position of an underlying lymph node on the surface of the skin.
- Provides intraoperative guidance for the surgeon to the lymph node during dissection.
- Verifies that the correct node has been biopsied.
- Helps the surgeon determine the possible presence of residual lymph nodes.
- Allows for lymph nodes to be harvested through a small incision as opposed to raising a skin flap.
- Can be rapidly and easily performed.

Adapted from Alex JC, Weaver DL, Fairbank JT, Rankin BS, Krag DN. Gamma-probe-guided lymph node localization in malignant melanoma. *Surg Oncol.* 1993 Oct; 2(5):303-8, with permission.

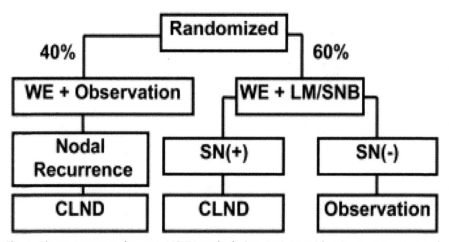

Fig. 1. Biopsy-proven melanoma. MSLT-I study design. Patients with primary cutaneous melanoma ≥1 mm or Clark level IV are assigned in a 60:40 distribution to wide excision plus lymphatic mapping and sentinel node biopsy, with immediate CLND for occult nodal metastases; or to wide excision plus observation, with delayed CLND or other treatment of palpable nodal metastases. All patients are followed up for disease-free and melanoma-specific survival. LM, lymphatic mapping; SNB, sentinel node biopsy; WE, wide excision. (Data from Morton DL, Thompson JF, Cochran AJ, Mozzillo N, Elashoff R, Essner R, Nieweg OE, Roses DF, Hoekstra HJ, Karakousis CP, Reintgen DS, Coventry BJ, Glass EC, Wang HJ; MSLT Group. Sentinel-node biopsy or nodal observation in melanoma. N Engl J Med. 2006 Sep 28; 355(13):1307-17.)

The primary end point of this study was melanoma-specific survival (MSS; survival until death from melanoma). The secondary end points included disease-free survival (DFS), survival with tumor-positive or tumor-negative sentinel nodes, and the incidence of sentinel node metastases, as compared with the incidence of clinically detected nodal metastases. Detailed results from the final trial report are listed in **Box 3**.[9]

Overall, patients with intermediate-thickness melanoma seemed to benefit the most with significant improvement in DFS in the biopsy group (**Box 4**). For patients with intermediate-thickness melanoma and subsequent nodal metastasis, MSS and DFS was improved for patients who underwent SLNB.

Several findings were published in a series of papers from the MSLT-1 group. Twelve years after accrual of the last patients, the final analysis was reported in 2014 and generated a lively and unfortunately, acerbic debate over the next few years.[13-17] Opponents took issue with the lack of difference seen in MSS indicating the procedure cannot be used as a therapeutic intervention.[13,15] MSLT-1 authors also performed several subgroup analyses to conclude that SLNB results in improved DFS. Critics argue that there is a clear lead time bias effect when patients who have already undergone nodal dissection are compared with those who have not when disease free is defined as the development of new nodal disease.[14] Some detractors even argue against the use of SLNB as standard of care for prognostication.[16]

The trial investigators responded in kind.[18-22] In the final report, they describe a clear and significant reduction in disease recurrence in the SLNB arm.[9] Furthermore, Faries and colleagues[12] demonstrated that those who underwent delayed nodal

---

Box 3
MSLT-I: final trial report results[9]

Survival data
- 10-year MSS: no difference for intermediate or thick melanomas when comparing SLNB with observation group.
- 10-year DFS: significantly higher in the SLNB versus observation group for intermediate (71.3% vs 64.7%) and thick (50.7% vs 40.5%) melanomas.

Prognostic significance of SLNB
- 10-year MSS for intermediate-thickness melanoma and SLNB-positive (62.1%) versus SLNB-negative (85.1%) (hazard ratio [HR] for death from melanoma, 3.09; 95% confidence interval [CI], 2.12–4.49; $P<.001$).
- 10-year MSS for thick melanoma and SLNB-positive (48.0%) versus SLNB-negative (64.6%) (HR for death from melanoma, 1.75; 95% CI, 1.07–2.87; $P = .03$).
- In multivariate analysis, sentinel node status was the strongest predictor of disease recurrence or death from melanoma.

Nodal metastasis (estimated cumulative incidence at 10 years) was the same between SLNB and observation group
- 20.0% for patients with intermediate-thickness melanoma.
- 41.4% for patients with thick melanoma.

In groups with nodal metastasis, survival advantages were seen in the intermediate-thickness group
- 10-year MSS was 62.1% (SLNB group) versus 41.5% (observation group) (HR for death from melanoma, 0.56; 95% CI, 0.37–0.84; $P = .006$).
- Distant DFS improved for patients with intermediate thickness (HR, 0.62; 95% CI, 0.42–0.91; $P = .02$).
- There were no differences seen in the patients with thick melanoma.

Post hoc latent-subgroup analysis performed to address lead time bias
- This subgroup specifically reviewed patients with intermediate-thickness melanoma that underwent immediate node dissection when SLNB-positive compared with those with delayed nodal development under observation.
- The estimated treatment effect on DFS (1.17; $P<.001$), distant DFS (0.73; $P = .04$), and MSS (0.68; $P = .05$). This translates to increases in survival times by factors of 3.2, 2.1, and 2.0, respectively.

Adapted from Morton DL, Thompson JF, Cochran AJ, Mozzillo N, Nieweg OE, Roses DF, Hoekstra HJ, Karakousis CP, Puleo CA, Coventry BJ, Kashani-Sabet M, Smithers BM, Paul E, Kraybill WG, McKinnon JG, Wang HJ, Elashoff R, Faries MB; MSLT Group. Final trial report of sentinel-node biopsy versus nodal observation in melanoma. *N Engl J Med.* 2014 Feb 13; 370(7):599-609, with permission.

---

dissection suffered from greater disease burden and increased morbidity. Data from other international groups also support these findings. Moncrieff and Garioch[20] showed a significantly increased risk of extracapsular spread (22.7% vs 42.7%; $P<005$; odds ratio, 253; 95% confidence interval, 126–514) in macroscopic compared with microscopic nodal metastases. Furthermore, data presented in the UK guidelines for management of cutaneous melanoma indicate that patients with macroscopic disease are likely to be offered more extensive resections and adjuvant radiotherapy as a result.[23]

In addressing the question of survival benefit, the authors admit that the trial was underpowered because of unexpected favorable outcomes among all patients enrolled. Their findings conclude that 80% of the patients with intermediate-thickness melanoma had no nodal metastasis and therefore early nodal excision would not improve survival in such a group, thus skewing survival results. Therefore,

---

Box 4
Suite of papers generated from MSLT-I data

1999: Validation of the accuracy of intraoperative lymphatic mapping and sentinel lymphadenectomy for early stage melanoma: a multicenter trial. This first report aimed to evaluate the accuracy of lymphatic mapping and SLNB and transferability of this technique worldwide. They compared rates of node identification in the MSLT-I group versus incidence of SN metastasis in a retrospective cohort at the organizing center (John Wayne Cancer Institute). Identification reached 97% in the MSLT cohort and incidence of metastasis approached that seen at John Wayne Cancer Institute. The paper concluded that lymphatic mapping and SLNB can be learned and applied in a standardized fashion.[10]

2005: Sentinel node biopsy for early stage melanoma: accuracy and morbidity in MSLT-I, an international multicenter trial. This article presented the learning phase each participating center had to complete before patient enrollment. All centers were required to present 30 consecutive cases where blue dye and radiocolloid injection were performed followed by lymphoscintigraphy. SLNB plus immediate CLND resulted in SN identification rate of 85%; each individual surgeon had to report at least 15 cases to show proficiency. Patients were then enrolled as noted in **Fig. 1**. This article demonstrated that lymphatic mapping and SLNB are safe and low-morbidity procedures for identifying nodes in the lymphatic basin.[11]

2006: Sentinel node biopsy or nodal observation in melanoma. This was the third interim analysis but first article from the MSLT-I working group to report detailed demographics, clinical results, and survival data for this multicenter trial. Pretrial statistical modeling indicated immediate versus delayed CLND could affect survival in intermediate-thickness melanoma (1.2–3.5 mm). This article evaluated 1269 patients with intermediate-thickness primary melanoma and demonstrated significantly higher DFS in the SLNB versus the observation group but no difference in MSS. When comparing SN-positive with SN-negative, survival curves widened significantly for DFS and MSS demonstrating the prognostic value of SLNB for intermediate-thickness melanoma.[8]

2010: The impact on morbidity and length of stay of early versus delayed complete lymphadenectomy in melanoma: results of the Multicenter Selective Lymphadenectomy Trial (I). This article demonstrated significantly worse lymphedema after delayed CLND compared with early CLND (for axillary and inguinal dissection). They also noted increased length of stay by 1.5–2 days in delayed CLND. No differences were seen with regards to other chronic toxicities, such as nerve dysfunction, motor weakness, or dysesthesias.[12]

2014: Final trial report of sentinel-node biopsy versus nodal observation in melanoma. *New England Journal of Medicine*. This was the fifth and final paper reporting 10-year findings (see **Box 3**).[9]

---

they performed cumulative rates of nodal metastasis after 10 years and noted that no differences were found in SLNB versus observation group countering the argument of "false-positive sentinel nodes." In addition, latent subgroup analysis was performed to exclude possible ascertainment bias in patients with SLNB-positive versus patients with delayed nodal development under observation. This statistical method estimated the treatment effect of performing immediate node dissection in the SLNB-positive group. For intermediate-thickness melanomas, DFS, distant DFS, and MSS all demonstrated significant increase in survival (see **Box 3**).[9]

Finally, the investigators correctly argue that accurate staging via SLNB is critical to timely referral for adjuvant therapies and enrollment in clinical trial. At the time of final report publication, available adjuvant treatments included completion node dissection and interferon gamma. These treatments were fraught with concerns regarding associated toxicity/morbidity and limited benefit. With the current success of immunotherapy for melanoma, the information garnered from SLNB is essential for establishing appropriate care for patients with advanced disease.[18,24,25]

HEAD AND NECK MELANOMA: A UNIQUE SUBSITE

Extensive lymphatics within HN have prompted questions and debate as to the accuracy and prognostic value of SLNB. The classic multi-institutional trials include few HN patients (eg, only 18% of MSLT-1 enrollees had HN melanoma)[9] and are thus underpowered with respect to definitive conclusions for this anatomic subsite. Some have argued that the conclusions drawn in these studies cannot be applied to HN patients without some qualifications.

Accuracy of SLNB for HN cases has been questioned. Interim analysis of MSLT-I in 2005 showed an SLNB success rate of 85% in HN cases compared with 98% for melanoma in other sites.[11] Since that time, several series have invalidated this concern. Erman and colleagues[26] studied 353 SLNB for HN melanoma performed in an academic otolaryngology setting. Accuracy was reported at 99.7%. Sentinel node involvement in this study was 19.6%.[26] These numbers match other large series, such as the Sunbelt Trial for melanoma at non-HN sites.[27] Multivariate analysis showed SLN status was the single most prognostic clinicopathologic factor taking into account Breslow depth and ulceration.[26]

There have been reports of increased false omission rates in HN cases compared with other sites.[28] This has been attributed to variable lymphatic drainage but also, drainage to several nodal basins, closeness to primary site, proximity to cranial nerves, and small sentinel nodes.[24,28] Roy and colleagues[24] analyzed 37 studies assessing accuracy of SLNB in HN melanoma. They report overall failure rates after melanoma surgery to be 3.3% to 6.9%, and false-negative rates from 10.4% to 24.5%. For HN melanoma, they noted a mean failure rate of 4.9% (0%–25%) and a false-negative rate of 20.6% (0%–50%). The wide incidence range reflects results from various institutions, many of which report low numbers of HN cases.[24]

Furthermore, the safety of SLNB in HN has been questioned because of complex cranial nerve anatomy and proximity to great vessels. Several large trials have disproven this and in fact have shown less morbidity overall for SLNB of HN. Wrightson and colleagues[29] reviewed complication after SLNB and demonstrated higher rates in the groin (8.1%) and axilla (4.4%) than HN (2.4%). The Sunbelt Melanoma Trial included greater than 300 HN patients and had no cases of permanent facial nerve paresis.[26]

Finally, similar to melanoma at other sites, SLN status remains the most important prognostic indicator in cN0 HN melanoma.[30] Hanks and colleagues[31] reviewed a 356-patient cohort of HN cutaneous melanoma cases over 10 years. They demonstrate 10-year overall survival (OS) and MSS (61%, 81%) for SLNB-negative patients dropped considerably in SLNB-positive patients (31%, 60.3%). In fact, 10-year OS, recurrence-free survival (RFS), regional RFS, distant DFS, PFS, and MSS all significantly diminished in patients with positive sentinel node status.[31] SLNB in HN melanoma is safe and accurate. It is now incorporated into the American Joint Committee on Cancer staging system, the National Comprehensive Cancer Network (NCCN) practice guidelines, and numerous national and international consensus statements.[30]

CURRENT INDICATIONS FOR SENTINEL LYMPH NODE BIOPSY

In 2018, the joint American Society of Clinical Oncology/Society of Surgical Oncology (ASCO-SSO) guidelines offered a systematic review of the literature regarding SLNB. This review included nine observational studies, two systematic reviews, and an updated randomized controlled trial of SLNB. Their recommendations are seen in **Box 5**. The rate of sentinel node metastasis in T1a and T1b lesions is 5.2% and 8%, respectively.[32] Despite this marginal difference, there does seem to be improved

---

Box 5
2018 ASCO-SSO practice guidelines[32]

Recommendation 1.1. Thin melanomas. Routine SLNB is not recommended for patients with melanomas that are T1a (nonulcerated lesions <0.8 mm in Breslow thickness). SLNB may be considered for T1b patients (0.8–1.0 mm Breslow thickness or <0.8 mm Breslow thickness with ulceration) after a thorough discussion with the patient of the potential benefits and risk of harms associated with the procedure.

Recommendation 1.2. Intermediate-thickness melanomas. SLN biopsy is recommended for patients with melanomas that are T2 or T3 (Breslow thickness of >1.0–4.0 mm).

Recommendation 1.3. Thick melanomas. SLNB may be recommended for patients with melanomas that are T4 (>4.0 mm in Breslow thickness), after a thorough discussion with the patient of the potential benefits and risks of harm associated with the procedure.

Data from Practice guidelines from Wong SL, Faries MB, Kennedy EB, Agarwala SS, Akhurst TJ, Ariyan C, Balch CM, Berman BS, Cochran A, Delman KA, Gorman M, Kirkwood JM, Moncrieff MD, Zager JS, Lyman GH. Sentinel Lymph Node Biopsy and Management of Regional Lymph Nodes in Melanoma: American Society of Clinical Oncology and Society of Surgical Oncology Clinical Practice Guideline Update. J Clin Oncol 2018;36(4):399-413.

---

prognosis for patients with T1b disease who have negative SLNB compared with those who do not undergo SLNB.

SLNB for intermediate-thickness melanoma generates the least controversy. Several studies reviewed demonstrate that SLNB imparts improved regional disease control and guides selection of adjuvant treatment. Prognostic significance of SLN status and the low rate of complications reveals that the benefits of performing SLNB outweigh the risks of observation (16%–20% expected metastatic rate).[32]

For thick melanomas, the lack of perceived benefit from SLNB because of assumed high rates of occult distant disease has led to fewer studies in this area. Most papers evaluating SLNB in thick melanomas have been published in the last few years and are retrospective.[33] A SEER database study found no difference in 5-year DSS with SLNB versus observation groups.[34] MSLT-I also described a cohort of thick melanomas with improved 10-year DFS but no difference in 10-year MSS between SLNB and observations groups (see **Box 3**).[9] Nonetheless, these studies have demonstrated that SLNB provides important prognostic information, in particular for SLNB-negative patients.[35] Results from SLNB can provide critical information to help guide treatment plans including intensity of surveillance and suitability for adjuvant treatments (**Box 6**).

MANAGEMENT OF THE NECK AFTER A POSITIVE SENTINEL NODE: THE NEW DEBATE

Although MSLT-I confirmed that SLNB is a reliable technique and that the pathologic status of the sentinel node is the most important predictor of survival outcome in patients with melanoma, important recent studies addressing the merits of CLND have further changed surgical practice. Although not without controversy, these studies also validate the importance of SLNB as a diagnostic tool and therapeutic intervention for many patients with melanoma.

THE GERMAN DERMATOLOGIC COOPERATIVE ONCOLOGY GROUP SELECTIVE LYMPHADENECTOMY TRIAL

DeCOG-SLT, a multicenter prospective randomized phase 3 trial published in June of 2016, compared CLND with observation in patients with sentinel node–positive

Box 6
SLNB contemporary technique: pearls

- Under optimal circumstances, WLE and SLNB should occur on the same day. This recommendation from NCCN attempts to minimize false-negative rates that might be elevated because of disrupted lymphatics from previous biopsy.

- The melanoma is injected with 2–4 aliquots of radiocolloid, usually in a four-quadrant fashion around the lesion.

- Acquisition of lymphoscintigraphy images may begin 3 minutes postinjection.

- Anatomic landmarks delineated by SPECT/CT are critical to the minimally invasive approach favored for HN.

- 1–3 mL of blue dye is injected through needles 25G or smaller. The bevel of the needle should be facing up and inserted nearly parallel to the skin. After injection, dermal lymphatics are seen arborizing around the lesion.

- Consideration must be given to where incisions for SLNB are placed and how that would affect future skin incisions should the patient need to return for completion lymphadenectomy.

- The radiotracer read of the node, usually a 10-second ex vivo count, should be documented. The bed from which the sentinel node was removed should have a radiotracer read of 10% or less of the ex vivo node.

- Sentinel nodes are labeled specifically as sentinel nodes when sent to pathology. This alerts the pathology team toward special handling. NCCN guidelines recommend submission of the entire node. Large nodes should be sliced at 2-mm intervals, whereas smaller nodes (<5 mm) should be submitted whole.

- If initial biopsy results indicate positive margins (MIS or invasive melanoma), staged reconstruction is recommended to allow for additional resection should this be necessary after return of the final pathology.

melanoma. It should be stated at the outset that this trial purposely excluded patients with HN melanoma because of the controversies discussed previously. That said, the trial's hypothesis that CLND would confer a survival benefit for positive SLNB patients was refuted. Distant metastasis-free survival (DMFS; the primary study end point), OS, and RFS were all comparable between the treatment groups. On multivariable analysis, sentinel node tumor burden ($\leq$1 mm including single cells vs >1 mm deposits) and primary melanoma tumor thickness ($\leq$2 mm vs >2 mm) were significant predictors of DMFS, OS, and RFS, whereas CLND, primary melanoma ulceration, number of positive sentinel nodes, and adjuvant interferon therapy were not. Further analysis of DMFS in the subgroups of positive sentinel node patients by nodal tumor burden was conducted, with no difference between the two treatment groups noted. The authors did note a small increase in regional disease control for patients treated with CLND, 8% versus 15% in the observation group. This was attended by a 24% "adverse event" rate in the CLND group, with lymphedema cited as the most common complication of further surgery.[36]

Based on these results, the DeCOG-SLT authors concluded that CLND may be avoided in patients whose sentinel node tumor burden is 1 mm or less. They remained open to the possibility that CLND is useful in patients with higher nodal burden, acknowledging that the 66% to 34% skew of low versus high nodal burden patients in their study impacts this recommendation.[36] The high rate of surgical complications in the study population likely influenced these recommendations. Having closed DeCOG-SLT early because of accrual challenges and power analyses impacted by better-than-expected survival of the study population, the authors looked to additional data from prospective trials being conducted elsewhere in the world. Even so, the final report by Leiter and colleagues[37] of the DeCOG-SLT, with updated analysis through 6 years of follow-up, did not shift their recommendations.

THE SECOND MULTICENTER SELECTIVE LYMPHADENECTOMY TRIAL

MSLT-II was designed to examine the benefit of immediate CLND versus serial clinical observation with ultrasonography in patients with melanoma with positive sentinel nodes. The randomized phase 3 trial was significantly larger than the DeCOG-SLT and was adequately powered to detect a difference between the treatment groups of 5% for the primary end point of MSS. The patients randomized to the observation arm of the trial were followed with clinical examination and regional nodal basin ultrasound every 4 months for the first 2 years, followed by every 6 months for years 3 and 4, and then annually thereafter. MSLT-II noted no significant differences in MSS, even after adjusting for other prognostic factors, between SLNB-positive patients undergoing immediate CLND and those observed by ultrasound. This was also true with respect to DMFS, but there was a small difference in DFS in favor of the CLND group (68 $\pm$ 1.7% vs 63 $\pm$ 1.7% in the observation group; $P = .05$). This was likely caused by improved regional control in a previously dissected nodal basin (92 $\pm$ 1.0% in dissection group vs 77 $\pm$ 1.5% in the observation group; $P<.001$). Nonsentinel node metastases were discovered on pathologic assessment of 11.5% of CLND patients; this increased over time to an actuarial rate of 17.9% (3 year) and 19.9% (5 year). In the observation arm, nonsentinel node metastases were located by ultrasound or physical examination in 22.9% (3 year) and 26.1% (5 year), a statistically significant difference between the two groups at both time points. Finally, the CLND group, much like that in the DeCOG-SLT trial, was more likely to experience an adverse event, with lymphedema noted in approximately 24% of patients postdissection.[38]

MSLT-II provides strong evidence that "no significant survival benefit" is provided by CLND to melanoma patients with positive sentinel nodes. The authors do, however, note that nodal dissection allows for complete staging and the opportunity to control regional metastasis; indeed, completion nodal dissection reduced the rate of regional nodal recurrence by almost 70%. Much like the DeCOG-SLT, most of the patients had a low nodal burden of metastatic melanoma; median diameter of largest tumor deposit was 0.61 mm in the dissection group and 0.67 mm in the observation group, and some nodes were deemed positive only through real-time polymerase chain reaction. As such, the authors caution against making conclusions about CLND in patients with higher nodal metastatic burden. They also note that it is unclear if avoiding CLND is safe in the absence of the rigorous follow-up schedule or in centers without specialized ultrasound services. MSLT-II confirmed the findings of MSLT-I that the pathologic status of the sentinel node is of critical prognostic value in melanoma, and additionally revealed that CLND, although offering additional prognostic information and improved regional control, does not impact MSS or DFS.[38]

TO DISSECT OR OBSERVE THE NECK?

With the new data provided by MSLT-II and DeCOG-SLT, CLND after positive SLNB is no longer the default decision for patients and surgeons. Both studies, including an updated final analysis of the DeCOG-SLT, demonstrate that survival is not impacted by additional surgery to remove remaining at-risk regional lymph nodes. Indeed, these studies provide additional evidence to MSLT-I that the survival benefit of surgery comes from SLNB itself. This point should be made abundantly clear to patients with positive sentinel nodes as they contemplate next steps in their treatment. Patients with surgically removed microscopic nodal disease should be offered close clinical observation, including ultrasound of the regional nodal basins, as one of their options, and be considered for available clinical trials and/or adjuvant therapy as part of a multidisciplinary approach to their ongoing melanoma care.

That completion nodal dissection reduces the regional recurrence rate should also be disclosed to the patient. Although this is not the same as providing a survival benefit, nodal dissection may be warranted in several circumstances. These include patients who are not able or interested in ongoing surveillance with serial ultrasounds at 4-month intervals for the first 2 years of surveillance. In their review of CLND after SLNB, Delman and Wong[39] argue that another subset of patients who might benefit from further surgery are those with significant projected life expectancy to avoid the development of clinically significant regional disease. Given the low but real risk of surgical morbidity from CLND, balancing this risk with the timing of surgery (immediate vs when nodal recurrence become evident) is important in a population where there is no survival benefit. This is particularly true in the era of tremendous developments in adjuvant therapy efficacy.[39]

There remain unanswered questions, however, for many HN surgical oncologists and their patients. Only 13.7% of the patients in the MSLT-II had melanomas of HN, and no HN melanoma patients were enrolled in the DeCOG-SLT. The surgical morbidity of axillary and groin nodal dissections is different from that of neck dissection, particularly with respect to lymphedema, which tends to be less common and less impactful than in the extremities. Risk to cranial nerves and major vasculature prompts concern for the sequelae of losing early opportunities to control regional disease for patients with HN melanoma, irrespective of their OS.[40] That positive nonsentinel nodes portend a poor prognosis leaves some surgeons reticent to adopt a watchful waiting approach; moreover, having this information early may lead to improved decisions around adjuvant therapies for patients at higher risk for poor survival outcomes. Finally, given that both prospective randomized trials noted a preponderance of low metastatic nodal burden in their study population, it remains uncertain whether observation protocols can be safely applied to patients with larger nodal metastatic deposits. The Minimal Sentinel Node Tumor Burden (MINITUB) trial of the European Organization for Research and Treatment of Cancer is examining small metastases and patterns of nodal burden (ie, subcapsular vs parenchymal location) in hopes of further defining the patients least likely to benefit from CLND; results are expected in 2023.

NCCN and the ASCO-SSO guidelines have been modified as a result of MSLT-II and DeCOG-SLT.[39,41] How HN surgeons adopt these guidelines remains to be seen. The University of Michigan recently looked at surgical activity during the year before, year after, and 2 years after MSLT-II; of the 235 consecutive SLNB-positive patients included over those 3 years, 67% underwent immediate CLND the year before, 33%, and 26%, respectively, after MSLT-II was published. Patients with HN melanoma were more likely to undergo completion nodal dissection compared with other primary sites (59% vs 33% [$P = .003$]; odds ratio, 5.22 [$P = .002$]), likely reflecting many of the aforementioned concerns. Patients with higher sentinel node tumor burden were also more likely to undergo further surgery (43% vs 10% for tumor burden $\geq$0.1 mm [$P<.001$]; odds ratio, 8.64 [$P = .002$]).[42]

This single institution's experience is a snapshot of the impact of MSLT-II overall: steady, progressive adoption of regional observation in appropriate SLNB-positive patients, coupled with reticence in applying the new recommendations to the group that was least represented in the MSLT-II cohort.[42] Low enrollment of HN patients in large melanoma trials is a common challenging issue and one that must be addressed in future trials. In the meantime, as the data evolve and surgeons gain experience with surveillance protocols, we must continue to make decisions with our patients based on the best available evidence.

SUMMARY

Over the last 60 years, SLNB has advanced from an interesting observation to the most precise and accurate staging technique performed for malignant melanoma. This is a result of international collaborations and technical innovations across subspecialties and systematic and methodical study of real-time clinical problems. Although there remain unanswered questions in this field, these extraordinary collective efforts continue to push toward less invasive, more informative and effective approaches to managing this deadly disease for patients.

DISCLOSURE

Nothing to disclose.

REFERENCES

1. Gould ED, Winship T, Philbin PH, et al. Observations on a "sentinel node" in cancer of the parotid. Cancer 1960;13:77–8.
2. Cabanas RM. An approach for the treatment of penile carcinoma. Cancer 1977; 39(2):456–66.
3. Morton DL. Overview and update of the phase III Multicenter Selective Lymphadenectomy Trials (MSLT-I and MSLT-II) in melanoma. Clin Exp Metastasis 2012; 29(7):699–706.
4. Morton DL, Wen DR, Wong JH, et al. Technical details of intraoperative lymphatic mapping for early stage melanoma. Arch Surg 1992;127(4):392–9.
5. Perissinotti A, Vidal-Sicart S, Nieweg O, et al. Melanoma and nuclear medicine. Melanoma Manag 2014;1(1):57–74.
6. Sherman AI. Ter-Pogossian M. Lymph-node concentration of radioactive colloidal gold following interstitial injection. Cancer 1953;6(6):1238–40.
7. Alex JC, Weaver DL, Fairbank JT, et al. Gamma-probe-guided lymph node localization in malignant melanoma. Surg Oncol 1993;2(5):303–8.
8. Morton DL, Thompson JF, Cochran AJ, et al, MSLT Group. Sentinel-node biopsy or nodal observation in melanoma. N Engl J Med 2006;355(13):1307–17.
9. Morton DL, Thompson JF, Cochran AJ, et al, MSLT Group. Final trial report of sentinel-node biopsy versus nodal observation in melanoma. N Engl J Med 2014;370(7):599–609.
10. Morton DL, Thompson JF, Essner R,. et al. Validation of the accuracy of intraoperative lymphatic mapping and sentinel lymphadenectomy for early-stage melanoma: a multicenter trial. Multicenter selective lymphadenectomy trial group. Ann Surg 1999;230(4):453–63 [discussion 463–5].
11. Morton DL, Cochran AJ, Thompson JF, et al. Multicenter selective lymphadenectomy trial group. Sentinel node biopsy for early-stage melanoma: accuracy and morbidity in MSLT-I, an international multicenter trial. Ann Surg 2005;242(3): 302–11 [discussion 311–3].
12. Faries MB, Thompson JF, Cochran A, et al. MSLT Cooperative Group. The impact on morbidity and length of stay of early versus delayed complete

lymphadenectomy in melanoma: results of the multicenter selective lymphade-nectomy trial (I). Ann Surg Oncol 2010;17(12):3324–9.

13. van Akkooi AC, Eggermont AM. Melanoma: MSLT-1–SNB is a biomarker, not a therapeutic intervention. Nat Rev Clin Oncol 2014;11(5):248–9.

14. van Akkooi AC. Sentinel node followed by completion lymph node dissection versus nodal observation: staging or therapeutic? Controversy continues despite final results of MSLT-1. Melanoma Res 2014;24(4):291–4.

15. Sladden M, Zagarella S, Popescu C, et al. No survival benefit for patients with melanoma undergoing sentinel lymph node biopsy: critical appraisal of the multi-center selective lymphadenectomy trial-I final report. Br J Dermatol 2015;172(3):566–71.

16. Yang JC, Sherry RM, Rosenberg SA. Melanoma: why is sentinel lymph node bi-opsy 'standard of care' for melanoma? Nat Rev Clin Oncol 2014;11(5):245–6.

17. Yang JC, Sherry RM. MSLT-I-response of clinical trial investigators. Nat Rev Clin Oncol 2014;11(11). https://doi.org/10.1038/nrclinonc.2014.65-c2.

18. Faries MB, Cochran AJ, Thompson JF. MSLT-I-response of clinical trial investiga-tors. Nat Rev Clin Oncol 2014;11(11). https://doi.org/10.1038/nrclinonc.2014.65-c1.

19. Faries MB, Cochran AJ, Elashoff RM, et al. Multicenter selective lymphadenec-tomy trial-I confirms the central role of sentinel node biopsy in contemporary mel-anoma management: response to 'No survival benefit for patients with melanoma undergoing sentinel lymph node biopsy: critical appraisal of the Multicenter Se-lective Lymphadenectomy Trial-I final report. Br J Dermatol 2015;172(3):571–3.

20. Moncrieff M, Garioch J. MSLT-I: it's all about the lymph nodes. Br J Dermatol 2015;173(2):626–7.

21. McGregor JM, Sasieni P. MSLT-I: it's all about the lymph nodes…: reply from the authors. Br J Dermatol 2015;173(2):627–8.

22. Ross MI, Gershenwald JE. How should we view the results of the multicenter se-lective lymphadenectomy trial-1 (MSLT-1)? Ann Surg Oncol 2008;15(3):670–3.

23. Marsden JR, Newton-Bishop JA, Burrows L, et al. Revised UK guidelines for the management of cutaneous melanoma 2010. British Association of Dermatologists (BAD) Clinical Standards Unit. J Plast Reconstr Aesthet Surg 2010;63(9):1401–19.

24. Roy JM, Whitfield RJ, Gill PG. Review of the tole of sentinel node biopsy in cuta-neous head and neck melanoma. ANZ J Surg 2016;86(5):348–55.

25. Wright FC, Souter LH, Kellett S, et al, Melanoma Disease Site Group. Primary excision margins, sentinel lymph node biopsy, and completion lymph node dissection in cutaneous melanoma: a clinical practice guideline. Curr Oncol 2019;26(4):e541–50.

26. Erman AB, Collar RM, Griffith KA, et al. Sentinel lymph node biopsy is accurate and prognostic in head and neck melanoma. Cancer 2012;118(4):1040–7.

27. McMasters KM, Egger ME, Edwards MJ, et al. Final results of the sunbelt mela-noma trial: a multi-institutional prospective randomized phase III study evaluating the role of adjuvant high-dose interferon Alfa-2b and completion lymph node dissection for patients staged by sentinel lymph node biopsy. J Clin Oncol 2016;34(10):1079–86.

28. de Rosa N, Lyman GH, Silbermins D, et al. Sentinel node biopsy for head and neck melanoma: a systematic review. Otolaryngol Head Neck Surg 2011;145(3):375–82.

29. Wrightson WR, Wong SL, Edwards MJ, et al. Complications associated with sentinel lymph node biopsy for melanoma. Ann Surg Oncol 2003;10:676–80.

30. Schmalbach CE, Bradford CR. Is sentinel lymph node biopsy the standard of care for cutaneous head and neck melanoma? Laryngoscope 2015;125(1): 153–60.

31. Hanks JE, Kovatch KJ, Ali SA, et al. Sentinel lymph node biopsy in head and neck melanoma: long-term outcomes, prognostic value, accuracy, and safety. Otolaryngol Head Neck Surg 2020;162(4):520–9.

32. Wong SL, Faries MB, Kennedy EB, et al. Sentinel lymph node biopsy and management of regional lymph nodes in melanoma: American Society of Clinical Oncology and Society of Surgical Oncology clinical practice guideline update. J Clin Oncol 2018;36(4):399–413.

33. Kachare SD, Singla P, Vohra NA, et al. Sentinel lymph node biopsy is prognostic but not therapeutic for thick melanoma. Surgery 2015;158:662–8.

34. Ribero S, Osella-Abate S, Sanlorenzo M, et al. Sentinel lymph node biopsy in thick-melanoma patients (N=350): what is its prognostic role? Ann Surg Oncol 2015;22:1967–73.

35. Monroe MM, Pattisapu P, Myers JN, et al. Sentinel lymph node biopsy provides prognostic value in thick head and neck melanoma. Otolaryngol Head Neck Surg 2015;153(3):372–8.

36. Leiter U, Stadler R, Mauch C, et al. German Dermatologic Cooperative Oncology Group (DeCOG). Complete lymph node dissection versus no dissection in patients with sentinel lymph node biopsy positive melanoma (DeCOG-SLT): a multicentre, randomised, phase 3 trial. Lancet Oncol 2016;17(6):757–67.

37. Leiter U, Stadler R, Mauch C, et al. German Dermatologic Cooperative Oncology Group. Final analysis of DeCOG-SLT trial: no survival benefit for complete lymph node dissection in patients with melanoma with positive sentinel node. J Clin Oncol 2019;37(32):3000–8.

38. Faries MB, Thompson JF, Cochran AJ, et al. Completion dissection or observation for sentinel-node metastasis in melanoma. N Engl J Med 2017;376(23):2211–22.

39. Delman KA, Wong SL. Completion node dissection after sentinel node biopsy in melanoma. JAMA Surg 2018;153(11):1045–6.

40. Schmalbach CE, Bradford CR. Completion lymphadenectomy for sentinel node positive cutaneous head & neck melanoma. Laryngoscope Investig Otolaryngol 2018;3(1):43.

41. Coit DG, Thompson JA, Albertini MR, et al. Cutaneous melanoma, version 2.2019, NCCN clinical practice guidelines in oncology. J Natl Compr Canc Netw 2019; 17(4):367–402.

42. Bredbeck BC, Mubarak E, Zubieta DG, et al. Management of the positive sentinel lymph node in the post-MSLT-II era. J Surg Oncol 2020. https://doi.org/10.1002/jso.26200.

Sentinel Node Biopsy for Nonmelanoma Skin Cancer of the Head and Neck

Rosh Sethi, MD, MPH[a], Kevin Emerick, MD[b],*

KEYWORDS

- Cutaneous squamous cell carcinoma • Merkel cell carcinoma
- Sebaceous cell carcinoma • Sentinel lymph node biopsy

KEY POINTS

- Sentinel lymph node biopsy should be considered for all cutaneous malignancy with a 10% risk of occult regional lymph node metastasis.
- Patients with regional metastasis from cutaneous malignancy have a poor survival; therefore, sentinel lymph node biopsy offers the potential to improve outcomes.
- Exact criteria to guide sentinel lymph node biopsy for cutaneous squamous cell carcinoma remains to be determined, but patients with multiple high-risk features should be considered.
- All patients with Merkel cell carcinoma greater than 1 cm diameter should undergo sentinel lymph node biopsy.

INTRODUCTION

Nonmelanoma skin cancer (NMSC) is the most prevalent cancer in the world.[1] Basal cell carcinoma makes up the vast majority of these cases, but is a low-risk cancer in terms of potential for regional and distant metastasis. Other NMSC, especially cutaneous squamous cell carcinoma (cSCC) and Merkel cell carcinoma (MCC), have a significant risk for regional metastasis and, therefore, sentinel lymph node biopsy (SLNB) is an important consideration in management. Sebaceous carcinoma and other adnexal tumors are also known to have regional metastasis. Sentinel lymph node biopsy is standard in the treatment of melanoma and this experience can provide a framework for how to approach SLNB for NMSC (**Table 1**).

Well-established clinical and pathologic data have allowed a risk stratification profile for patients with melanoma. These pathologic features define the patient's risk of occult lymph node metastasis and need for SLNB or observation. In a prospective

[a] Brigham and Women's Hospital, 75 Francis Street, Boston, MA 02115, USA; [b] Massachusetts Eye and Ear Infirmary, 243 Charles Street, Boston, MA 02114, USA
* Corresponding author.
E-mail address: Kevin_emerick@meei.harvard.edu

Otolaryngol Clin N Am 54 (2021) 295–305
https://doi.org/10.1016/j.otc.2020.11.005
0030-6665/21/© 2020 Elsevier Inc. All rights reserved.

oto.theclinics.com

Table 1	
Nonmelanoma sentinel lymph biopsy summary guide	
Histology	**Criteria for SLNB Consideration**
Squamous cell carcinoma	1. BWH T2b ($\geq$2 of the following: >2 cm, poorly differentiated, PNI, deep invasion beyond subcutaneous fat) 2. $\geq$3 of the following: >2 cm, poorly differentiated, deep invasion beyond fat, >5 mm depth of invasion, PNI, LVI, recurrent, occurring in scar, sarcomatoid/spindle feature, immunocompromised patient
MCC	1. All lesions >1 cm 2. Lesions <1 cm but LVI and high mitoses
Sebaceous carcinoma	>2 cm, LVI (discuss for all tumors given small existing data)
Others	Anticipated/estimated risk of occult metastasis >10%

randomized trial, MSLT-1, a survival benefit was demonstrated for patients who have microscopic regional metastasis identified by SLNB compared with those who present with macroscopic disease.[2] Additionally, SLNB has a practical benefit, helping to guide adjuvant treatment and surveillance. This framework can be applied to SLNB for NMSC. In this article, we consider cSCC as well as other rare tumors such as MCC and sebaceous carcinoma.

CONSIDERATIONS FOR CUTANEOUS SQUAMOUS CELL CARCINOMA
Rationale for Sentinel Lymph Node Biopsy

Cutaneous SCC is the second most common skin cancer.[1] It has a continually increasing incidence approaching almost 400 cancers per 100,000 people per year in Australia and more than 700,000 cases per year in the United States.[3–5] It disproportionately affects the head and neck region because of its chronic sun exposure. The vast majority of cSCC is cured with excision and 95% of all cSCC fall into this low-risk category.[6] However, owing to the high prevalence of cSCC patients, there are still an estimated 5604 to 12,572 patients per year who develop regional lymph node metastasis. These regional metastases lead to approximately 3932 to 8791 deaths per year from cSCC.[7] To put this in context, this is similar to the number of deaths per year from melanoma (6850).[8]

Although the overall survival from low-risk cSCC is in the very high 90s, once a patient has a regional metastasis, survival significantly decreases.[6] In a series from Australia in 2005 involving 181 patients, Clark and colleagues[9] reported a 39% disease-specific survival for patients with regional metastasis. Similarly, in 2017 Amoils and colleagues[10] reported a similar 5-year survival of less than 40% for patients with regional metastasis. Creighton and colleagues[11] published a series of 62 patients in 2018 showing a 56% overall survival. One of the best survival outcomes was reported in a prospective clinical trial also published in 2018. Porceddu and colleagues[12] reported a 5-year overall survival of 76% when comparing adjuvant radiation and chemoradiation. This study highlights the potentially improved survival in patients receiving the optimal and close care associated with a clinical trial. The regional lymph node basin is the first site of metastasis in approximately 85% of all cases. These survival statistics highlight the potential impact of SLNB.

Risk Factors for Occult Metastasis

Histopathologic melanoma data identified the group of lesions with at least a 10% risk of occult lymph node metastasis and therefore the recommendation for SLNB. For cSCC, defining such a criterion has been more difficult. One of the most frequently cited criteria is from the Brigham and Women's Hospital. In 2013 Jambusaria-Pahlajani and colleagues[13] reported a retrospective cohort study identifying 4 features predicting a higher risk of regional metastasis: size greater than 2 cm, deep invasion beyond the subcutaneous fat, perineural invasion (PNI), and poor tumor differentiation. Twenty percent of patients with more than 1 risk factor developed regional metastasis. Other retrospective cohort studies and case reviews reported additional histopathologic features, such as lymphovascular invasion (LVI), depth of invasion greater than 6 mm, bone invasion, and spindle or sarcomatoid features.[10,11,14,15] Less well-defined clinical features such as rapid growth, growth within the previous scar, and recurrence after previous treatment have also been shown to carry significance.[14–16] Practitioners are well aware that immunosuppressed patients have a large number of cSCC lesions and more high-risk lesions. Elghouche and colleagues[17] performed a meta-analysis assessing the impact of immunosuppression and found a hazard ratio of 2.2 for the risk of local and regional recurrence as well as a 3.61 ratio for disease-specific survival. It is likely that all of these features play a role in the risk profile for occult metastasis. Future research to better understand and quantify these risks will be key to defining the role of SLNB.

Review of Sentinel Lymph Node Biopsy Literature

Unlike melanoma, SLNB experience with cSCC is limited to single institution experiences. Wu and colleagues[16] published a prospective series of 83 SLNB patients based on the Brigham and Women's stage T2b criteria. Only 10% of biopsies in the T2b group were positive. Four patients developed a recurrence after a negative biopsy; however, all of these events occurred in the setting of a local recurrence following SLNB. Durham and associates[14] published a case review series from the University of Michigan, where they performed SLNB on 53 patients with a positivity rate of 15.1%. The criteria for their series was less well-defined in terms of specific inclusion criteria for SLNB. However, assessment of the data shows that LVI, PNI, and overall clinical size are associated with the presence of lymph node metastasis. This series identified 5 patients who underwent a more thorough processing of the tissue, including use of immunohistochemical staining, and 2 of the 5 cases reviewed were found to have microscopic disease initially considered negative. Unlike melanoma, the processing of SLNB tissue has not yet been standardized. This report suggests that immunohistochemical staining may be more accurate. Mooney and colleagues[15] recently published a prospective series from Sydney Australia. They reported on 105 patients with a 10% SLNB positive rate and a 14.3% total subclinical nodal metastasis. Similar to the series at the University of Michigan, a specific criterion for study enrollment was not defined. However, the data demonstrated several key factors to identify patients who may benefit from SLNB. No patient had a positive node with depth of invasion of less than 5 mm.

Additionally, the risk of metastasis further increased for tumors greater than 10 mm in thickness. When combining this depth of invasion with the presence of PNI the rate of lymph node metastasis increased to 28%. This group reported patients with 4 or more risk factors (size >2 cm, invasion into subcutaneous fat, depth of invasion >5 mm, poor tumor differentiation, PNI, PNI, local recurrence, ear or lip location, immunocompromised status, and carcinoma in a preexisting scar) having a greater than 20% risk of occult lymph node metastasis. The SLNB experience to date supports consideration of a broad inclusion criteria of risk factors and the importance of multiple high-risk factors increases risk for occult metastasis.

Impact of Sentinel Lymph Node Biopsy on Outcome and Management

The impact of SLNB on outcomes and clinical care remain to be determined. From a practical standpoint, SLNB can be used to help determine the need for follow-up and adjuvant radiation therapy. The SLNB series mentioned elsewhere in this article report a relatively high risk—approximately 10%—of local recurrence, in-transit metastasis, and even distant metastasis.[15,16] Therefore, patients who meet the criteria for considering SLNB should be closely monitored for 2 to 3 years, regardless of SLNB outcome.

For those with a positive SLNB, potential next steps in management include observation, completion lymphadenectomy, and radiation. Ebrahimi and colleagues[18] reported a large series that showed patients with a single lymph node metastasis of less than 3 cm without ECS treated only surgically had 100% survival at 5 years. This finding suggests a limited benefit for adjuvant radiation after a single positive SLNB. In patients without local recurrence, lymph node recurrence after a negative SLNB is very low, limiting any benefit from adjuvant radiation.[15,16]

Consideration for completion lymph node dissection (CLND) is more complex. The SLNB series reported were not collected and managed in a manner to provide any clear guidance on this management. Melanoma data have shown approximately a 15% rate of nonsentinel lymph nodes identified at time of completion node dissection.[19] Durham and colleagues[14] reported 2 of 5 patients who underwent completion node dissection had positive nodes. Given the limited morbidity and potential to improve regional control, lymphadenectomy is a reasonable management option after a positive SLNB. Lymphadenectomy should be based on the primary lesion location and its expected at risk lymph node regions. The mapping from SLNB should also be used to help to guide this dissection.[20,21] Patients not undergoing completion lymphadenectomy need close observation with serial imaging.

The impact of SLNB on survival cannot be determined from the current literature. There has not been a study designed to answer this question. Series to date have reported survival rates of 20% to 100% at 3 years for positive SLNB.[14,15,22] This disparate experience makes any comparison with existing survival data on macroscopic lymph node metastasis impossible. However, given the poor survival reported for patients with macroscopic lymph node metastasis there is a potential opportunity to improve outcomes by detecting micrometastasis. A future clinical trial will be needed to answer this question.

The emerging role of immunotherapy is likely to have an impact on adjuvant treatment. Checkpoint inhibitors in the adjuvant setting are currently being explored in a clinical trial. Based on future data, the decision to give adjuvant immunotherapy could be determined by SLNB. This type of treatment could have a more significant impact on recurrence at the primary site, regionally, as well as distantly, thereby improving disease-specific and overall survival.

CONSIDERATIONS FOR MERKEL CELL CARCINOMA

MCC is a rare and aggressive cutaneous malignancy of neuroendocrine origin that predominantly occurs in the head and neck (43%) and upper limbs and shoulder (24%).[23] Regional lymph node metastasis is clearly associated with worse outcomes, and assessment of lymph node status is important from a prognostic and treatment planning perspective. SLNB is considered an important staging tool in patients with clinically node-negative MCC and is recommended by the National Comprehensive Cancer Network MCC practice guidelines.[24]

Risk Factors for Occult Metastasis

Although the majority of patients with MCC present without clinically evident nodal involvement, up to 40% of patients may ultimately develop regionally metastasis.[25] Several tumor factors are associated with increased risk of occult nodal metastasis, including tumor thickness, diameter, location, mitotic rate, LVI, and tumor-infiltrating lymphocyte burden.

Within the head and neck, anatomic subsite may independently predict risk of nodal metastasis and survival. A retrospective analysis of the Surveillance Epidemiology and End Results (SEER) database found that lip tumors are associated with the highest rates of local invasion (13.7%), whereas ear tumors had the highest rate of nodal metastasis (63.2%).[26]

Tumor depth and diameter have been identified as independent prognostic factors for SLNB status, as well as overall and disease-specific survival. In their study of 191 patients who underwent SLNB for MCC, Smith and colleagues[27] reported 31% SLNB positivity across all primary tumor sites. They found that the odds of SLNB positivity increased 1.4 times as tumor depth doubled and 1.7 times as tumor diameter doubled. In a study of 2104 patients with head and neck and non–head and neck MCC, tumor extension beyond the dermis was identified as a unique factor associated with worse disease-specific survival.[28] Stokes and colleagues[29] in their retrospective review of 213 patients who underwent SLNB or lymph node dissection found that only 4% of patients with tumors less than 1 cm had clinically evident regional lymph node metastasis at the time of presentation compared with 24% in patients who had tumors greater than 1 cm in size, suggesting that patients with MCC less than 1 cm may have a low risk of occult metastasis.

Additional prognostic factors have been associated with SLN positivity in retrospective reviews. In 1 study of 153 patients who underwent SLNB, Fields and colleagues[30] identified tumor size greater than 2 cm and the presence of LVI as independent factors associated with SLNB positivity. In their review of 95 patients with clinically node-negative MCC at the University of Michigan, Schwartz and colleagues[31] identified increased tumor thickness, infiltrative (vs circumscribed) growth pattern, and increased mitotic rate as independent predictors of SLN positivity in multivariable models. Notably, no subgroup in their study was identified as having less than a 15% risk of SLN positivity.[31] Tumor-associated immune infiltrates at the tumor margin have also been identified as a prognostic indicator.[32]

Review of the Sentinel Lymph Node Biopsy Literature

Sentinel lymph node biopsy has been used widely among institutions who care for patients with MCC. A large systematic review of 721 patients with tumors in any location from 36 published studies found that SLNB positivity was 29.6% with a false-negative rate of 17.1%.[33] In a systematic review of 136 patients with head and neck MCC from 29 publications, SLNB positivity was 30.9% with a false-negative rate of 19.2%.[34]

Unique to head and neck MCC, complex lymph node drainage patterns may limit its reliability and prognostic value owing to the higher risk of false-negative results.[35] However, other studies have shown SLNB in the head and neck to be very reliable, with false-negative rates of less than 5%.[14,15] Discordant drainage pathways have historically limited widespread use of SLNB across many cancer subtypes; however, several single-institution studies have supported the use of SLNB in the workup of patients with clinically node-negative MCC of the head and neck.[25,36–39] This discrepancy may be the result of a different biologic behavior of MCC or potentially a different set of head and neck experiences among surgeons performing SLNB for MCC.

Large series are uncommon owing to the inherent rarity of MCC. In a review of 122 clinically node-negative patients at the Dana-Farber Cancer Institute, a 32% SLNB positivity rate was reported.[40] In a series of 76 patients with clinically node-negative MCC who underwent SLNB, Harounian and colleagues[41] identified SLN positivity in 29% of patients. Of note, this series did not identify an association between primary tumor site, diameter, patient age, sex, or immune status with SLNB positivity.[41,42]

Impact of Sentinel Lymph Node Biopsy on Outcome and Management

The impact of SLNB on MCC disease-specific and overall survival has been assessed across multiple studies, although findings are variable, in large part owing to differences in SLNB techniques, histologic analysis, false-negative SLNB rates, center-specific treatment paradigms based on SLNB results, and multiple lymph node positivity. Several studies demonstrated an association between SLNB status and disease-free and overall survival. A National Cancer Database analysis of 1174 patients who underwent SLNB found a significant association between SLN positivity and decreased overall survival.[41] A multicenter observational trial from Europe of 87 patients with clinically node-negative MCC who underwent SLNB found significantly increased overall and disease-free survival among patients with a negative SLNB. Notably, all patients in this series underwent wide local excision with adjuvant radiation to the primary site, and node-positive patients additionally underwent lymph node dissection and regional adjuvant radiation therapy.[43] A 2003 to 2009 SEER registry review of 1193 patients, of which 474 underwent SLNB, found that a negative SLNB was associated with a significantly improved 5-year disease-specific survival.[44]

However, several other studies failed to demonstrated any association between SLNB status and survival outcomes. In their review of 150 patients treated at the Mayo Clinic, Sims and colleagues[45] found no significant difference in disease-specific survival at 1, 3, or 5 years among patients with a positive versus a negative SLNB status. Among patients with a positive SLNB who received treatment to the nodal basin, disease-specific survival and overall survival were also similar to patients with negative SLNB. Fields and colleagues[30] found no significant difference in recurrence or disease-free survival between SLNB-positive and -negative patients in their cohort of 153 patients who underwent SLNB; however, the majority of SLNB-positive patients received radiation or chemotherapy. In their SEER registry database analysis of 721 patients with cutaneous head and neck MCC who underwent SLNB, Fritsch and colleagues[46] found an SLN positivity rate of 23.1% and no association between survival outcomes and SLN positivity.

There are additional conflicting reports in the literature as to whether SLNB itself may be associated with a decreased risk of recurrence or disease progression. In a SEER study of 1193 patients with stage I and II MCC, 474 underwent SLNB and 719 were observed in the regional lymph node basin. Patients who underwent SLNB had a 5-year disease-specific survival benefit when compared with those who were observed.[44] Single-institution studies, however, have not demonstrated any survival benefit associated with SLNB itself.[47] At present, SLNB remains a diagnostic rather than therapeutic tool in the workup and management of MCC.

Although it is not clear that SLNB positivity is strongly associated with overall survival outcomes, current guidelines strongly advocate for the use of SLNB in clinically node-negative MCC as an important prognostic and staging tool. Unlike melanoma, and similar to cSCC, prior studies have not identified primary tumor subgroups with a lower than 15% risk of SLNB positivity; therefore, SLNB is advocated for all patients.[31] Patients with lesions less than 1 cm and no LVI may be the exception to this recommendation.

Among patients with SLNB positivity, current guidelines support CLND, regional radiation therapy, or both. An National Cancer Database analysis of 447 MCC SLNB-positive patients compared survival outcomes for CLND alone versus CLND with adjuvant radiation or adjuvant radiation alone. CLND alone was associated with worse survival outcomes compared with the other treatment regimens.[48] Lee and colleagues[49] compared CLND alone with radiation therapy alone in their cohort of 163 patients and reported no difference in disease-specific 5-year survival (71% vs 64%) or disease-free survival (52% vs 61%). Perez and colleagues[50] similarly found no difference in overall survival between patients who underwent CLND alone, radiation alone, or CLND with radiation at Moffitt Cancer Center. Morbidity was low across all treatment groups (lymphedema and surgical site infections).

Among patients with SLNB negativity, providers may consider observation, elective radiation, or elective CLND to the nodal basin.[51] Elective radiation may be used in higher risk patients, for example, those in whom appropriate immunohistochemistry was not performed or patients in whom the primary lesion was excised without an adequate assessment of high-risk features. Of note, there is potentially an increased risk of false-negative SLNB result in the head and neck owing to the complex lymph node drainage.[21] Nontraditional SLNB locations must be carefully assessed to appropriately guide further treatment. Further analysis of elective treatment of SLN-negative patients is necessary, including an assessment of disease and overall survival parameters.

CONSIDERATIONS FOR OTHER NONMELANOMA SKIN CANCERS

Sebaceous cell carcinoma is a rare malignant tumor that arises from the sebaceous glands, most commonly occurring in the head and neck, particularly in the eyelids, where it may arise from the meibomian glands. SLNB has been reported in a small retrospective series, although it remains relatively uncommon.[52–54] In a study of 10 patients with eyelid sebaceous cell carcinoma who underwent SLNB, no positive SLN were identified; however, 2 of 10 patients went on to develop recurrence in regional lymph nodes, raising concern for a high false-negative rate and reinforcing the risk for regional metastasis. Imaging or SLNB should be considered.[52] Sentinel lymph node biopsy for sebaceous carcinoma has been successfully used in a larger series with other periocular lesions. These series highlight the feasibility of SLNB for periocular tumors and the occurrence of occult metastasis. However, studies did not identify a clear criterion for performing SLNB or demonstrated a survival benefit given the relatively small sample size.[54,55]

SUMMARY

When considering SLNB for any cutaneous tumor, it is important to assess the prognostic value, false-negativity rate, and implications for treatment planning. The technique itself has been well-described and with imaging adjuncts is a safe and efficient procedure in the head and neck. Therefore, applying a broad consideration of any tumor with a greater than 10% risk of occult metastasis, SLNB should be considered. SLNB for MCC is an established important diagnostic and prognostic procedure. It should be discussed for all patients with MCC. Although the role for SLNB in cSCC remains to be defined, SLNB does offer the potential for important diagnostic information that can be used to personalize care. Additional data are needed to define who needs this procedure and how its outcome directs additional care. Clinical experience and multidisciplinary discussions remain key to identifying patients who may benefit from SLNB.

CLINICS CARE POINTS

- Disease survival from regionally metastatic cSCC is approximately 50% based on multiple studies.
- BWH stage T2b has approximately a 10-20% risk of occult regional lymph node metastasis.
- MCC has a high rate (>40%) of regional metastasis and survival is dramatically decreased in those with regional metastasis.
- MCC has a higher rate of false negative SLNB and those with negative SLNB need continued close surveillance.

DISCLOSURE

R. Sethi – No disclosures. K. Emerick – Consultant; Regeneron and Sanofi; This work does not directly relate to sentinel lymph node biopsy and this content. Work does relate to systemic therapy for cSCC.

REFERENCES

1. Rogers HW, Weinstock MA, Coldiron BM, et al. Incidence estimate of nonmelanoma skin cancer (keratinocyte carcinomas) in the U.S. population, 2012. JAMA Dermatol 2015;151:1081–6.
2. Morton DL, Thompson JF, Cochran AJ, et al. Sentinel-node biopsy or nodal observation in melanoma. N Engl J Med 2006;355:1307–17.
3. Muzic JG, Schmitt AR, Baum CL, et al. Incidence and trends of basal cell carcinoma and cutaneous squamous cell carcinoma: a population-based study in Olmsted County, Minnesota, 2000 to 2010. Mayo Clin Proc 2017;92:890–8.
4. Staples MP, Elwood M, Burton RC, et al. Non-melanoma skin cancer in Australia: the 2002 national survey and trends since 1985. Med J Aust 2006;184:6–10.
5. Rogers HW, Weinstock MA, Harris AR, et al. Incidence estimate of nonmelanoma skin cancer in the United States, 2006. Arch Dermatol 2010;146:283–7.
6. Alam M, Ratner D. Cutaneous squamous cell carcinoma. N Engl J Med 2001; 344(13):975–83.
7. Karia PS, Han J, Schmults CD. Cutaneous squamous cell carcinoma: estimated incidence of disease, nodal metastasis, and deaths from disease in the United States, 2012. J Am Acad Dermatol 2013;68:957–66.
8. Siegel RL, Miller KD, Jemal A. Cancer statistics 2020. CA Cancer J Clin 2020; 70(1):7–30.
9. Clark J, Li W, Smith G, et al. Outcome of treatment for advanced cervical metastatic squamous cell carcinoma. Head Neck 2005;27(2):87–94.
10. Amoils M, Lee CS, Sunwoo J, et al. Node-positive cutaneous squamous cell carcinoma of the head and neck: survival, high-risk features, and adjuvant chemoradiotherapy outcomes. Head Neck 2017;39(5):881–5.
11. Creighton F, Lin A, Leavitt E, et al. Factors affecting survival and locoregional control in head and neck cSCCA with nodal metastasis. Laryngoscope 2018;128(8): 1881–6.
12. Porceddu SV, Bressel M, Poulsen MG, et al. Postoperative concurrent chemoradiotherapy versus postoperative radiotherapy in high-risk cutaneous squamous cell carcinoma of the head and neck: the randomized phase III TROG 05.01 trial. J Clin Oncol 2018;36(13):1275–83.

13. Jambusaria-Pahlajani A, Kanetsky PA, Karia PS, et al. Evaluation of AJCC tumor staging for cutaneous squamous cell carcinoma and a proposed alternative tumor staging system. JAMA Dermatol 2013;149(4):402–10.

14. Durham A, Lowe L, Malloy K, et al. Sentinel lymph node biopsy for cutaneous squamous cell carcinoma of the head and neck. JAMA Otolaryngol Head Neck Surg 2016;142(12):1171–6.

15. Mooney CP, Martin RCW, Dirven R, et al. Sentinel node biopsy in 105 high-risk cutaneous SCCs of the head and neck: results of a multicenter prospective study. Ann Surg Oncol 2019;26:4481–8.

16. Wu MP, Sethi R, Emerick K. Sentinel lymph node biopsy for high-risk squamous cell carcinoma of the head and neck. Laryngoscope 2020;130(1):108–14.

17. Elghouche AN, Pflum Z, Schmalbach CE. Immunosuppression impact on head and neck cutaneous squamous cell carcinoma: a systematic review with meta-analysis. Otolaryngol Head Neck Surg 2019;160:439–46.

18. Ebrahimi A, Clark JR, Veness MJ, et al. Metastatic head and neck cutaneous squamous cell carcinoma: defining a low-risk patient. Head Neck 2012;34:365–70.

19. Faries MB, Thompson JF, Cochran AJ, et al. Completion dissection or observation for sentinel-node metastasis in melanoma. N Engl J Med 2017;376(23):2211–22.

20. Remenschneider AK, Dilger AE, Wang Y, et al. The predictive value of single-photon emission computed tomography/computed tomography for sentinel lymph node localization in head and neck cutaneous malignancy. Laryngoscope 2015;125:877–82.

21. Creighton F, Bergmark R, Emerick K. Drainage patterns to nontraditional nodal regions and level IIB in cutaneous head and neck malignancy. Otolaryngol Head Neck Surg 2016;155:1005–11.

22. Takahashi A, Imafuku S, Nakayama J, et al. Sentinel node biopsy for high-risk cutaneous squamous cell carcinoma. Eur J Surg Oncol 2014;40(10):1256–62.

23. Harms KL, Healy MA, Nghiem P, et al. Analysis of prognostic factors from 9387 Merkel cell carcinoma cases forms the basis for the new 8th edition AJCC staging system. Ann Surg Oncol 2016;23:3564–71.

24. National comprehensive cancer network. Merkel Cell Carcinoma (Version 1. 2020). Available at: https://www.nccn.org/professionals/physician_gls/pdf/mcc.pdf. Accessed September 15, 2020.

25. Schmalbach CE, Lowe L, Teknos TN, et al. Reliability of sentinel lymph node biopsy for regional staging of head and neck Merkel cell carcinoma. Arch Otolaryngol Head Neck Surg 2005;131:610–4.

26. Smith VA, MaDan OP, Lentsch EJ. Tumor location is an independent prognostic factor in head and neck Merkel cell carcinoma. Otolaryngol Head Neck Surg 2012;146:403–8.

27. Smith FO, Yue B, Marzban SS, et al. Both tumor depth and diameter are predictive of sentinel lymph node status and survival in Merkel cell carcinoma. Cancer 2015;121:3252–60.

28. Smith VA, Camp ER, Lentsch EJ. Merkel cell carcinoma: identification of prognostic factors unique to tumors located in the head and neck based on analysis of SEER data. Laryngoscope 2012;122:1283–90.

29. Stokes JB, Graw KS, Dengel LT, et al. Patients with Merkel cell carcinoma tumors < or = 1.0 cm in diameter are unlikely to harbor regional lymph node metastasis. J Clin Oncol 2009;27:3772–7.

30. Fields RC, Busam KJ, Chou JF, et al. Recurrence and survival in patients undergoing sentinel lymph node biopsy for Merkel cell carcinoma: analysis of 153 patients from a single institution. Ann Surg Oncol 2011;18:2529–37.

31. Schwartz JL, Griffith KA, Lowe L, et al. Features predicting sentinel lymph node positivity in Merkel cell carcinoma. J Clin Oncol 2011;29:1036–41.

32. Feldmeyer L, Hudgens CW, Ray-Lyons G, et al. Density, distribution, and composition of immune infiltrates correlate with survival in Merkel cell carcinoma. Clin Cancer Res 2016;22:5553–63.

33. Gunaratne DA, Howle JR, Veness MJ. Sentinel lymph node biopsy in Merkel cell carcinoma: a 15-year institutional experience and statistical analysis of 721 reported cases. Br J Dermatol 2016;174:273–81.

34. Karunaratne YG, Gunaratne DA, Veness MJ. Systematic review of sentinel lymph node biopsy in Merkel cell carcinoma of the head and neck. Head Neck 2018;40: 2704–13.

35. O'Brien CJ, Uren RF, Thompson JF, et al. Prediction of potential metastatic sites in cutaneous head and neck melanoma using lymphoscintigraphy. Am J Surg 1995; 170:461–6.

36. Patel M, Newlands C, Whitaker S. Single-centre experience of primary cutaneous Merkel cell carcinoma of the head and neck between 1996 and 2014. Br J Oral Maxillofac Surg 2016;54:741–5.

37. Kwan K, Ghazizadeh S, Moon AS, et al. Merkel cell carcinoma: a 28-year experience. Otolaryngol Head Neck Surg 2020;163:364–71.

38. Ricard AS, Sessiecq Q, Siberchicot F, et al. Sentinel lymph node biopsy for head and neck Merkel cell carcinoma: a preliminary study. Eur Ann Otorhinolaryngol Head Neck Dis 2015;132:77–80.

39. Dwojak S, Emerick KS. Sentinel lymph node biopsy for cutaneous head and neck malignancies. Expert Rev Anticancer Ther 2015;15:305–15.

40. Gupta SG, Wang LC, Penas PF, et al. Sentinel lymph node biopsy for evaluation and treatment of patients with Merkel cell carcinoma: the Dana-Farber experience and meta-analysis of the literature. Arch Dermatol 2006;142:685–90.

41. Harounian JA, Molin N, Galloway TJ, et al. Effect of sentinel lymph node biopsy and LVI on Merkel cell carcinoma prognosis and treatment. Laryngoscope 2020. https://doi.org/10.1002/lary.28866.

42. Conic RRZ, Ko J, Saridakis S, et al. Sentinel lymph node biopsy in Merkel cell carcinoma: predictors of sentinel lymph node positivity and association with overall survival. J Am Acad Dermatol 2019;81:364–72.

43. Servy A, Maubec E, Sugier PE, et al. Merkel cell carcinoma: value of sentinel lymph-node status and adjuvant radiation therapy. Ann Oncol 2016;27:914–9.

44. Kachare SD, Wong JH, Vohra NA, et al. Sentinel lymph node biopsy is associated with improved survival in Merkel cell carcinoma. Ann Surg Oncol 2014;21: 1624–30.

45. Sims JR, Grotz TE, Pockaj BA, et al. Sentinel lymph node biopsy in Merkel cell carcinoma: the Mayo Clinic experience of 150 patients. Surg Oncol 2018; 27:11–7.

46. Fritsch VA, Camp ER, Lentsch EJ. Sentinel lymph node status in Merkel cell carcinoma of the head and neck: not a predictor of survival. Head Neck 2014;36: 571–9.

47. Tarantola TI, Vallow LA, Halyard MY, et al. Prognostic factors in Merkel cell carcinoma: analysis of 240 cases. J Am Acad Dermatol 2013;68:425–32.

48. Cramer JD, Suresh K, Sridharan S. Completion lymph node dissection for Merkel cell carcinoma. Am J Surg 2020. https://doi.org/10.1016/j.amjsurg.2020.02.018.

49. Lee JS, Durham AB, Bichakjian CK, et al. Completion lymph node dissection or radiation therapy for sentinel node metastasis in Merkel cell carcinoma. Ann Surg Oncol 2019;26:386–94.
50. Perez MC, Oliver DE, Weitman ES, et al. Management of sentinel lymph node metastasis in Merkel cell carcinoma: completion lymphadenectomy, radiation, or both? Ann Surg Oncol 2019;26:379–85.
51. Pellitteri PK, Takes RP, Lewis JS Jr, et al. Merkel cell carcinoma of the head and neck. Head Neck 2012;34:1346–54.
52. Wilson MW, Fleming JC, Fleming RM, et al. Sentinel node biopsy for orbital and ocular adnexal tumors. Ophthal Plast Reconstr Surg 2001;17:338–44 [discussion 344–35].
53. Ho VH, Ross MI, Prieto VG, et al. Sentinel lymph node biopsy for sebaceous cell carcinoma and melanoma of the ocular adnexa. Arch Otolaryngol Head Neck Surg 2007;133:820–6.
54. Owen JL, Kibbi N, Worley B, et al. Sebaceous carcinoma: evidence-based clinical practice guidelines. Lancet Oncol 2019;20:e699–714.
55. Freitag SK, Aakalu VK, Tao JP, et al. Sentinel lymph node biopsy for eyelid and conjunctival malignancy: a report by the American academy of ophthalmology. Ophthalmology 2020. https://doi.org/10.1016/j.ophtha.2020.07.031.

Radiation Therapy for Cutaneous Malignancies of the Head and Neck

Rohan Katipally, MD[a],*, Nishant Agrawal, MD[b],
Aditya Juloori, MD[a]

KEYWORDS

- Radiotherapy • Radiation therapy • Skin cancer • Keratinocyte carcinoma
- Basal cell carcinoma • Squamous cell carcinoma • Melanoma
- Merkel cell carcinoma

KEY POINTS

- Radiation therapy (RT) plays an integral role in the definitive and adjuvant management of cutaneous cancers of the head and neck, including basal cell carcinoma, cutaneous squamous cell carcinoma, melanoma, and Merkel cell carcinoma.
- RT may serve as an appropriate alternative to surgery for basal cell carcinoma and squamous cell carcinoma in cosmetically and functionally sensitive areas.
- Various RT modalities are available in the treatment of cutaneous malignances (ranging from low-energy x-rays, to megavoltage electrons or photons, to brachytherapy).

INTRODUCTION

Radiation therapy (RT) plays a significant role in the management of cutaneous cancers of the head and neck, which include basal cell carcinoma (BCC), cutaneous squamous cell carcinoma (SCC), melanoma, and Merkel cell carcinoma (MCC). Commonly used RT modalities include kilovoltage photons, megavoltage electrons, megavoltage photons, and low-dose-rate and high-dose-rate (HDR) brachytherapy. Kilovoltage (ie, low-energy) photons include orthovoltage, superficial, contact, and soft x-rays and deposit most dose superficially with little dose penetrating into deeper tissues, which is advantageous for superficial skin tumors. Megavoltage electrons penetrate more deeply but still show rapid dose decrease with increasing tissue depth. Megavoltage photons are suitable for larger, deeply invasive tumors. Brachytherapy involves the

[a] Department of Radiation and Cellular Oncology, Duchossois Center for Advanced Medicine, University of Chicago Medicine, 5758 South Maryland Avenue, MC 9006, Chicago, IL 60637, USA; [b] Department of Surgery, Section of Otolaryngology-Head and Neck Surgery, University of Chicago Medicine, 5841 South Maryland Avenue, Chicago, IL 60637, USA
* Corresponding author.
E-mail address: rohan.katipally@uchospitals.edu

Otolaryngol Clin N Am 54 (2021) 307–327
https://doi.org/10.1016/j.otc.2020.11.009
oto.theclinics.com

use of applicators to bring the source of radiation close to the tumor, which may provide a more desirable dose distribution for highly nonuniform skin surfaces. It includes both radionuclide brachytherapy (frequently using iridium-192) and electronic brachytherapy (using electronically generated x-rays).[1]

BASAL CELL CARCINOMA

Indications for definitive RT include[1,2]:

- Primary BCC in patients who are not candidates for surgery
- Primary BCC located in specific anatomic locations that would result in unacceptable cosmetic/functional outcomes with surgery (medial canthus, eyelid)

Discussion

Surgery and definitive RT were compared in an older randomized controlled trial at the Gustave Roussy Institute.[3] From 1982 to 1988, patients with BCC of the face were randomized to surgery or RT (with interstitial brachytherapy, superficial contact therapy, or conventional RT). Although techniques studied in this trial do not reflect modern RT, the 4-year local recurrence (LR) was 0.7% for surgery and 7.5% for RT. Cosmetic outcomes, as evaluated by the patients, dermatologist, and photographic assessment, generally favored surgery, with 87% of patients receiving surgery grading their cosmesis as good compared with 69% with RT.

However, multiple meta-analyses have shown strong local control with definitive RT. An older meta-analysis (published in 1989) of primary treatment of BCC published a 5-year LR of 8.7% with RT, compared with 1.0% with Mohs micrographic surgery and 10.1% with surgical excision.[4] In 2017, Zaorsky and colleagues[5] published a meta-analysis of 21 studies using hypofractionated RT (predominantly T1–T2 SCCs and BCCs) with a median 1-year LR rate of 2% and 5-year LR of 14%.

Individual retrospective series (**Table 1**) report excellent local control (LC) and elucidate multiple risk factors for recurrence (such as tumor location, size, histology, and previously untreated vs recurrent setting). In general, higher LC is reported for BCC than SCC. A Washington University retrospective series showed a 94% LC for previously untreated BCC and 86% for recurrent (median follow-up 5.8 years).[6] In a retrospective series of BCC and SCC treated with soft x-rays, the crude LR was 4.5% for BCC (with mean follow-up of 77 months) and the 15-year LR rate was 6.1%.[7] A retrospective study of 604 BCCs in Spain showed a 5-year cure rate of 94.4% and 15-year cure rate of 84.8%.[8] Tumor location on the nasolabial fold and tumor size greater than or equal to 1 cm predicted for recurrence. Regarding histology, Zagrodnik and colleagues[9] reported a lower 5-year LR for nodular subtypes (8.2%) and a higher 5-year LR for sclerosing subtypes (27.7%).

Based on multiple institutional series, the cosmesis after primary RT is generally very good. In one series, cosmesis was rated as poor/fair in only 5.9% of previously untreated BCCs, and recurrent BCCs did not show a higher rate of poor/fair cosmesis.[6] Another series of 127 BCCs using orthovoltage x-rays showed good to excellent cosmetic outcome in 98%, using total doses ranging from 25 to 60 Gy.[10]

Tumors of the medial canthus and eyelids are at risk of poor cosmesis after surgery. Multiple retrospective series show strong LC with good cosmetic outcomes with RT, making them an acceptable alternative to excision. For eyelid, interstitial brachytherapy showed 96.7% LC, with a low rate of unsatisfactory functional and cosmetic outcomes (8.3%).[11] Late toxicities included nasolacrimal duct stenosis (6.7%), chronic epiphora (5%), ectropion (5%), and cataract (3.3%). Another series using kilovoltage

Table 1
Selected studies of primary radiation therapy for basal cell carcinoma

Series	Study Design	N	Intervention	Outcomes	Toxicity
Avril et al,[3] 1997	Randomized, controlled trial	347	Arm 1: surgery Arm 2: RT (radionuclide interstitial brachytherapy, ELS, conventional)	4-y LR: 0.7% (surgery) vs 7.5% (RT)	Good cosmesis: 87% (surgery) vs 69% (RT)
Locke et al,[6] 2001	Retrospective	389	Electrons, ELS, MV photons (<2%)	LC: 94% (previously untreated) and 86% (recurrent)	Fair/poor cosmesis: 5.9% Soft tissue necrosis: 2%
Schulte et al,[7] 2005	Retrospective	1019	ELS	Crude LR: 4.5% 5-y LR: 4.2% 10-y LR: 6.1% 15-y LR: 6.1%	Pooled BCC and SCC Hypopigmentation: 72.7% Telangiectasias: 51.5% Erythema: 44.5% Hyperpigmentation: 23.4%
Zagrodnik et al,[9] 2003	Retrospective	175	ELS	5-y LR: 15.8% (all histologies), 8.2% (nodular subtype), 26.1% (superficial subtype), 27.7% (sclerosing subtype)	Not reported
Seegenschmiedt et al,[10] 2001	Retrospective	127	ELS	LR: 1.6%	Acute grade 1: 100% Acute grade 2: 54% Acute grade 3: 30% Late toxicity: 2.4%
Guix et al,[19] 2000	Retrospective	102	Radionuclide interstitial brachytherapy	5-y LR: 2.0%	Pooled BCC and SCC 6-wk ulceration present: 10.3% 4-mo ulceration present: 0% 6-mo good/excellent cosmesis: 98%

(continued on next page)

Table 1
(continued)

Series	Study Design	N	Intervention	Outcomes	Toxicity
Krengli et al,[11] 2014	Retrospective	52	Radionuclide interstitial brachytherapy	LC: 3.8%	Pooled histologies Nasolacrimal duct stenosis: 6.7% Chronic epiphora: 5% Ectropion: 5% Unilateral cataract: 3.3% Optimal cosmetic and functional outcome: 68.3% Unsatisfactory cosmetic and functional outcome: 8.3%

Abbreviations: ELS, electronically generated low-energy radiation sources (typically low-energy kilovoltage photons); LC, local control; MV, megavoltage.
Data from Refs.[3,6,7,9–11,19]

photons for medial canthus BCC showed chronic epiphora in 21%, chronic dry eye in 3%, and severe complications (including vision loss) in 0%.[12]

Indications for adjuvant RT include[1,2]:

- Postoperative bed ± cranial nerve pathways for gross perineural tumor spread
- Postoperative bed for close or positive margins not amenable to further resection
- Postoperative bed for recurrence after prior margin negative resection
- Postoperative bed for locally advanced tumors involving bone or muscle
- Nodal basins for N2 disease after lymphadenectomy

Discussion

Perineural involvement or neurotropism is a frequently used term that refers to both microscopic perineural invasion (PNI), which reflects the histologic finding of tumor infiltration of nerves and is often incidental, and perineural tumor spread (PNTS), which reflects gross tumor involvement along a nerve and is often clinically or radiographically apparent.[13] Although perineural involvement is more common in SCC, it is still considered a risk factor for LR in BCC (see **Table 3**), and the extent of perineural involvement is associated with worse locoregional control (LRC). A retrospective review of 135 patients with perineural involvement from the University of Florida included both BCC (22%) and SCC (78%).[14] Patients with clinically apparent PNTS showed a 5-year LRC of 56%, compared with 80% for patients with only microscopic PNI. However, outcomes for BCC specifically were not explicitly reported. The radiographic extent of PNTS was associated with both worse 5-year LC (25% for macroscopic disease radiographically vs 76% for negative imaging) and 5-year overall survival (OS) (58% vs 90%) in both BCC and SCC.[15]

Adjuvant RT can be considered for positive/close margins not amenable to re-excision, because positive margins have been associated with increased 5-year LR (26% compared with 14% with negative margins).[16] Based on a series where normal skin was marked and the tumor was excised with Mohs surgery, a 4-mm resection margin using conventional excision would be required to eliminate the subclinical tumor extent in tumors less than 2 cm.[17] However, this may not always be feasible in cosmetically/functionally sensitive locations.

CUTANEOUS SQUAMOUS CELL CARCINOMA

Indications for definitive RT include[1,2]:

- Primary SCC in patients who are not candidates for surgery
- Primary SCC located in specific anatomic locations that would result in unacceptable cosmetic/functional outcomes with surgery (eg, eyelids, medial canthus)

Discussion

Multiple retrospective studies show excellent LC with primary RT for SCC (**Table 2**). In the aforementioned Washington University series, the LCs were 89% and 68% in the previously untreated and recurrent settings, respectively (median follow-up 5.8 years).[6] In the series by Schulte and colleagues,[7] the crude LR was 6.9% for SCC (mean follow-up of 77 months) and the 15-year LR was 12.8%.

Primary RT has not been compared with surgery for SCC in a randomized trial. In an older meta-analysis by Rowe and colleagues[18] published in 1992, RT was associated with a 6.7% LR in studies with follow-up less than 5 years and a 10.0% LR in studies

Table 2
Selected studies of primary radiation therapy for squamous cell carcinoma

Series	Study Design	N	Intervention	Outcomes	Toxicity
Locke et al,[6] 2001	Retrospective	142	Electrons, superficial therapy, MV photons (<2%)	LC: 89% (previously untreated) and 68% (recurrent)	Fair/poor cosmesis: 13% Soft tissue necrosis: 9%
Schulte et al,[7] 2005	Retrospective	245	ELS	Crude LR: 6.9% 5-y LR: 6.0% 10-y LR: 10.5% 15-y LR: 12.8%	Pooled BCC and SCC Hypopigmentation: 72.7% Telangiectasias: 51.5% Erythema: 44.5% Hyperpigmentation: 23.4%
Guix et al,[19] 2000	Retrospective	34	Radionuclide interstitial brachytherapy	5-y LR: 2.9%	Pooled BCC and SCC 6-wk ulceration present: 10.3% 4-mo ulceration present: 0% 6-mo good/excellent cosmesis: 98%

Data from Refs.[6,7,19]

with follow-up greater than or equal to 5 years, compared with 5.7% and 8.1%, respectively, for surgical excision. Mohs had an LR of 3.1% with follow-up greater than or equal to 5 years, the lowest across all treatment modalities. Factors associated with LR across all treatment modalities included size greater than 2 cm, higher grade, location on the ear or lip, perineural spread, recurrent disease, and immunosuppression.

Cosmesis is a relevant outcome after RT that historically favored surgery rather than primary RT. However, subsequent modern retrospective series demonstrated good cosmetic outcomes. In the retrospective series by Locke and colleagues,[6] cosmetic outcome was rated as good or excellent in 92% of patients, based on retrospective evaluation of telangiectasia, pigment change, and fibrosis of the skin. Cosmesis was worse (ie, poor or fair) when receiving greater than 50 Gy at less than 3 Gy per fraction. Furthermore, higher rates of poor or fair cosmesis were seen in SCC (13%) than in BCC (5.9%), attributable to higher doses administered. Brachytherapy also shows excellent cosmetic outcomes. In a series of SCC and BCC of the face using HDR brachytherapy and custom-made surface molds, only 10% had ulcerations at the 6-week follow-up and all ulcerations were healed by the 4-month follow-up (with 5-year LC 98%).[19] After 6 months, cosmesis was rated as good or excellent in 98% of patients.

The benefit of RT for particular anatomic locations (eg, eyelids and medial canthus) was previously described in relation to BCC and applies to SCC as well.

Indications for adjuvant RT include[1,2]:

- Postoperative bed ± cranial nerve pathways for gross perineural tumor spread or microscopic PNI (extensive or involving large-caliber nerve)
- Postoperative bed for close or positive margins not amenable to further resection
- Postoperative bed for recurrence after prior margin negative resection plus or minus additional resection
- Postoperative bed for T3/T4 tumors
- Postoperative bed for desmoplastic/infiltrative tumors in the setting of chronic immunosuppression
- Nodal basins for N2 disease after lymphadenectomy
- Nodal basins for clinically node-negative patients at high risk of nodal metastasis

Discussion

Clinically or radiographically apparent perineural tumor spread (PNTS) warrants adjuvant RT to improve LRC (**Table 3**). A retrospective series of BCC and SCC with clinical PNTS showed high rates of local failure with 5-year recurrence-free survival (RFS) of 39%.[20] Tumors involving cranial nerves V1/V2 or invading multiple nerves had worse RFS. Of all failures, 87% were local, underscoring the role of adjuvant local therapy. Another study of postoperative RT with clinical PNTS showed a 5-year RFS of 62%, disease-free survival (DFS) of 75%, and OS of 64%.[21] Notably, when classifying extent of PNTS into zones, less extensive spread (zone 1) had a 5-year RFS of 88%, whereas more extensive spread (zones 2 and 3) had a 5-year RFS of 51%.

Microscopic PNI that warrants adjuvant RT must involve a large-caliber nerve (nerve sheath measuring at least 0.1 mm in caliber or located deeper than the dermis). A retrospective cohort study of SCC showed that tumors with large nerve (≥0.1 mm) invasion were associated with increased risk of nodal metastasis (hazard ratio [HR], 5.6) and death from disease (HR, 4.5), but invasion of small nerves (<0.1 mm) was not associated with worse outcomes.[22] Extensive PNI is another microscopic finding that may increase risk of recurrence. A University of Michigan series defined extensive

Table 3
Selected studies of adjuvant radiation therapy for basal cell carcinoma and squamous cell carcinoma

Series	Study Population	Study Design	N	Intervention	Outcomes	Toxicity
Garcia-Serra et al,[14] 2003	Microscopic PNI and clinical PNTS (BCC and SCC)	Retrospective	135	Adjuvant or primary RT (ELS, electrons, MV photons)	5-y LC: 87% (microscopic PNI) vs 55% (clinical PNTS) 5-y LRC: 72% vs 50%	Overall RT complications: 10% (microscopic PNI) vs 33% (clinical PNTS) Soft tissue necrosis: 5.1% vs 9.2% Transient CNS disorder: 0% vs 3% Osteoradionecrosis: 1.7% vs 1.3%
Lin et al,[20] 2013	Clinical PNTS (BCC and SCC)	Retrospective	56	Adjuvant or primary RT (electrons, MV photons)	5-y RFS: 48% (all), 39% (SCC) vs 80% (BCC)	Severe blindness: 4 of 30 (receiving RT to orbit)
Warren et al,[21] 2014	Clinical PNTS (SCC)	Retrospective	50	Adjuvant RT	5-y RFS: 62% 5-y DSS: 75% 5-y OS: 64%	Orbital exenteration: 2 of 50 (eye complications, precluded IMRT)
Carter et al,[22] 2013	Microscopic PNI (SCC)	Retrospective	114	Surgery ± adjuvant RT (18%)	Large-caliber PNI (≥0.1 mm): disease-specific death HR 4.5 and nodal metastasis HR 5.6	Not reported
Sapir et al,[23] 2016	Extensive microscopic PNI (SCC)	Retrospective	102	Adjuvant RT (MV photons with IMRT or 3DCRT, electrons) or observation	RFS: 94% (RT) vs 25% (no RT)	Not reported
Strassen et al,[26] 2017	Recurrent SCC	Retrospective	67	Adjuvant RT or observation	5-y RFS: 78% (RT) vs 30% (no RT) 5-y OS: 79% vs 46%	Not reported
Kim et al,[27] 2018	T3/T4 (BCC and SCC)	Retrospective	71	Adjuvant or primary RT	3-y DSS: 86% (BCC with adjuvant RT), 93% (SCC with adjuvant RT)	Not reported
Manyam et al,[28] 2017	Immuno-suppression (SCC)	Retrospective	205	Adjuvant RT (electrons, MV photons with 3DCRT or IMRT)	2-y PFS: 38.7% (immunosuppressed) vs 71.6% (immunocompetent) 2-y OS: 60.9% vs 78.1%	Not reported

Study						
Wang et al,[30] 2012	SCC with nodal metastases	Retrospective	122	Surgery ± adjuvant RT (MV photons, electrons)	5-y DFS: 74% (RT) vs 34% (no RT), 5-y OS: 66% vs 27%	Not reported
Ebrahimi et al,[31] 2012	SCC with nodal metastases (N1)	Retrospective	168	Surgery ± adjuvant RT	(N1 disease) 5-y LRC: 87% (RT) vs 91% (no RT), 5-y DFS: 90% vs 97%	Not reported

Abbreviations: 3DCRT, three-dimensional conformal RT; CNS, central nervous system; DSS, disease-specific survival; HR, hazard ratio; IMRT, intensity-modulated RT; RFS, recurrence-free survival.
Data from Refs.[14,20–23,26–28,30,31]

PNI as involvement of more than 2 nerves.[23] RFS in the nerves (94% vs 25%) and overall DFS (73% vs 40%) were improved with adjuvant RT. In contrast, adjuvant RT did not improve outcomes for focal PNI (1–2 nerves involved).

For positive/close margins not amenable to reexcision, adjuvant RT has been shown to improve RFS (9% relapse with adjuvant RT compared with 57% without, using ≤2 mm to define close margins).[24] With conventional excision, surgical margins greater than 4 mm have been recommended (>6 mm if high-risk features are present, based on size, grade, invasion, and location), based on assessment of subclinical tumor extension.[25]

For recurrent disease, adjuvant RT may improve locoregional control, with 1 series noting improved 5-year RFS (78% vs 30%) and OS (79% vs 46%) compared with no adjuvant treatment.[26] Multiple series show that tumor size greater than 2 cm and T3/T4 tumors are associated with high recurrence rates.[18,27] However, with surgery followed by adjuvant RT for SCC, Memorial Sloan Kettering reported 3-year disease-specific survival (DSS) of 92.9%.[27]

Immunosuppression is associated with worse outcomes, even with bimodality therapy. Manyam and colleagues[28] published a retrospective analysis of head and neck SCC receiving surgery and postoperative RT showing that immunosuppressed patients had a worse 2-year locoregional RFS compared with immunocompetent patients (47.3% vs 86.1%) and a trend for worse 2-year OS (60.9% vs 78.1%). Furthermore, desmoplastic histology was strongly associated with LR (HR, 16.11), based on a prospective cohort of SCC undergoing surgery.[29]

In patients with regional lymph node metastases undergoing therapeutic lymphadenectomy, adjuvant RT is recommended for N2 or greater disease. A retrospective series of SCC with nodal metastases showed that adjuvant RT was associated with a higher 5-year DFS than surgery alone (74% vs 34%) and higher 5-year OS (66% vs 27%).[30] However, with a single nodal metastasis less than or equal to 3 cm (N1), 5-year DSS was 97%, making this subgroup suitable for omitting adjuvant RT.[31] For clinically node-negative patients, factors associated with increased risk of metastasis were tumor thickness (HR, 4.79), tumor horizontal size (HR, 2.22), tumor location at ear (HR, 3.61), and immunosuppression (HR, 4.32).[29] Although these risk factors are well defined, the indication for elective nodal irradiation must be balanced against possible toxicities. Thus, ASTRO (American Society for Radiation Oncology) Clinical Practice Guidelines conditionally recommend elective nodal RT when at high risk of nodal metastasis and undergoing RT to the primary site with overlap of an adjacent nodal basin.[2]

Technique for Basal Cell Carcinoma and Squamous Cell Carcinoma

Based on the ASTRO Clinical Practice Guideline, all RT modalities (eg, kilovoltage/megavoltage photons, electrons, brachytherapy) result in similar in LC and cosmesis, supported by multiple retrospective studies.[2,6,7,19] Modality choice should be individualized to specific tumor characteristics and normal tissue constraints. The American Brachytherapy Society (ABS) consensus statement recommends that electronic brachytherapy only be used on a prospective clinical trial or registry, requiring more mature follow-up to understand late toxicity, and recommends radionuclide brachytherapy as an option for T1 to T2 tumors (using radionuclide-based applicators, molds/flaps, or interstitial catheters).[1]

A wide array of appropriate doses and fractionation schemes are appropriate per ASTRO and ABS guidelines.[1,2] With definitive RT, conventional fractionation (1.8–2.0 Gy/fraction) regimens should have a biologically effective dose (BED_{10}) of 70 to 93.5 Gy and hypofractionated (2.1–5.0 Gy/fraction) regimens should have a BED_{10}

of 56 to 88 Gy. With postoperative RT, conventional fractionation (1.8–2.0 Gy/fraction) regimens should have a biologically effective dose (BED_{10}) of 70 to 93.5 Gy and hypofractionated (2.1–5.0 Gy/fraction) regimens should have a BED_{10} of 56 to 88 Gy. Adjuvant RT to nodal basins after lymphadenectomy should be 60 to 66 Gy at 1.8 to 2.0 Gy/fraction and elective nodal RT should typically be 50 to 54 Gy at 1.8 to 2.0 Gy/fraction.

For large-caliber or extensive PNI or clinical/radiographic PNTS, target volumes typically include involved cranial nerve pathways (frequently CN V and CN VII) located retrograde (toward the base of skull).[13] For clinical/radiographic PNTS, volumes should include anterograde coverage (nerve pathways away from the base of skull) and include communicating interconnections between cranial nerves.[13]

CUTANEOUS MELANOMA

Indications for definitive RT include:

- Lentigo maligna or lentigo maligna melanoma in patients who are not candidates for surgery

Discussion

RT is typically not recommended in the definitive management of malignant melanoma. However, definitive RT is considered for lentigo maligna and lentigo maligna melanoma in patients who are not candidates for surgery (**Table 4**). A meta-analysis of 9 studies using definitive RT for lentigo maligna reported a 5% LR (18 recurrences among 349 assessable patients with a median follow-up time of 3 years).[32] Only 5 patients (1.4%) experienced progression to lentigo maligna melanoma. Another retrospective series of lentigo maligna and early lentigo maligna melanoma showed 88% complete clearance after 1 treatment course (involving treatments twice weekly over 3 weeks to total doses for 100–160 Gy using Grenz rays).[33]

Technique

The optimal dose prescription and modality have not been established, although Fogarty and colleagues[32] recommend 54 to 60 Gy in 2-Gy fractions prescribed to a 5-mm depth.

Indications for adjuvant RT include:

- Postoperative bed for desmoplastic histology with high-risk features, which include head and neck location, extensive neurotropism, close margins where re-resection is unfeasible, or locally recurrent disease
- Nodal basins for high-risk features after lymphadenectomy (specifically gross or microscopic extranodal extension, ≥1 parotid node, ≥2 cervical nodes, ≥2–3-cm cervical node size)

Discussion

Although there are no strong indications for adjuvant RT in melanoma (**Table 5**), desmoplastic variants display low predisposition for regional lymph node or distant metastasis, so increased risk of LR may drive morbidity and mortality. A retrospective series of 130 patients with nonmetastatic desmoplastic melanoma (62% located in head and neck) showed a 24% LR rate for surgery alone and 7% for surgery followed by RT (median follow-up of 6.6 years).[34] In tumors with PNI, postoperative RT was associated with improved 10-year LC (91% vs 63%), whereas there was no benefit in tumors without any neurotropism. Another series from Moffitt Cancer Center also

Table 4
Selected studies of primary radiation therapy for melanoma

Series	Study Population	Study Design	N	Intervention	Outcomes	Toxicity
Fogarty et al,[32] 2013	Lentigo maligna	Systematic review	349	ELS (superficial RT and Grenz rays)	Pooled LR: 5%	Not pooled
Hedblad et al,[33] 2012	Lentigo maligna	Retrospective	593	ELS (Grenz rays)	LR: 9.8%	Hypopigmentation: 15% Hyperpigmentation: 20% Severe acute dermatitis: 2%

Data from Fogarty GB, Hong A, Scolyer RA, et al. Radiotherapy for lentigo maligna: a literature review and recommendations for treatment. Br J Dermatol. 2014;170(1):52-58. https://doi.org/10.1111/bjd.12611; and Hedblad M-A, Mallbris L. Grenz ray treatment of lentigo maligna and early lentigo maligna melanoma. J Am Acad Dermatol. 2012;67(1):60-68. https://doi.org/10.1016/j.jaad.2011.06.029.

Table 5
Selected studies of adjuvant radiation therapy for melanoma

Series	Study Population	Study Design	N	Intervention	Outcomes	Toxicity
Guadagnolo et al,[34] 2013	Desmoplastic melanoma	Retrospective	130	Surgery ± adjuvant RT (electrons, MV photons)	Crude LR: 7% (RT) vs 24% (no RT) 10-y LR if PNI present: 91% (RT) vs 63% (no RT)	RT complications: 21% Osteoradionecrosis: 4.2% Nonhealing wound: 2.8%
ANZMTG 01. 02/TROG 02.01[36]	High-risk, node-positive melanoma	Randomized controlled trial	217	Arm 1: adjuvant RT Arm 2: observation	LN relapse: 21% (RT) vs 36% (no RT) 5-y OS: 40% vs 45%	Among head and neck sites RT toxicity: All grade 2: 63% All grade 3: 11% All grade 4: 7% Grade 2–4 fibrosis: 54% (RT) vs 34% (no RT) Grades 2–4 pain: 24% vs 10%
Agrawal et al,[38] 2009	High-risk, node-positive melanoma	Retrospective	615	Surgery ± RT	Regional recurrence: 10.2% (RT) vs 40.6% (no RT) 5-y regional control (cervical nodes only): 93% vs 43% 5-y DSS: 51% vs 30%	Grade 2–3 treatment-related morbidity: 16% 5-y treatment-related morbidity: 20% (RT) vs 13% (no RT) 5-y lymphedema rate: 1% (cervical) vs 44% (inguinal)
EORTC 1325 (KEYNOTE-054)[39]	Resected stage III melanoma	Randomized controlled trial	1019	Arm 1: surgery + pembrolizumab Arm 2: surgery + placebo No RT	1-y RFS: 75.4% (pembrolizumab) vs 61.0% (placebo)	Grades 3–5: 14.7% (pembrolizumab) vs 3.4% (placebo)

Abbreviation: EORTC, European Organisation for Research and Treatment of Cancer.
Data from Refs.[34,36,38,39]

showed that adjuvant RT improved LC in the setting of positive margins (LR, 14% vs 54%) or negative margins with high-risk features (head and neck location, Breslow depth >4 mm, Clark level V).[35] Almost all patients in both studies received 30 Gy in 5 fractions (twice weekly over 2.5 weeks). The benefit of adjuvant RT for neurotropic melanoma of the head and neck is currently being investigated in the ongoing ANZMTG (Australia and New Zealand Melanoma Trials Group) 01.09/TROG (Trans-Tasman Radiation Oncology Group) 08.09 (RTN2) randomized trial.

Treatment of the regional lymph nodes can be considered in patients at high risk for nodal recurrence. The benefit was best shown in the ANZMTG 01.02/TROG 02.01 randomized trial of clinically node-positive melanoma with high-risk features after lymphadenectomy (defined as ≥ 1 parotid, ≥ 2 cervical/axillary, ≥ 3 inguinofemoral nodes, extranodal extension, or maximum node diameter ≥ 3 cm for cervical or ≥ 4 cm for an axillary or inguinal node).[36] The risk of nodal relapse was reduced with adjuvant RT (HR, 0.56), but there was no difference in RFS or OS. Longer follow-up (median follow-up 73 months) confirmed a decreased risk of lymph node relapse with adjuvant RT (21% vs 36%; HR, 0.52), again with no difference in RFS or OS.[37]

The decreased rate of nodal relapse was also reported in a large retrospective series from MD Anderson and Roswell Park.[38] In patients with high-risk nodal disease (eg, ≥ 2 cm size of largest cervical node, ≥ 2 cervical nodes, or the presence of extranodal extension), adjuvant RT was associated with a lower regional recurrence rate than lymphadenectomy alone (10.2% vs 40.6%). Furthermore, there was improved 5-year distant metastasis–free survival (43% vs 28%) and DSS (51% vs 30%) with adjuvant RT.

In addition, adjuvant immunotherapy plays an increasing role in the treatment of resected high-risk melanoma.[39] The role of regional nodal RT is unclear in this setting, and further prospective study is needed to determine the population of patients who remain at high risk of locoregional relapse in the setting of immunotherapy.

Technique

When treating the postoperative bed, the recommended fractionation is 30 Gy in 5 fractions delivered twice weekly using either electrons or photons per the MD Anderson series.[34] For regional lymph nodes, the recommended dose is 48 Gy delivered in 20 fractions starting within 12 weeks of lymph node dissection, per the ANZMTG 01.02/TROG 02.01 trial. The treatment volume included the dissected nodal basins and the lymphadenectomy scar. Another regimen used is 30 Gy in 5 fractions delivered twice weekly over 2.5 weeks per the MD Anderson/Roswell Park series.[38]

MERKEL CELL CARCINOMA

Indications for definitive RT include:

- Primary MCC in patients who are not candidates for surgery

Discussion

Primary management of MCC is typically surgical, and definitive RT is reserved for patients that are not surgical candidates. The efficacy of primary RT is supported by small retrospective series (**Table 6**). Gunaratne and colleagues[40] published a meta-analysis of 23 studies encompassing 264 patients showing that primary RT can provide adequate locoregional control. Mean RT dose was 48.7 ± 13.2 Gy to the primary and 49.4 Gy ± 10.1 Gy to the regional nodes. Rates of recurrence were 7.6% for primary sites and 16.3% for regional sites.

Table 6
Selected studies of primary radiation therapy for Merkel cell carcinoma

Series	Study Design	N	Intervention	Outcomes	Toxicity
Gunaratne et al,[40] 2017	Systematic review	23 (studies) 332 (sites)	Dose: 49.1 Gy ± 11.7 Gy Primary site RT (51.5%), regional nodal RT (48.2%)	In-field recurrence: 11.7% Primary site recurrence: 7.6% Regional site recurrence: 16.3%	Not reported
Wright and Holtzmann,[41] 2018	NCDB	2454	Primary surgery or primary RT	Median OS (stage I/II): 76 mo (surgery) vs 25 mo (RT) 5-y OS (stage I/II): 61% vs 32% Median OS (stage III): 30 mo vs 15 mo 5-y OS (Stage III): 34% vs 19%	Not reported

Abbreviation: NCDB, National Cancer Database.
Data from Gunaratne DA, Howle JR, Veness MJ. Definitive radiotherapy for Merkel cell carcinoma confers clinically meaningful in-field locoregional control: A review and analysis of the literature. J Am Acad Dermatol. 2017;77(1):142-148.e1. https://doi.org/10.1016/j.jaad.2017.02.015; and Wright GP, Holtzman MP. Surgical resection improves median overall survival with marginal improvement in long-term survival when compared with definitive radiotherapy in Merkel cell carcinoma: A propensity score matched analysis of the National Cancer Database. Am J Surg. 2018;215(3):384-387. https://doi.org/10.1016/j.amjsurg.2017.10.045.

The quality of evidence comparing surgery versus definitive RT is poor, because surgery has been the historical standard of care. In a National Cancer Database (NCDB) analysis comparing surgery (39% receiving postoperative RT) and definitive RT, median OS was better in the surgery group for both stage I/II patients (76 vs 25 months) and stage III disease (30 vs 15 months).[41] However, despite propensity-score matching, surgery was recommended but not performed in only 8% of patients receiving primary RT and the cohorts still differed in terms of primary site of origin and tumor size. The University of Wisconsin also showed a worse OS with nonsurgical management on univariate analysis with HR 4.4 (although limited by a multivariate analysis not being performed).[42]

Technique

The recommended dose regimen is 60 to 66 Gy at 2 Gy/fraction, typically with wide margins (5 cm) and the use of electrons with bolus to optimize skin dose. Retrospective data suggest excellent in-field control with greater than or equal to 55 Gy for gross disease and greater than or equal to 50 Gy for microscopic disease.[43]

Indications for adjuvant RT include:

- Postoperative bed for all cases (although it is reasonable to observe small ≤1 cm, low-risk tumors)
- Postoperative bed in the setting of chronic immune suppression, LVSI, or positive margins not amenable to further surgery
- Nodal basins for clinically node-positive disease (with or without lymphadenectomy)
- Nodal basins in the setting of positive sentinel lymph node biopsy (SLNB) but no lymphadenectomy is performed
- Nodal basins for clinically node-negative disease when no SLNB is performed but there is high risk of nodal disease

Discussion

Although limited to heterogeneous retrospective series, adjuvant RT generally decreases LR and may improve progression-free survival (PFS), but improvements in OS are less certain (**Table 7**). The British Columbia Cancer Agency showed that adjuvant RT to the primary site decreased locoregional recurrence in the setting of less than 1-cm margins (5.3% vs 25%).[44] Recurrence rates were low with margins greater than or equal to 1 cm with RT (6.7%) and without RT (7.7%). However, 5-year cancer-specific survival was not improved by adjuvant RT.

Although observation is considered for small low-risk tumors, adjuvant RT may still decrease LR in this group. The University of Washington published a series of low-risk head and neck MCCs (tumor size ≤2 cm, negative margins, negative SLNB, and no immunosuppression) where RT significantly decreased LR (0% vs 26%). Still, DSS and OS were not affected.[45] All 6 patients experiencing a recurrence were successfully salvaged (all receiving RT).

Historically, the benefit of elective RT to regional nodal basins in stage I MCC was supported by a French randomized trial, but the ability to generalize to modern practice is limited because this preceded the use of SLNB and PET for staging.[46] Patients were randomized to regional nodal RT or observation. The regional recurrence rate was reduced with adjuvant nodal irradiation (0% vs 16.7%) but there was no difference in PFS or OS. This trial was ultimately closed prematurely because of the widespread adoption of SLNB.

Table 7
Selected studies of adjuvant radiation therapy for Merkel cell carcinoma

Series	Study Population	Study Design	N	Intervention	Outcomes	Toxicity
Harrington and Kwan,[44] 2015	Margins <1 cm	Retrospective	179	Surgery ± adjuvant RT	LR (margin <1 cm): 4.9% (RT) vs 25% (no RT) LR (margin >1 cm): 7.1% (RT did not improve) 5-y DSS: 77% (RT did not improve)	Not reported
Takagishi et al,[45] 2016	Low-risk MCC	Retrospective	46	Surgery ± RT (electrons, MV photons)	LR: 0% (RT) vs 26% (no RT) DSS and OS not improved with RT	Significant late toxicity: 0% (RT)
Jouary et al,[46] 2011	Elective nodal RT for stage I MCC (preceding SLNB era)	Randomized controlled trial	83	Arm 1: surgery + adjuvant RT (primary and nodal) Arm 2: surgery + adjuvant RT (primary only)	Regional recurrence: 0% (nodal RT) vs 16.7% (no nodal RT) 3-y PFS: 89.7% vs 81.2% 3-y OS: 92.3% (nodal RT did not improve)	Grade 1 skin: 19.3% Grade 2 skin: 7.2% Nodal RT did not affect toxicity
Strom et al,[47] 2016	MCC, including node positive	Retrospective	171	Surgery ± adjuvant RT	Node positive: 3-y LC: 91.2% (RT) vs 76.9% (no RT) 3-y LRC: 79.5% vs 59.1% 3-y DSS: 57.0% vs 30.2% 3-y OS: 73% vs 66%	Not reported

Data from Refs.[44–47]

A Moffitt Cancer Center series showed improved 3-year LC (91.2% vs 76.9%), LRC (79.5% vs 59.1%), and OS (73% vs 66%) with adjuvant RT among pathologically node-positive patients.[47] Another small retrospective series showed that nodal RT decreases regional recurrence in node-positive patients (18% vs 33%), which included patients receiving SLNB, SLNB followed by lymphadenectomy, and upfront lymphadenectomy.[48]

Technique

Adjuvant RT should begin as soon as possible (within 4 weeks) because rapid recurrences occur with treatment delays.[49] Dose regimens to the tumor bed are typically 50 to 56 Gy after negative margins, 56 to 60 Gy with microscopic positive margins, and 60 to 66 Gy with grossly positive margins at 2 Gy/fraction. Dose regimens to the regional nodal basins are 60 to 66 Gy for gross lymphadenopathy, 50 to 60 Gy after lymphadenectomy or positive SLNB (with higher doses for extracapsular extension), and 46 to 50 Gy for elective nodal irradiation at 2 Gy/fraction.

SUMMARY

RT plays an integral role in the management of head and neck cutaneous cancers. In BCC and SCC, it shows excellent outcomes in the definitive setting, serving as an appropriate alternative in cosmetically and functionally sensitive areas, or when patient comorbidities preclude safe surgery. Although definitive RT plays a smaller role in melanoma and MCC, adjuvant RT improves locoregional control in specific clinical contexts across BCC, SCC, melanoma, and MCC. These improvements in locoregional control do not always translate to improvements in DSS or OS, which underscores the importance of individualized clinical judgment weighing risks and benefits for each patient. In addition, the wide array of modalities available (ranging from low-energy x-rays to megavoltage electrons or photons to brachytherapy) exemplify the versatile application of RT to cutaneous cancer treatment and inspire many future directions of study.

DISCLOSURES

None.

REFERENCES

1. Shah C, Ouhib Z, Kamrava M, et al. The American brachytherapy society consensus statement for skin brachytherapy. Brachytherapy 2020;19(4):415–26.
2. Likhacheva A, Awan M, Bhatnagar A, et al. Definitive and postoperative radiation therapy for basal and squamous cell cancers of the skin: an ASTRO clinical practice guideline. Pract Radiat Oncol 2020;10(1):8–20.
3. Avril M-F, Auperin A, Margulis A, et al. Basal cell carcinoma of the face: surgery or radiotherapy? Results of a randomized study. Br J Cancer 1997;76(1):100–6.
4. Rowe DE, Carroll RJ Jr, Day CL. Long-term recurrence rates in previously untreated (Primary) basal cell carcinoma: implications for patient follow-up. J Dermatol Surg Oncol 1989;15(3):315–28.
5. Zaorsky NG, Lee CT, Zhang E, et al. Hypofractionated radiation therapy for basal and squamous cell skin cancer: a meta-analysis. Radiother Oncol 2017;125(1): 13–20.
6. Locke J, Karimpour S, Young G, et al. Radiotherapy for epithelial skin cancer. Int J Radiat Oncol 2001;51(3):748–55.

7. Schulte K-W, Lippold A, Auras C, et al. Soft x-ray therapy for cutaneous basal cell and squamous cell carcinomas. J Am Acad Dermatol 2005;53(6):993–1001.

8. Hernández-Machin B, Borrego L, Gil-García M, et al. Office-based radiation therapy for cutaneous carcinoma: evaluation of 710 treatments: office-based radiation therapy. Int J Dermatol 2007;46(5):453–9.

9. Zagrodnik B, Kempf W, Seifert B, et al. Superficial radiotherapy for patients with basal cell carcinoma: recurrence rates, histologic subtypes, and expression of p53 and Bcl-2. Cancer 2003;98(12):2708–14.

10. Seegenschmiedt MH, Oberste-Beulmann S, Lang E, et al. Radiotherapy for basal cell carcinoma. Local control and cosmetic outcome. Strahlenther Onkol Organ Dtsch Rontgengesellschaft Al 2001;177(5):240–6.

11. Krengli M, Masini L, Comoli AM, et al. Interstitial brachytherapy for eyelid carcinoma: outcome analysis in 60 patients. Strahlenther Onkol 2014;190(3):245–9.

12. Swanson EL, Amdur RJ, Mendenhall WM, et al. Radiotherapy for basal cell carcinoma of the medial canthus region: RT for medial canthus basal cell carcinoma. Laryngoscope 2009;119(12):2366–8.

13. Bakst RL, Glastonbury CM, Parvathaneni U, et al. Perineural invasion and perineural tumor spread in head and neck cancer. Int J Radiat Oncol Biol Phys 2019;103(5):1109–24.

14. Garcia-Serra A, Hinerman RW, Mendenhall WM, et al. Carcinoma of the skin with perineural invasion. Head Neck 2003;25(12):1027–33.

15. Galloway TJ, Morris CG, Mancuso AA, et al. Impact of radiographic findings on prognosis for skin carcinoma with clinical perineural invasion. Cancer 2005; 103(6):1254–7.

16. Nagore E, Grau C, Molinero J, et al. Positive margins in basal cell carcinoma: relationship to clinical features and recurrence risk. A retrospective study of 248 patients. J Eur Acad Dermatol Venereol 2003;17(2):167–70.

17. Wolf DJ, Zitelli JA. Surgical margins for basal cell carcinoma. Arch Dermatol 1987;123(3):340–4.

18. Rowe DE, Carroll RJ, Day CL. Prognostic factors for local recurrence, metastasis, and survival rates in squamous cell carcinoma of the skin, ear, and lip. J Am Acad Dermatol 1992;26(6):976–90.

19. Guix B, Finestres F, Tello J-I, et al. Treatment of skin carcinomas of the face by high-dose-rate brachytherapy and custom-made surface molds. Int J Radiat Oncol Biol Phys 2000;47(1):95–102.

20. Lin C, Tripcony L, Keller J, et al. Cutaneous carcinoma of the head and neck with clinical features of perineural infiltration treated with radiotherapy. Clin Oncol 2013;25(6):362–7.

21. Warren TA, Panizza B, Porceddu SV, et al. Outcomes after surgery and postoperative radiotherapy for perineural spread of head and neck cutaneous squamous cell carcinoma: Cutaneous SCC with perineural spread. Head Neck 2016;38(6):824–31.

22. Carter JB, Johnson MM, Chua TL, et al. Outcomes of primary cutaneous squamous cell carcinoma with perineural invasion: an 11-year cohort study. JAMA Dermatol 2013;149(1):35.

23. Sapir E, Tolpadi A, McHugh J, et al. Skin cancer of the head and neck with gross or microscopic perineural involvement: Patterns of failure. Radiother Oncol 2016; 120(1):81–6.

24. Najim M, Cross S, Gebski V, et al. Early-stage squamous cell carcinoma of the lip: The Australian experience and the benefits of radiotherapy in improving outcome

in high-risk patients after resection. Head Neck 2012. https://doi.org/10.1002/hed.23148.

25. Brodland DG, Zitelli JA. Surgical margins for excision of primary cutaneous squamous cell carcinoma. J Am Acad Dermatol 1992;27(2):241–8.

26. Strassen U, Hofauer B, Jacobi C, et al. Management of locoregional recurrence in cutaneous squamous cell carcinoma of the head and neck. Eur Arch Otorhinolaryngol 2017;274(1):501–6.

27. Kim SK, Barker CA. Outcomes of radiation therapy for advanced T3/T4 nonmelanoma cutaneous squamous cell and basal cell carcinoma. Br J Dermatol 2018; 178(1):e30–2.

28. Manyam BV, Garsa AA, Chin R-I, et al. A multi-institutional comparison of outcomes of immunosuppressed and immunocompetent patients treated with surgery and radiation therapy for cutaneous squamous cell carcinoma of the head and neck: immune status and cutaneous malignancy. Cancer 2017;123(11): 2054–60.

29. Brantsch KD, Meisner C, Schönfisch B, et al. Analysis of risk factors determining prognosis of cutaneous squamous-cell carcinoma: a prospective study. Lancet Oncol 2008;9(8):713–20.

30. Wang JT, Palme CE, Morgan GJ, et al. Predictors of outcome in patients with metastatic cutaneous head and neck squamous cell carcinoma involving cervical lymph nodes: Improved survival with the addition of adjuvant radiotherapy. Head Neck 2012;34(11):1524–8.

31. Ebrahimi A, Clark JR, Lorincz BB, et al. Metastatic head and neck cutaneous squamous cell carcinoma: defining a low-risk patient. Head Neck 2012;34(3): 365–70.

32. Fogarty GB, Hong A, Scolyer RA, et al. Radiotherapy for lentigo maligna: a literature review and recommendations for treatment. Br J Dermatol 2014; 170(1):52–8.

33. Hedblad M-A, Mallbris L. Grenz ray treatment of lentigo maligna and early lentigo maligna melanoma. J Am Acad Dermatol 2012;67(1):60–8.

34. Guadagnolo BA, Prieto V, Weber R, et al. The role of adjuvant radiotherapy in the local management of desmoplastic melanoma: radiotherapy for Desmoplastic Melanoma. Cancer 2014;120(9):1361–8.

35. Strom T, Caudell JJ, Han D, et al. Radiotherapy influences local control in patients with desmoplastic melanoma. Cancer 2014;120(9):1369–78.

36. Burmeister BH, Henderson MA, Ainslie J, et al. Adjuvant radiotherapy versus observation alone for patients at risk of lymph-node field relapse after therapeutic lymphadenectomy for melanoma: a randomised trial. Lancet Oncol 2012;13(6): 589–97.

37. Henderson MA, Burmeister BH, Ainslie J, et al. Adjuvant lymph-node field radiotherapy versus observation only in patients with melanoma at high risk of further lymph-node field relapse after lymphadenectomy (ANZMTG 01.02/TROG 02.01): 6-year follow-up of a phase 3, randomised controlled trial. Lancet Oncol 2015; 16(9):1049–60.

38. Agrawal S, Kane JM, Guadagnolo BA, et al. The benefits of adjuvant radiation therapy after therapeutic lymphadenectomy for clinically advanced, high-risk, lymph node-metastatic melanoma. Cancer 2009;115(24):5836–44.

39. Eggermont AMM, Blank CU, Mandala M, et al. Adjuvant pembrolizumab versus placebo in resected stage III melanoma. N Engl J Med 2018;378(19):1789–801.

40. Gunaratne DA, Howle JR, Veness MJ. Definitive radiotherapy for Merkel cell carcinoma confers clinically meaningful in-field locoregional control: a review and analysis of the literature. J Am Acad Dermatol 2017;77(1):142–8.e1.
41. Wright GP, Holtzman MP. Surgical resection improves median overall survival with marginal improvement in long-term survival when compared with definitive radiotherapy in Merkel cell carcinoma: a propensity score matched analysis of the National Cancer Database. Am J Surg 2018;215(3):384–7.
42. Liang E, Brower JV, Rice SR, et al. Merkel cell carcinoma analysis of outcomes: a 30-year experience. PLoS One 2015;10(6):e0129476.
43. Foote M, Harvey J, Porceddu S, et al. Effect of radiotherapy dose and volume on relapse in Merkel cell cancer of the skin. Int J Radiat Oncol Biol Phys 2010;77(3): 677–84.
44. Harrington C, Kwan W. Radiotherapy and conservative surgery in the locoregional management of Merkel cell carcinoma: the British Columbia cancer agency experience. Ann Surg Oncol 2016;23(2):573–8.
45. Takagishi SR, Marx TE, Lewis C, et al. Postoperative radiation therapy is associated with a reduced risk of local recurrence among low risk Merkel cell carcinomas of the head and neck. Adv Radiat Oncol 2016;1(4):244–51.
46. Jouary T, Leyral C, Dreno B, et al. Adjuvant prophylactic regional radiotherapy versus observation in stage I Merkel cell carcinoma: a multicentric prospective randomized study. Ann Oncol 2012;23(4):1074–80.
47. Strom T, Carr M, Zager JS, et al. Radiation therapy is associated with improved outcomes in Merkel Cell carcinoma. Ann Surg Oncol 2016;23(11):3572–8.
48. Hoeller U, Mueller T, Schubert T, et al. Regional nodal relapse in surgically staged Merkel cell carcinoma. Strahlenther Onkol 2015;191(1):51–8.
49. Tsang G, O'Brien P, Robertson R, et al. All delays before radiotherapy risk progression of Merkel cell carcinoma. Australas Radiol 2004;48(3):371–5.

The Role of Systemic Therapy in Advanced Cutaneous Melanoma of the Head and Neck

Melissa A. Wilson, MD, PhD[a], Leslie A. Fecher, MD[b],*

KEYWORDS

• Melanoma • BRAF • MEK • Immunotherapy • Checkpoint inhibitor

KEY POINTS

• Immunotherapy and BRAF/MEK targeted therapy have improved survival in advanced unresectable melanoma.

INTRODUCTION

The treatment of advanced melanoma has dramatically changed over the last decade. With the discovery of activating *BRAF* mutations and the advent of targeted therapies and checkpoint inhibitors, the overall survival of patients with advanced melanoma has increased. Survival for advanced unresectable melanoma previously averaged less than 1 year. In the era of checkpoint inhibitors such as antibodies against cytotoxic T-lymphocyte antigen (CTLA)-4 and programmed death (PD) receptor-1, and targeted therapies, such as BRAF and MEK inhibitors, 5-year overall survival rates as high as 55% have been reported.[1,2] Indeed, the most recent update of the American Joint Committee on Cancer staging system deferred major revisions in the stage IV category owing to the dramatic improvement in outcomes and the need for ongoing evaluation.[3] Here we provide an overview of systemic therapies, including the pivotal agents that have led to these advances. Advanced unresectable melanoma refers to patients with melanoma involving nodal and/or in-transit disease or distant metastases not amenable to complete resection. It is important to distinguish this population from the resected stage III/IV population, for whom adjuvant therapy can be considered. Neoadjuvant paradigms are also being studied intensely. Unfortunately, not all patients respond to these treatments and relapses still occur. Noncutaneous melanomas (uveal and mucosal) have not shown the same degree of response, and ongoing research seeks to improve outcomes for all subsets of melanoma.

[a] Sidney Kimmel Cancer Center, Thomas Jefferson University, 1025 Walnut Street, Suite 700, Philadelphia, PA 19107, USA; [b] University of Michigan, Rogel Cancer Center, C343 MIB, 1500 East Medical Center Drive, SPC 5848, Ann Arbor, MI 48109-5848, USA
* Corresponding author.
E-mail address: lfecher@med.umich.edu

Otolaryngol Clin N Am 54 (2021) 329–342
https://doi.org/10.1016/j.otc.2020.11.006
0030-6665/21/© 2020 Elsevier Inc. All rights reserved.

SYSTEMIC THERAPY

Melanoma, typically of cutaneous origin in the United States, often affects the head and neck. Head and neck melanomas carry a worse prognosis compared with other primary sites.[4] In 2020, there will be an estimated 100,350 new cases and 6850 deaths.[5] However, over the last decade there has been a dramatic decrease in mortality owing to advancements in systemic therapies.

Chemotherapy and immunotherapies were a mainstay of treatment of advanced melanoma before more recent advances. A number of chemotherapy regimens exist that offer clinical response and palliation, but no regimen has demonstrated improvement in overall survival. The first treatment approved by the US Food and Drug Administration (FDA) for metastatic melanoma was dacarbazine (DTIC), an alkylating agent, in 1975 based on phase I and II studies that demonstrated a maximum 28% response rate[6] (**Fig. 1**). Temozolomide, an analog of DTIC, has also been used in the treatment of melanoma and has similar activity to DTIC. A randomized phase III trial demonstrated no difference in response rate between patients with melanoma treated with DTIC (12.1%) and temozolomide (13.5%) ($P = .20$).[7] The major advantage to temozolomide is its oral administration and ability to cross into the central nervous system, which is attractive in advanced melanoma given the high incidence of brain metastases.[8] A number of additional single-agent chemotherapies have been used, including carmustine, carboplatin, taxanes, and combination platinums and taxanes.[9–12]

Combination regimens of chemotherapies and chemotherapies with immunotherapies have been investigated and include CVD (cisplatin, vinblastine or vindesine, DTIC), the Dartmouth regimen (carmustine (BCNU), DTIC, cisplatin, and tamoxifen), and biochemotherapy (cisplatin, vinblastine or vindesine, DTIC + Interferon -α + Interleukin-2).[13–15] Although smaller trials seemed to favor combination regimens, results from larger randomized trials did not demonstrate reproducibly increased response rates or overall survival, and DTIC remained the standard of care. Chemotherapy remains a treatment option for patients with relapsed or refractory melanoma after newer approved standard therapies.

Immunotherapies have been a foundation of treatment for melanoma for years based on an intimate relationship between the immune system and melanoma, including reports of spontaneous regression of tumors and vitiligo.[16,17] Before checkpoint inhibitor development, immunotherapies included cancer vaccines, cytokine

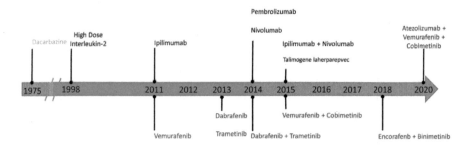

Fig. 1. Timeline of FDA-approved agents, coded by drug category: chemotherapy, immunotherapy, targeted therapy, and combination immunotherapy and targeted therapy.

therapies such as IFN and IL-2, and adoptive T-lymphocyte therapy.[18–21] High-dose IL-2 received FDA approval in 1998 (see **Fig. 1**). IL-2, an activator of T-lymphocytes as well as of other immune effector cells, administered at high doses yields response rates of approximately 16%, including 6% complete response rates (where response rate is composed of complete responses and partial responses).[20,21] Although the numbers were low, the durability of response was notable. Unfortunately, this treatment is challenging to administer and receive owing to capillary leak syndrome, multi-organ dysfunction that requires inpatient management, and strict eligibility criteria; other IL-2 molecules are in development.[22,23]

Molecularly Targeted Therapies

Genetic and molecular studies have discovered a number of somatic mutations involved in the pathogenesis of melanoma. These mutations have been identified at various stages of melanoma progression, including early tumor development, tumor metastasis, or both. These breakthroughs have led to an understanding of the mechanisms involved in melanoma tumorigenesis and to the development of targeted therapy in the treatment of melanoma.[24] Notable somatic mutations identified in melanoma include BRAF, NRAS, KIT, PTEN, and GNA11/GNAQ.

BRAF is mutated in 40% to 60% of melanomas, with the most common BRAF mutation at codon 600, resulting in substitution of glutamic acid for valine (V600 E).[25] The BRAF V600 E mutation results in constitutive kinase activity of BRAF and subsequent signaling through the downstream mitogen-activated protein kinase (MAPK) pathway.[26] Additional BRAF V600 mutations have been observed in melanoma tumor samples and melanoma cell lines.[27,28] Occasionally, mutations have been identified in BRAF in the loop domain (exon 11).[27] Interestingly, BRAF has been shown to be mutated in a significant percentage of benign nevi, suggesting that BRAF mutations are early events in the progression to melanoma.[29] BRAF mutations are associated with truncal melanomas and younger age, although BRAF V600 K have been associated with older patients and in areas of increased sun exposure.[30]

Activating mutations in NRAS have been identified in approximately 15% to 20% of melanoma tumors.[31,32] The most common NRAS mutation is in exon 3 at codon 61, specifically substitution of leucine for glutamine (Q61 L), although other amino acid changes are observed.[33] Q61 mutations result in a constitutively active form of the protein leading to uncontrolled cellular proliferation. Additional NRAS mutations have been identified in exon 2 at codons 12 and 13.[34] NRAS mutations are associated with nodular melanomas, chronically sun-damaged skin, thicker melanomas, and an increased mitotic rate.[35]

KIT mutations have been demonstrated to be associated with melanomas arising from acral skin, mucosa, and chronically sun-damaged skin.[36] KIT is mutated or amplified in approximately 30% of these melanoma tumor types. There is no one predominant KIT mutation and mutations are found in exons 9, 11, 12, 13, and 17. Data indicate that not all mutations result in functional dependence on KIT or correspond with sensitivity to KIT inhibitors.[37]

Recent clinical trials have demonstrated the benefit of targeting mutant BRAF with specific inhibitors, vemurafenib and dabrafenib.[38,39] Moreover, the use of MEK inhibitors, either alone or in combination with BRAF inhibitors, has demonstrated clinical response in patients with the BRAF V600 mutation.[40–42] After the dose-finding phase I study, the BRIM phase II trial (BRAF in melanoma) demonstrated an impressive 53% response rate in a population of pretreated patients with melanoma.[43] The BRIM 3 study was a randomized phase III clinical trial with 675 previously untreated patients with melanoma investigating vemurafenib (960 mg orally twice daily) versus DTIC,

1000 mg/m^2 intravenously (IV) every 3 weeks.[38] Treatment with vemurafenib resulted in a response rate of 48% compared with a 5% response rate for DTIC; moreover, at 6 months, the overall survival for patients treated with vemurafenib was 84% compared with 64% in patients treated with DTIC, and a relative reduction of risk of death of 63% (P<.001). An extended survival analysis of BRIM3 later reported a median overall survival of 13.6 months for patients treated with vemurafenib compared with 9.7 months for patients treated with DTIC.[44] Interestingly, the overall survival curves converged over time (>3 years), thought to be due to treatment crossover and subsequent therapies.

Dabrafenib was also evaluated in patients with metastatic melanoma with a BRAF V600 E or K mutation (BREAK studies). The single arm, phase II BREAK-2 trial evaluated safety and response of dabrafenib at 150 mg orally twice daily.[45] Seventy-six patients with BRAF V600 E melanoma and 16 patients with BRAF V600 K melanoma were enrolled and treated with tolerable toxicities. In the BRAF V600 E patients, the median progression-free survival was 6.3 months and the median overall survival was 13.1 months, although these rates were lower in the BRAF V600 K patients: the median progression-free survival was 4.5 months and the median overall survival was 12.9 months. Dabrafenib in BRAF V600 E/K mutant melanoma was further evaluated in a phase III randomized clinical trial of 250 treatment-naïve patients randomized (3:1) to dabrafenib or DTIC.[39] The median progression-free survival was 5.1 months for patients treated with dabrafenib compared with 2.7 months for patients treated with DTIC (hazard ratio [HR], 0.3; P<.0001). The long-term follow-up analysis of the BREAK-2 and BREAK-3 studies demonstrated that some patients maintained lasting responses with 5-year overall survival rates of 24% and 22% for dabrafenib and DTIC, respectively.[46] All DTIC patients progressed and received subsequent treatment.

Trametinib was first developed as a single agent to target MEK in solid tumors. MEK is a molecule in the MAPK pathway, located directly downstream of BRAF. In vitro studies demonstrated that inhibition of MEK decreased cell proliferation and increased apoptosis. MEK inhibitors are not mutation dependent and inhibit the wild-type MEK protein. An initial phase I study evaluated the safety and toxicity of trametinib and determined the recommended phase II dose via escalation and cohort expansions in select tumor types.[40,41] Patients with melanoma were enrolled in all cohorts, 97 in total, and 36 were BRAF mutant. Of the BRAF mutant patients, 30 had no prior treatment with a BRAF inhibitor. In this subgroup, 2 patients experienced a complete response, 8 patients experienced a partial response, and 19 patients experienced reduction in their tumors with a median duration of response of 5.6 months.[40] The most common side effect was rash, but gastrointestinal side effects (nausea, vomiting, and diarrhea), fatigue, peripheral edema, and decreased left ventricular ejection fraction (n = 7) were also reported. A phase III study in patients with BRAF mutant melanoma compared the recommended trametinib dose of 2 mg/d orally with chemotherapy, either DTIC 1000 mg/m^2 IV every 3 weeks or paclitaxel 175 mg/m^2 IV every 3 weeks; 322 patients with up to 1 previous line of therapy were randomized 2:1.[47] Trametinib improved the median progression-free survival to 4.8 months compared with 1.5 months in chemotherapy-treated patients and the 6-month overall survival to 81% compared with 67%, respectively. Common side effects included rash, diarrhea, and peripheral edema. Rare side effects included ocular toxicity and decreased ejection fraction.

Even though patients with BRAF mutant melanoma experienced benefits from treatment with single agent BRAF and MEK inhibitors, disease relapse and progression occurred in almost all patients. Research identified a number of mechanisms of treatment resistance, including MEK reactivation and reactivation of the MAPK pathway. Thus, investigation of the combination of the BRAF inhibitor, dabrafenib, and the MEK inhibitor, trametinib was begun. A combined phase I and phase II clinical trial evaluated pharmacokinetics and safety of this combination with a cohort expansion at the recommended phase II dosing and compared it with single agent dabrafenib.[42] The maximum tolerated dose of the combination of dabrafenib and trametinib was 150 mg orally twice daily and 2 mg/d orally, respectively. Pyrexia was observed more frequently in patients receiving the combination compared with single agent dabrafenib (71% vs 26%, respectively), whereas the development of cutaneous squamous cell carcinoma was decreased with the combination (7% vs 19%). Outcomes were improved in patients who received combination dabrafenib and trametinib compared with single agent dabrafenib with a median progression-free survival of 9.4 months compared with 5.8 months, respectively (HR, 0.39; $P<.001$). Improved response rate and survival rates with combination dabrafenib and trametinib were also demonstrated when compared against the FDA-approved single agent BRAF inhibitor, vemurafenib.[48] Seven hundred and four patients were randomized in this open-label, phase III trial. At the preplanned interim analysis, the 12-month overall survival was 72% for the combination compared with 65% for the single agent (HR; 0.69; $P = .005$). A median progression-free survival of 11.4 months was also improved for the combination compared with 7.3 months for vemurafenib. Analyses in various disease subsets all favored treatment with combination with side effects being similar in both cohorts. A 5-year overall survival rate of 34% was reported for a combined 563 patients from these 2 trials who received combination dabrafenib and trametinib.[1]

The addition of the MEK inhibitor, cobimetinib, to the BRAF inhibitor, vemurafenib, also increased progression-free survival to 9.9 months compared with single agent vemurafenib at 6.2 months as well as response rates (68% vs 45%) in a randomized phase III trial.[49] There was increased toxicity observed in patients receiving combination vemurafenib and cobimetinib treatment, however, compared with single agent vemurafenib. Recently, a third BRAF and MEK inhibitor combination was shown to be superior to single agent BRAF inhibitor. The combination of encorafenib (a BRAF inhibitor) and binimetinib (a MEK inhibitor) demonstrated an improved median progression-free survival of 14.9 months compared with a median progression-free survival of 7.3 months with single agent vemurafenib (HR, 0.54; $P<.0001$).[50] Treatment with this combination is tolerable with increased gamma glutamyl transferase and creatinine kinase, and hypertension as common side effects, but decreased pyrexia and photosensitivity compared with each single agent, encorafenib or vemurafenib. Overall, treatment with BRAF mutant-specific inhibitors led to an increase in overall survival in patients with melanoma, which had been lacking with previous melanoma therapies.

The targeting of mutations other than BRAF has not achieved the same success in melanoma. NRAS mutations signal through multiple intracellular pathways including the MAPK pathway. MEK inhibitors have been used most recently in clinical trials in an attempt to target NRAS mutant melanoma.[51–53] In a recent study, patients with melanoma with an NRAS mutation were randomized to treatment with single agent binimetinib or DTIC.[51] Results demonstrated that median progression-free survival for patients treated with binimetinib was 2.8 months compared with 1.5 months in patients treated with DTIC, with an objective response rate of 15% compared with 7%, respectively. These results highlight the need for ongoing development in the treatment of NRAS-mutant melanoma. The use of KIT inhibitors, imatinib, dasatinib, and nilotinib has demonstrated responses in some isolated cases, primarily stable disease and partial responses.[37,54–56] The continued discovery of somatic mutations in melanoma will allow for the ongoing development of specific therapies directed toward individual mutations and for the development of personalized medicine.

Checkpoint inhibitors

Tumor cells attempt to evade detection and destruction by the immune system through a variety of mechanisms.[57,58] CTLA-4 is a protein that can translocate to the cell surface of T lymphocytes to inhibit T-cell costimulation and activation when bound to B7.1 (CD80) and B7.2 (CD86).[57] Programmed death receptor ligand (PD-L1) (B7-H1) is expressed on many cell types, including multiple types of cancer, and negatively regulates antitumor cytotoxic T-cell responses when bound by PD-1.[58] Checkpoint inhibitors refer to therapies that interfere with these regulatory mechanisms of T cell activation. The current agents approved by the FDA for the treatment of advanced melanoma are antagonistic antibodies against CTLA-4, PD-1, and PD-L1 and are administered IV.

Ipilimumab, a human IgG1 monoclonal antagonistic antibody against CTLA-4, was the first agent to show an improvement in overall survival in melanoma in a randomized controlled trial that led to its FDA approval in 2011[59] (see **Fig. 1**). This trial randomized 676 patients 3:1:1 to ipilimumab in combination with a glycoprotein 100 (gp100) peptide vaccine versus ipilimumab alone versus gp100 alone. There was an increase in median overall survival from 6.4 months (95% confidence interval [CI], 5.5–8.7) for gp100 alone to 10 months (95% CI, 8.5–11.5) in patients who received ipilimumab with gp100 and to 10.1 months (95% CI, 8.0–13.8) with ipilimumab alone. The overall survival at 24 months was 14% for gp100 alone versus 24% and 22% for ipilimumab alone and with gp100, respectively. Ipilimumab is currently approved at a dose of 3 mg/kg every 3 weeks for 4 doses. Ipilimumab also has demonstrated activity in the brain.[60] The durability of benefit of ipilimumab was further supported in a pooled patient data analysis of 12 prospective and retrospective trials that included 1861 patients with melanoma.[61] Patients were treated at different doses and schedules of ipilimumab and included treatment-naïve and previously treated patients. The median overall survival was 11.4 months (95% CI, 10.7–12.1 months). A 3-year overall survival rate of 22% was reported for all patients that was accompanied by a plateau in the survival curve; notably, a 17% overall survival rate at 7 years was also reported. This finding supported the concept that, if a response was obtained, it would be maintained.

Two PD-1 inhibitors were studied simultaneously and received FDA approval for the treatment of advanced unresectable melanoma in 2014: pembrolizumab, a humanized IgG4 monoclonal antibody, and nivolumab, a human IgG4 monoclonal antibody (**see Fig. 1**). A multicenter phase Ib trial, Keynote-001, evaluated pembrolizumab in multiple cancers, including 655 patients with melanoma at 3 doses: 2 mg/kg every 3 weeks, 10 mg/kg every 2 weeks, or 10 mg/kg every 3 weeks.[62–64] This trial included previously treated and treatment-naïve patients, as well as randomized and nonrandomized cohorts. The initial FDA approval was for previously treated patients at a dose of 2 mg/kg every 3 weeks based on the initial report of durable response rate. Several updates have been published to this study, including an objective response rate of 33% (95% CI, 30%–37%) with a median overall survival of 23 months (95% CI, 20–29) and a 24-month overall survival rate of 49% (95% CI, 44%–53%) for the entire melanoma population.[64] The most recent update for this study reported an estimated 5-year overall survival rate of 34% for all patients and a median overall survival of 23.8 months. At 55 months of follow-up, 73% of all responses were ongoing.[65]

Keynote 002, a randomized phase II trial, compared pembrolizumab with chemotherapy in ipilimumab-refractory patients with melanoma.[66] Five hundred forty patients were randomized 1:1:1 to pembrolizumab 2 mg/kg or 10 mg/kg every 3 weeks or investigator choice chemotherapy (ICC). This work demonstrated an improved progression-free survival (primary end point) and response rate for both pembrolizumab cohorts compared with ICC. Although not powered for comparison, the authors interpreted the data for the 2 pembrolizumab doses to be similar and 2 mg/kg every 3 weeks was recommended. Final analysis reported median overall survival and 2-year overall survival rates for the 3 respective arms of 13.4 months and 36%, 14.7 months and 38%, and 11.0 months and 30%.[67] Overall survival differences were not significant, possibly owing to crossover. Keynote 006, a randomized phase III trial, compared pembrolizumab at 10 mg/kg every 2 or 3 weeks or ipilimumab 3 mg/kg every 3 weeks for 4 doses in 834 patients with melanoma.[68] In this study, the 2 pembrolizumab-treated groups evidenced improved estimated 12-month overall survival rates (74.1% vs 68.4% vs 58.2%), response rates (33.7% vs 32.9% vs 11.9%), and estimated 6-month progression-free survival rates (47.3% vs 46.4% vs 26.5%), respectively. At a median follow-up of 57.7 months, the authors reported results for the 2 combined pembrolizumab arms and ipilimumab: a median overall survival rate of 32.7 months (95% CI, 24.5–41.6) and 15.9 months (95% CI, 13.3–22.0), respectively.[69] The FDA approval of pembrolizumab was later expanded to include first-line treatment.

Nivolumab was also evaluated in a large phase I study in multiple cancer types, which enrolled 107 patients with melanoma.[70] Nivolumab was administered every 2 weeks with doses ranging from 0.1 to 10.0 mg/kg. Across all doses, an overall response rate of 31% was seen in the patients with melanoma with an estimated median duration of response of 2 years. The median overall survival was 16.8 months with a 2-year overall survival rate of 43%. At the 3 mg/kg FDA-approved dose, the response rate was 41% with a median overall survival of 20.3 months. The most recent update reported an estimated 5-year overall survival rate of 34.2%.[71] A phase III trial, Checkmate 037, randomized (2:1) 405 patients with melanoma progressed through ipilimumab, and through BRAF inhibitor therapy if *BRAF* mutant, to nivolumab 3 mg/kg every 2 weeks versus ICC.[72] The objective response rate per independent radiologic review and overall survival were coprimary end points. This study reported an overall response rate of 31.7% versus 10.6% at the first interim analysis, which led to nivolumab receiving accelerated approval from the FDA for previously treated melanoma (see **Fig. 1**). The authors provided an updated report in 2017 with overall survival data.[73] The overall response rate was 27% versus 10% for nivolumab versus ICC, the median duration of response was 32 months versus 13 months, and the median overall survival was 16 months versus 14 months, respectively. Next, treatment-naïve, *BRAF* wild-type patients with melanoma were randomized in another phase III trial, Checkmate-066, to nivolumab or DTIC.[74] In this study of 418 patients, overall survival was the primary end point and a significant improvement in 1-year overall survival was reported: 72.9% (95% CI, 65.5–78.9) for nivolumab versus 42.1% (95% CI, 33.0–50.9) for DTIC. An improved response rate and progression-free survival were also reported for nivolumab.

Treatment with anti-PD1 agents typically is continued to maximal toxicity, progression, maximal benefit, or up to 2 years. PD-L1 expression in tumor tissue can be evaluated, but is not required for treatment with PD1 inhibitor therapy given limited predictive value.[75] Patients without PD-L1 expression can still respond to PD1 inhibitor therapy. Antagonistic PD-1/PD-L1 antibodies were evaluated as weight-based doses in trials. More recently, the FDA labels have been modified for flat dosing given simulations by a population pharmacokinetics model that determined that a clinically meaningful effect on safety and efficacy between the 2 doses was unlikely.[76] Pembrolizumab is approved at 200 mg every 3 weeks and nivolumab at 240 mg every 2 weeks. Additional mathematical modeling has also led to approval of alternative doses and schedules: nivolumab 480 mg every 4 weeks and pembrolizumab 400 mg every 6 weeks.[77–79]

Combination immunotherapy with ipilimumab and nivolumab was then evaluated in a phase I study evaluating various doses and schedules (concurrent and sequential) in 8 cohorts.[80] Ipilimumab 3 mg/kg and nivolumab 1 mg/kg every 3 weeks for 4 doses, followed by single agent nivolumab was selected for further study because these were the maximum doses with an acceptable level of adverse events. Patients treated in this cohort evidenced an overall response rate of 53% (9/17), which included 3 complete responses; all 9 had a tumor reduction of 80% or greater at the first tumor assessment. This regimen has been further studied in phase II and phase III trials.[81,82] Checkmate 067, a phase III double-blind trial, randomized 945 treatment naive patients (1:1:1) to ipilimumab with nivolumab, nivolumab alone, or ipilimumab alone.[82] This study was designed to evaluate progression-free survival and overall survival as coprimary end points. The FDA-approved combination ipilimumab and nivolumab at this dosing schedule in October 2015 for the treatment of advanced, unresectable melanoma based on a significant improvement in median progression-free survival: 11.5 months (95% CI, 8.9–16.7) for ipilimumab with nivolumab versus 2.9 months (95% CI, 2.8–3.4) for ipilimumab alone with an overall response rate of 58% versus 19% for the combination versus ipilimumab alone (see **Fig. 1**). Further, nivolumab demonstrated an improved median progression-free survival of 6.9 months (95% CI, 4.3–9.5) compared with ipilimumab with an HR of 0.57 (99.5% CI, 0.43–0.76), as well as an overall response rate of 44%. The study was not designed for a formal statistical comparison of combination therapy to nivolumab.

Several updates of this study have been published. Notably, the 5-year overall survival rates were 52% for ipilimumab with nivolumab, 44% for nivolumab alone, and 26% for ipilimumab alone.[2] These response rates were similar to those initially reported and included complete response rates of 22%, 19%, and 6% for ipilimumab with nivolumab, nivolumab alone, and ipilimumab alone, respectively. The authors also reported outcomes after treatment: rates of subsequent systemic therapy (46% for ipilimumab with nivolumab, 59% for nivolumab alone, and 75% for ipilimumab alone), as well as the treatment-free interval, defined as the time from the last dose of the trial drug to subsequent systemic therapy or the last known date alive. The median treatment-free interval for ipilimumab with nivolumab was 18.1 months, 1.9 months for ipilimumab alone, and 1.8 months for nivolumab alone. Further, of the patients alive at 5 years, 74% of the combination treatment patients were not on treatment compared with 58% of the nivolumab group and 45% of the ipilimumab group. This result speaks to the durability of response after completing treatment, as well as to the risk/incidence of toxicities for each of these treatment groups, where more patients stop treatment in the combination arm owing to toxicity. This regimen has also shown intracranial responses in patients with asymptomatic, nonirradiated brain metastases.[83]

The majority of side effects related to checkpoint inhibitors are due to immune attack on normal parts of the body, termed immune-related adverse events.[84] There is ongoing research to understand the mechanisms of action and optimal management. These toxicities are unpredictable regarding severity, timing, and presentation, and require a high level of suspicion. Most commonly, the skin, bowels, and endocrine glands can be effected; however, any organ may be impacted. Most require holding immunotherapy, often temporarily, but sometimes permanently depending on the grade and the affected organ. They typically do not resolve on their own and require treatment with steroids, often at high doses, for no less than 4 weeks' duration.

Occasionally, additional immunosuppressive agents are needed and toxicities can rebound and can be fatal, although rarely. Guidelines have been developed to facilitate their management.[85] Side effects are graded according to the common toxicity criteria; grade 3 and 4 toxicities are more severe and grade 5 is fatal.[86] Patients with altered immune systems at baseline, such as patients with preexisting autoimmune conditions or immunosuppression, seem to be at greater risk.

The reported treatment related grade 3 or 4 toxicity rates for ipilimumab, nivolumab, and combination ipilimumab and nivolumab are 27%, 16%, and 55%, respectively.[82] The combination toxicity rate is for ipilimumab 3 mg/kg with nivolumab 1 mg/kg every 3 weeks for 4 doses followed by single agent nivolumab. Given this rate of toxicity, alternative combination regimens are under investigation. One phase IIIb/IV randomized, controlled trial, Checkmate 511, evaluated the rate of treatment-related grade 3 to 5 adverse events in patients with melanoma treated with 2 different regimens of ipilimumab with nivolumab.[87] Three hundred and sixty patients were randomized 1:1 to ipilimumab 1 mg/kg with nivolumab 3 mg/kg (I1N3) every 3 weeks for 4 doses or ipilimumab 3 mg/kg with nivolumab 1 mg/kg (I3N1—standard dosing) every 3 weeks for 4 doses. All patients who tolerated therapy then received nivolumab 480 mg every 4 weeks until disease progression or unacceptable toxicity. This regimen showed a lower grade 3 to 5 immune-related adverse event rate for I1N3 of 34% compared with 48% for I3N1. The efficacy seemed to be similar, with an overall response rate of 46% and 51% for the 2 arms, respectively, but additional investigation is needed.

The optimal therapy sequence or combination across mechanisms of action is also an ongoing area of discussion and research. Many investigators believe that there is a greater potential for durable response and treatment-free period with immunotherapy and often recommend this in the first- line setting.[75] Combination regimens of BRAF/MEK inhibitors with PD1/PDL1 antagonistic antibodies are also being pursued. The FDA recently approved the regimen of vemurafenib, cobimetinib, and atezolizumab, a PD-L1 antagonistic antibody, for the treatment of *BRAF* V600–mutant melanoma given a significantly improved progression-free survival (15.1 months vs 10.6 months) compared with vemurafenib/cobimetinib alone[88] (see **Fig. 1**). This regimen and other combination regimens come with a high rate of grade 3 and 4 treatment-related adverse events (79%). How this regimen will fit into current practice is being determined. Most in the melanoma community agree that treatment decisions must be tailored to the features of the patient and their melanoma.

SUMMARY

Survival in advanced melanoma is consistently improving with the development and deployment of effective systemic therapies. However, there are still relapses and not all melanomas respond to these therapies. Ongoing research into novel pathways and combination strategies is continuing. Toxicities do come with these agents and must be balanced with cancer control.

CLINICS CARE POINTS

- Immunotherapy and BRAF/MEK targeted therapy have improved survival in advanced unresectable melanoma.
- Immunotherapy offers the potential for improved survival with time free from treatment.
- The optimal sequence or combination of therapies remain to be determined and is often tailored to patient and disease burden.

COI

M.A. Wilson: Clinical trial funding: Ascentage, Bristol Myers Squibb, Iovance; L.A. Fecher: Clinical trial funding: Merck, Incyte, Bristol-Myers-Squibb, EMD Serono, Pfizer, Array, Kartos; Consulting Elsevier (Melanoma Co-chair: Via Oncology Pathways).

REFERENCES

1. Robert C, Grob JJ, Stroyakovskiy D, et al. Five-year outcomes with dabrafenib plus trametinib in metastatic melanoma. N Engl J Med 2019;381:626–36.
2. Larkin J, Chiarion-Slieni V, Gonzalez R, et al. Five-year survival with combined nivolumab and ipilimumab in advanced melanoma. N Engl J Med 2019;381: 1535–46.
3. Gershenwald JE, Scolyer RA, Hess KR, et al. Melanoma staging: evidence based changes in the AJCC 8th Ed. Cancer staging manual. Ca Cancer J Clin 2017; 67(6):472–92.
4. Lachiewicz AM, Berwick M, Wiggins CL, et al. Survival differences between patients with scalp or neck melanoma and those with melanoma of other sites in the surveillance, epidemiology, and end results (SEER) program. Arch Dermatol 2008;144(4):515–21.
5. Siegel RL, Miller KD, Jemal A. Cancer statistics, 2020. CA Cancer J Clin 2020; 70(1):7–30.
6. Crosby T, Fish B, Coles B, et al. Systemic treatments for metastatic cutaneous melanoma. Cochrane Database Syst Rev 2018;(2):CD001215.
7. Middleton MR, Grob JJ, Aaronson N, et al. Randomized phase III study of temozolomide versus dacarbazine in the treatment of patients with advanced metastatic malignant melanoma. J Clin Oncol 2000;18:158–66.
8. Yung WK, Albright RE, Olson J, et al. A phase II study of temozolomide vs procarbazine in patients with glioblastoma multiforme at first relapse. Br J Cancer 2000;83(5):588–93.
9. Hill GJ 2nd, Ruess R, Berris R, et al. Chemotherapy of malignant melanoma with dimethyl traizeno imidazole carboxamide (DITC) and nitrosourea derivatives (BCNU, CCNU). Ann Surg 1974;180(2):167–74.
10. Evans LM, Casper ES, Rosenbluth R. Phase II trial of carboplatin in advanced malignant melanoma. Cancer Treat Rep 1987;71(2):171–2.
11. Legha SS, Ring S, Papadopoulos N, et al. A phase II trial of taxol in metastatic melanoma. Cancer 1990;65(11):2478–81.
12. Flaherty KT, Lee SJ, Zhao F, et al. Phase III trial of carboplatin and paclitaxel with or without sorafenib in metastatic melanoma. J Clin Oncol 2013;31(3):373–9.
13. Legha SS, Ring S, Papadopoulos N, et al. A prospective evaluation of a triple-drug regimen containing cisplatin, vinblastine, and dacarbazine (CVD) for metastatic melanoma. Cancer 1989;64(10):2024–9.
14. McClay EF, Mastrangelo MJ, et al. Effective combination chemo/hormonal therapy for malignant melanoma: experience with three consecutive trials. Int J Cancer 1992;50(4):553–6.
15. Atkins MB, Hsu J, Lee S, et al. Phase III trial comparing concurrent biochemotherapy with cisplatin, vinblastine, dacarbazine, interleukin-2, and interferon alfa-2b with cisplatin, vinblastine, and dacarbazine alone in patients with metastatic malignant melanoma (E3695): a trial coordinated by the Eastern cooperative oncology group. J Clin Oncol 2008;26(35):5748–54.

16. Boon T, Coulie PG, Eynde BJ, et al. Human T cell responses against melanoma. Annu Rev Immunol 2006;24:175–208.
17. Byrne KT, Turk MJ. New perspectives on the role of vitiligo in immune responses to melanoma. Oncotarget 2011;2(9):684–94.
18. Hersey P, Gallagher SJ, Kirkwood JM, et al. Melanoma vaccines. In: Balch CM, et al, editors. Cutaneous melanoma. 6th edition. Switzerland: Springer Nature AG; 2019. p. 1–23.
19. Rosenberg SA, Restifo N. Adoptive cell transfer as personalized immunotherapy for human cancer. Science 2015;348(6230):62–8.
20. Atkins M, Lotze MT, Dutcher JP, et al. High-dose recombinant interleukin 2 therapy for patients with metastatic melanoma: analysis of 270 patients treated between 1985 and 1993. J Clin Oncol 1999;17(7):2105.
21. Atkins MB, Kunkel L, Sznol M, et al. High-dose recombinant interleukin-2 therapy in patients with metastatic melanoma: long-term survival update. Cancer J Sci Am 2000;6(Suppl 1):S11–4.
22. Schwartzentruber DJ. Guidelines for the safe administration of high-dose interleukin-2. J Immunother 2001;24(4):287–93.
23. Hurwitz ME, Cho DC, Balar AV, et al. Baseline tumor-immune signatures associated with response to bempegaldesleukin (NKTR-214) and nivolumab. J Clin Oncol 2019;37. suppl; abstr 2623.
24. Dhomen N, Marais R. BRAF signaling and targeted therapies in melanoma. Hematol Oncol Clin North Am 2009;23(3):529–45.
25. Davies H, Bignell GR, Cox C, et al. Mutations of the BRAF gene in human cancer. Nature 2002;417:949–54.
26. Sebolt-Leopold JS, Herrera R. Targeting the mitogen-activated protein kinase cascade to treat cancer. Nat Rev Cancer 2004;4(12):937–47.
27. Omholt KA, Platz A, Kanter L, et al. NRAS and BRAF mutations arise early during melanoma pathogenesis and are preserved throughout tumor progression. Clin Cancer Res 2003;9(17):6483–8.
28. Greshock JK, Nathanson K. Distinct patterns of DNA copy number alterations associate with BRAF mutations in melanomas and melanoma-derived cell lines. Genes Chromosomes Cancer 2009;48(5):419–28.
29. Pollock PM, Harper UL, Hansen KS, et al. High frequency of BRAF mutations in nevi. Nat Genet 2003;33(1):19–20.
30. Long GV, Menzies AM, Nagrial AM, et al. Prognostic and clinicopathologic associations of oncogenic BRAF in metastatic melanoma. J Clin Oncol 2011;29(10): 1239–46.
31. Edlundh-Rose E, Egyhazi S, Omholt K, et al. NRAS and BRAF mutations in melanoma tumors in relation to clinical characteristics: a study based mutation screening by pyrosequencing. Melanoma Res 2006;16(6):471–8.
32. Goel VK, Lazar AJ, Warneke CL, et al. Examination of mutations in BRAF, NRAS, and PTEN in primary cutaneous melanoma. J Invest Dermatol 2006;126(1): 154–60.
33. Saldanha G, Potter L, Daforno P, et al. Cutaneous melanoma subtypes show different BRAF and NRAS mutation frequencies. Clin Cancer Res 2006;12(15): 4499–505.
34. Ball NJ, Yohn JJ, Morelli JG, et al. Ras mutations in human melanoma: a marker of malignant progression. J Invest Dermatol 1994;102(3):285–90.
35. Devitt B, Liu W, Salemi R, et al. Clinical outcome and pathological features associated with NRAS mutation in cutaneous melanoma. Pigment Cell Melanoma Res 2011;24(4):666–72.

36. Curtin JA, Busam K, Pinkel D, et al. Somatic activation of KIT in distinct subtypes of melanoma. J Clin Oncol 2006;24(26):4340–6.

37. Carvajal RD, Antonescu CR, Wolchok JD, et al. KIT as a therapeutic target in metastatic melanoma. JAMA 2011;305(22):2327–34.

38. Chapman PD, Hauschild A, Robert C, et al. Improved survival with vemurafenib in melanoma with BRAF V600E mutation. N Engl J Med 2011;364(26):2507–16.

39. Hauschild A, Grob JJ, Demidov LV, et al. Dabrafenib in BRAF-mutated metastatic melanoma: a multicentre, open-label, phase 3 randomised controlled trial. Lancet 2012;380(9839):358–65.

40. Falchook GS, Lewis KD, Infante JR, et al. Activity of the oral MEK inhibitor trametinib in patients with advanced melanoma: a phase 1 dose-escalation trial. Lancet 2012;13:782–9.

41. Infante JR, Fecher LA, Falchook GS, et al. Safety, pharmacokinetic, pharmacodynamic, and efficacy data for the oral MEK inhibitor trametinib: a phase I dose-escalation trial. Lancet Oncol 2012;13(8):773–81.

42. Flaherty K, Infante J, Daud A, et al. Combined BRAF and MEK inhibition in melanoma with BRAF V600 Mutations. N Engl J Med 2012;367(18):1694–703.

43. Sosman JA, Kim KB, Schuchter L, et al. Survival in BRAF V600-mutant advanced melanoma treated with vemurafenib. N Engl J Med 2012;366:707–14.

44. Chapman PD, Robert C, Larkin J, et al. Vemurafenib in patients with BRAF V600 mutations-positive metastatic melanoma: final overall survival results of the randomized BRIM-3 Study. Ann Oncol 2017;28(10):2581–7.

45. Ascierto P, Minor D, Ribas A, et al. Phase II trial (BREAK-2) of the BRAF inhibitor dabrafenib (GSK2118436) in patients with metastatic melanoma. J Clin Oncol 2013;31(26):3205–11.

46. Hauschild A, Ascierto P, Schadendorf D, et al. Long term outcomes in patients with BRAF V600 mutant metastatic melanoma receiving dabrafenib monotherapy analysis from phase 2 and p3 clinical trials. Eur J Cancer 2020;125:114–20.

47. Flaherty K, Robert C, Hersey P, et al. Improved survival with MEK Inhibition in BRAF-mutated melanoma. N Engl J Med 2012;367(2):107–14.

48. Robert C, Karaszewska B, Schachter J, et al. Improved overall survival in melanoma with combined dabrafenib and trametinib. N Engl J Med 2015;372(1):30–9.

49. Larkin J, Ascierto PA, Dreno B, et al. Combined vemurafenib and cobimetinib in BRAF-mutated melanoma. N Engl J Med 2014;371(20):1867–76.

50. Dummer R, Ascierto PA, Gogas HJ, et al. Encorafenib plus binimetinib versus vemurafenib or encorafenib in patients with BRAF-mutant melanoma (COLUMBUS): a multicentre, open-label, randomised phase 3 trial. Lancet Oncol 2018;19(5):603–15.

51. Dummer R, Schadendorf D, Ascierto PA, et al. Binimetinib versus dacarbazine in patients with advanced NRAS-mutant melanoma (NEMO): a multicentre, open-label, randomised, phase 3 trial. Lancet Oncol 2017;18(4):435–45.

52. Atefi M, Bjoern T, Avramis E, et al. Combination of Pan-RAF and MEK inhibitors in NRAS mutant melanoma. Mol Cancer 2015;14(1):27.

53. Grimaldi AM, Simeone E, Ascierto PA. The role of MEK inhibitors in the treatment of metastatic melanoma. Curr Opin Oncol 2014;26(2):196–203.

54. Hodi FS, Friedlander P, Corless CL, et al. Major response to imatinib mesylate in KIT-mutated melanoma. J Clin Oncol 2008;26(12):2046–51.

55. Woodman SE, Trent JC, Stemke-Hale K, et al. Activity of dasatnib against L576P KIT mutant melanoma: molecular, cellular, and clinical correlates. Mol Cancer Ther 2009;8(8):2079–85.

56. Tran A, Tawbi HA. A potential role for nilotinib in KIT-mutated melanoma. Expert Opin Investig Drugs 2012;21(6):861–9.
57. Peggs KS, Quezada SA, Korman AJ, et al. Principles and use of anti-CTLA4 antibody in human cancer immunotherapy. Curr Opin Immunol 2006;18(2):206–13.
58. Zou W, Chen L. Inhibitory B7-family molecules in the tumour microenvironment. Nat Rev Immunol 2008;8(6):467–77.
59. Hodi FS, O'Day SJ, McDermott DF, et al. Improved survival with ipilimumab in patients with metastatic melanoma. N Engl J Med 2010;363(8):711.
60. Margolin K, Ernstoff MS, Hamid O, et al. Ipilimumab in patients with melanoma and brain metastases: an open-label, phase 2 trial. Lancet Oncol 2012;13: 459–65.
61. Schadendorf D, Hodi FS, Robert C, et al. Pooled analysis of long-term survival data from phase II and Phase III trials of ipilimumab in unresectable or metastatic melanoma. J Clin Oncol 2015;33(17):1889–94.
62. Hamid O, Robert C, Daud A, et al. Safety and tumor responses with lambrolizumab (Anti–PD-1) in melanoma. N Engl J Med 2013;369:134–44.
63. Robert C, Ribas A, Wolchok JD, et al. Anti-programmed-death-receptor-1 treatment with pembrolizumab in ipilimumab-refractory advanced melanoma: a randomised dose-comparison cohort of a phase 1 trial. Lancet 2014;384(9948): 1109–17.
64. Ribas A, Hamid O, Daud A, et al. Association of pembrolizumab with tumor response and survival among patients with advanced melanoma. JAMA 2016; 315:1600–9.
65. Hamid O, Robert C, Daud A, et al. Five-year survival outcomes for patients with advanced melanoma treated with pembrolizumab in KEYNOTE-001. Ann Oncol 2019;30:582–8.
66. Ribas A, Puzanov I, Dummer R, et al. Pembrolizumab versus investigator choice chemotherapy for ipilimumab-refractory melanoma (KEYNOTE-002): a randomized, controlled, phase 2 trial. Lancet Oncol 2015;16:908–18.
67. Hamid O, Puzanov I, Dummer R, et al. Final analysis of a randomized trial comparing pembrolizumab versus investigator-choice-chemotherapy for ipilimumab-refractory advanced melanoma. Eur J Cancer 2017;86:37–45.
68. Robert C, Schachter J, Long GV, et al. Pembrolizumab versus ipilimumab in advanced melanoma. N Engl J Med 2015;372:2521–32.
69. Robert C, Ribas A, Schachter J, et al. Pembrolizumab versus ipilimumab in advanced melanoma (Keynote-006): post-hoc 5-year results from an open-label, multicentre, randomized, controlled, phase 3 study. Lancet Oncol 2019; 20(9):1239–51.
70. Topalian SL, Sznol M, McDermott DF, et al. Survival, durable tumor remission, and long-term safety in patients with advanced melanoma receiving nivolumab. J Clin Oncol 2014;32(10):1020–30.
71. Topalian SL, Hodi FS, Brahmer JR, et al. Five-year survival and correlates among patients with advanced melanoma, renal cell carcinoma, or non-small cell lung cancer treated with nivolumab. JAMA Oncol 2019;5(10):1411–20.
72. Weber JS, D'Angelo SP, Minor D, et al. Nivolumab versus chemotherapy in patients with advanced melanoma who progressed after anti-CTLA-4 treatment (CheckMate 037): a randomised, controlled, open-label, phase 3 trial. Lancet Oncol 2015;16(4):375–84.
73. Larkin J, Minor D, D'Angelo S, et al. Overall survival in patients with advanced melanoma who received nivolumab versus investigator's choice chemotherapy

in CheckMate 037: a randomized, controlled, open-label phase III trial. J Clin Oncol 2018;36(4):383–90.

74. Robert C, Long GV, Brady B, et al. Nivolumab in previously untreated melanoma without BRAF mutation. N Engl J Med 2015;372(4):320–30.

75. Pavlick AC, Fecher L, Ascierto P, et al. Frontline therapy for BRAF-mutated metastatic melanoma: how do you choose, and is there one correct answer? Am Soc Clin Oncol Educ Book 2019;39:564–71.

76. Zhao X, Suryawanshi S, Hruska M, et al. Assessment of nivolumab benefit-risk profile of a 240-mg flat dose relative to a 3-mg/kg dosing regimen in patients with advanced tumors. Ann Oncol 2017;28(8):2002–8.

77. Bi Y, Liu J, Furmanski B, et al. Model-informed drug development approach supporting approval of the 4-week (Q4W) dosing schedule for nivolumab (Opdivo) across multiple indications: a regulatory perspective. Ann Oncol 2019;30(4):644–51.

78. Lala M, Akala O, Chartash E, et al. Pembrolizumab 400 mg Q6W dosing: first clinical outcomes data from KEYNOTE-555 cohort B in metastatic melanoma patients. 2020 AACR Virtual Meeting. Abstract CT042. Presented April 28, 2020.

79. Lala M, Li TR, de Alwis DP, et al. A six-weekly dosing schedule for pembrolizumab in patients with cancer based on evaluation using modelling and simulation. Eur J Cancer 2020;131:68–75.

80. Wolchok, Harriet K, Margaret KC, et al. Nivolumab plus ipilimumab for advanced melanoma. N Engl J Med 2013;369:122–33.

81. Postow MA, Chesney J, Pavlick AC, et al. Nivolumab and ipilimumab versus ipilimumab in untreated melanoma. N Engl J Med 2015;372:2006–17.

82. Larkin J, Hodi FS, Wolchok JD. Combined nivolumab and ipilimumab or monotherapy in untreated melanoma. N Engl J Med 2015;373(13):1270–1.

83. Tawbi H, Forsyth P, Algazi A, et al. Combined nivolumab and ipilimumab in melanoma metastatic to the brain. N Engl J Med 2018;379(8):722–30.

84. Postow M, Sidlow R, Hellman M. Immune-related adverse events associated with immune checkpoint blockade. N Engl J Med 2018;378:158–68.

85. Puzanov I, Diab A, Abdallah K, et al. Managing toxicities associated with immune checkpoint inhibitors: consensus recommendations from the Society for Immunotherapy of Cancer (SITC) Toxicity Management Working Group. J Immunother Cancer 2017;5(1):95.

86. Available at: https://ctep.cancer.gov/protocoldevelopment/electronic_applications/docs/CTCAE_v5_Quick_Reference_8.5x11.pdf. Accessed October 1, 2020.

87. Lebbe C, Meyer N, Mortier L, et al. Evaluation of two dosing regimens for nivolumab in combination with ipilimumab in patients with advanced melanoma: results from the phase IIIb/IV CheckMate 511 trial. J Clin Oncol 2019;37:867–75.

88. Gutzmer R, Stroyakovskiy D, Gogas H, et al. Atezolizumab, vemurafenib, and cobimetinib as first-line treatment for unresectable advanced BRAFV600 mutation-positive melanoma (IMspire150): primary analysis of the randomised, double-blind, placebo-controlled, phase 3 trial. Lancet 2020;395(10240):1835–44.

The Role of Systemic Therapy in Advanced Cutaneous Squamous Cell Carcinoma

Caitlin P. McMullen, MD[a],*, Thomas J. Ow, MD, MS[b,c]

KEYWORDS

- Squamous cell cancer • Skin cancers • Cancer treatment protocols
- Immunotherapy

KEY POINTS

- Systemic therapy for head and neck cutaneous squamous cell carcinoma (HNCSCC) generally is reserved for patients with unresectable or distant metastatic disease.
- The agents used most commonly currently include platinum-based cytotoxic agents, agents targeting the epidermal growth factor receptor (EGFR) pathway, and programmed cell death protein 1 receptor (PD-1) immune checkpoint inhibitors.
- Although clinical trials studying systemic therapy for cutaneous squamous cell carcinoma (CSCC) have been limited, recent studies have led to US Food and Drug Administration approval of the PD-1 inhibitors cemiplimab and pembrolizumab for patients with locally advanced or metastatic disease.
- Recent data suggest that cisplatin-based concurrent chemoradiation does not provide benefit compared with radiation alone in the postoperative setting.
- Current clinical studies are examining PD-1 inhibitors as neoadjuvant and adjuvant therapy.

INTRODUCTION

Systemic therapy largely has been reserved for palliative treatment of cutaneous squamous cell carcinoma (CSCC) that cannot be treated with local therapy, but systemic agents have been employed in the adjuvant setting for very high-risk lesions. Until recently, data to guide the appropriate application have been limited. Efforts to

[a] Department of Head and Neck – Endocrine Oncology Program, Moffit Cancer Center, 12902 USF Magnolia Drive, Tampa, FL 33612, USA; [b] Department of Otorhinolaryngology–Head and Neck Surgery, Montefiore Medical Center/Albert Einstein College of Medicine, 3400 Bainbridge Avenue, 3rd Floor Medical Arts Pavilion, Bronx, NY 10467, USA; [c] Department of Pathology, Montefiore Medical Center/Albert Einstein College of Medicine, 3400 Bainbridge Avenue, 3rd Floor Medical Arts Pavilion, Bronx, NY 10467, USA
* Corresponding author.
E-mail address: caitlin.mcmullen@moffitt.org

Otolaryngol Clin N Am 54 (2021) 343–355
https://doi.org/10.1016/j.otc.2020.11.007
0030-6665/21/© 2020 Elsevier Inc. All rights reserved.

develop large-scale clinical trials and the advent of immune checkpoint therapy have changed the landscape of systemic therapy for CSCC. This article defines advanced CSCC, because systemic therapy is reserved mostly for this subset of patients. Commonly used agents and the specific settings for which systemic therapy has either an established or potential benefit are discussed. Included is a review of immunotherapy in CSCC, discussing indications, outcomes, and new applications and clinical trials for advanced CSCC that are under way at the time of this publication.

DEFINITION OF ADVANCED CUTANEOUS SQUAMOUS CELL CARCINOMA

The discussion of systemic therapy in this review is relevant to advanced head and neck CSCC (HNCSCC). It is important to differentiate "high risk" from "advanced." High-risk features include location (ie, all areas of the head and neck are considered either moderate risk or high risk), poor differentiation, perineural invasion, immunosuppressed status of the patient, lymphatic or vascular invasion, and high-risk subtypes (ie, acantholytic, adenosquamous, desmoplastic, or metaplastic).[1] A patient may have high-risk features but not an advanced HNCSCC. Advanced HNCSCC suggests disease that has invaded to an extensive degree locally or has demonstrated regional and/or distant metastatic spread. These lesions carry significantly worse prognosis. A clear definition of advanced HNCSCC is debated, but it can be defined based on lesions that are deemed stage III or stage IV based on the American Joint Committee on Cancer (AJCC) staging guidelines. Physical examination and imaging for a suspected advanced CSCC are necessary to determine clinical stage prior to treatment. Features of stage III and stage IV disease, as defined by AJCC, 8th edition, are summarized in **Table 1**. These staging groups encompass patients with extensive local disease, who have developed lymph node spread, or who have distant metastasis. **Fig. 1** provides examples of patients with locally advanced and regionally and distant metastatic HNCSCC.

SYSTEMIC AGENTS USED TO TREAT ADVANCED CUTANEOUS SQUAMOUS CELL CARCINOMA

Until recently, data supporting a role for systemic therapy for patients with CSCC has been based mostly on small retrospective series and a few early clinical trials. Patients with unresectable or widely metastatic disease often require systemic therapy to mitigate their advanced disease, and thus agents have been chosen based on information extrapolated from other cancer types and/or hypothetical activity based on the biological properties of a given drug and the known biology of CSCC. In 2018, a phase I trial with an expansion phase II cohort of patients with advanced CSCC studying the immune checkpoint inhibitor, cemiplimab, demonstrated promising response rates,[2] which led to the rapid US Food and Drug Administration (FDA) approval of this agent for unresectable/metastatic CSCC. This event has dramatically changed the approach toward systemic treatment of this disease. This article reviews drugs that have been used to treat CSCC, including cytotoxic agents, molecular targeted agents, and immune checkpoint inhibitors.

Cytotoxic Agents

Various cytotoxic drugs have been utilized to treat advanced CSCC, including platinum-based agents, taxanes, vinca alkaloids, bleomycin, 5-fluorouracil (5-FU), methotrexate, doxorubicin, gemcitabine, and ifosfomide.[3] A majority of these agents, however, have been examined only in small series using a variety of regimens; thus, the responses to these agents are varied and not well characterized. Generally, limited

Table 1
Factors associated with advanced cutaneous squamous cell carcinoma

Features of Local Disease	American Joint Committee on Cancer Stage
Greatest tumor dimension ≥4 cm	T3
Minimal erosion of bone	T3
Perineural invasion in nerves >0.1 mm, deeper than dermis	T3
Clinical or radiologic evidence of nerve involvement	T3
Invasion depth >6 mm or deeper than subcutaneous fat	T3
Extensive cortical or medullary bone involvement	T4a
Invasion of the cranial base	T4b
Invasion through cranial foramen	T4b

Features of Metastatic Disease	American Joint Committee on Cancer Stage
Metastasis to an isolated ipsilateral lymph node, ≤3 cm in greatest dimension, ENE(−)	N1
Metastasis to an isolated ipsilateral lymph node, 3–6 cm in greatest dimension, ENE(−)	N2a
Metastasis to multiple ipsilateral lymph nodes, none >6 cm in greatest dimension, ENE(−)	N2b
Metastasis to bilateral or contralateral lymph nodes, none >6 cm in greatest dimension, ENE(−)	N2c
Metastasis to any lymph node, >6 cm in greatest dimension, ENE(−)	N3a
Metastasis to any lymph node, ENE(+)	N3b
Distant metastasis	M1

responses with early recurrence/progression have been typical.[3] Strategies that include platinum, alone or with other agents, have been employed most often. Outcomes reported across multiple small observational studies have been modest, with partial responses or stable disease reported in the 15% to 50% range.[3–6]

Molecular Targeted Agents

The molecular target that has received the most attention in CSCC is the epidermal growth factor receptor (EGFR) and its downstream pathways. EGFR is a transmembrane receptor among the ErbB family of receptors. EGFR is activated by extracellular epidermal growth factor (EGF) ligands, such as EGF and transforming growth factor-α. Activated EGFR triggers several tyrosine kinase cascades, including the mitogen-activated protein kinase (MAPK)/extracellular signal-regulated (ERK) pathway, and phosphoinositide 3-kinase (PI3K) pathways.[7] EGFR has been shown to be overexpressed in CSCC, and an association with aggressive features has been reported.[8] EGFR inhibitors, including antibodies that block the EGFR receptor, and small molecules that block EGFR tyrosine kinase activity, have been employed and studied in small trials studying CSCC.[9–21] Cetuximab, a monoclonal antibody to EGFR, showed

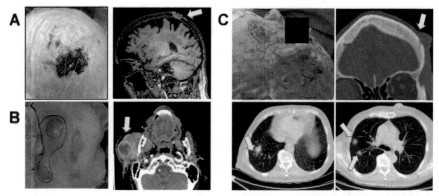

Fig. 1. Examples of patients with advanced CSCC. (*A*) Patient with advanced scalp squamous cancer, with evidence of bone invasion through the calvarium on T1 contrast MR imaging (*arrow*). (*B*) Patient with advanced regional metastasis to the parotid gland (*arrow*), on CT imaging with contrast, and upper neck lymph nodes. This patient presented with facial nerve paralysis consistent with clinical perineural invasion. (*C*) Patient with a left temple squamous cancer recurrent after surgery and radiation. Left temple exhibited minor bone invasion (*right upper panel* [*arrow*]). He developed pulmonary metastases in the right lung, noted as spiculated lesions on CT imaging (*lower panels* [*arrows*]).

substantial activity as a single agent in CSCC, with a disease control rate of 69% and response rate of 28%. Another monoclonal antibody to EGFR, panitumumab, has shown a similar response rate.[10] Cetuximab also has been implemented concurrently with radiation (RT),[15] with platinum therapy,[17] and more recently in active trials in combination with immune checkpoint inhibitors.[22] Small molecule EGFR tyrosine kinase inhibitors, such as erlotinib and gefitinib, as well as a multikinase inhibitor that includes EGFR, lapatinib, also have been evaluated—results resemble those of anti-EGFR antibodies.[11–14,19,21]

Agents targeting signaling molecules downstream of EGFR also are under active investigation. Cobimetinib is a small molecule inhibitor of MEK, a downstream MAPK/ERK signaling molecule that is being actively studied in CSCC.[22] mTOR inhibitors are an area of interest for patients with CSCC—because many of these lesions arise among patients who require immunosuppression for organ transplant survival, the concurrent antineoplastic properties of mTOR inhibitors, perhaps coupled with other PI3K inhibitors, are an area of active study.[23,24] Overall, targeting EGFR and downstream pathways carries substantial promise in CSCC; however, more robust clinical trials are necessary to establish definitive benefit in the appropriate settings.

Immune Checkpoint Inhibitors—Programmed Cell Death Protein 1 Receptor Pathway Blockade

Immune checkpoint inhibitors are drugs that block molecules that typically repress the immune response. There is strong rationale for these agents in CSCC. CSCCs are common among immunosuppressed individuals, and this disease has been shown to carry a high mutation burden[25]—a biomarker for response to immune checkpoint inhibitors in several different cancer types.[26] A key immune checkpoint is the programmed cell death protein 1 receptor (PD-1), which is expressed on cytotoxic T-lymphocytes and activated by its ligands, programmed death ligand 1 (PD-L1) and programmed death ligand 2 (PD-L2). PD-1 activation leads to T-cell apoptosis and repression of the immune response. Tumor cells can up-regulate these ligands, typically PD-L1, to evade immune surveillance. Recently, several drugs have been developed that target this pathway. As discussed previously, cemiplimab, a monoclonal antibody that targets PD-1, demonstrated a 47% response rate among patients with locally advanced or metastatic CSCC, with a large proportion of these patients exhibiting benefit for over 6 months.[2] These results led to FDA approval of this agent for patients with unresectable/metastatic CSCC. More recently, pembrolizumab, another anti–PD-1 antibody, demonstrated a 34% objective response rate, a 52% disease control rate, and a median progression-free survival of 6.9 months among 105 patients with recurrent or metastatic advanced CSCC,[27] also leading to FDA approval. The PD-1 inhibitor, nivolumab, and the PD-L1 inhibitor atezolizumab, also are under active investigation for patients with CSCC.[22] These agents are showing substantial promise, especially for patients with HNCSCC, where locoregionally advanced disease often poses significant challenges among patients with multiply recurrent disease, second primary disease burden, and advanced age. Immune checkpoint inhibitors are being studied further in new combination approaches as well as in the neoadjuvant and adjuvant settings.[22]

INDICATIONS AND APPLICATIONS FOR SYSTEMIC THERAPY FOR ADVANCED CUTANEOUS SQUAMOUS CELL CARCINOMA

Curative treatment of HNCSCC relies on surgical resection and/or radiation therapy (RT) to ablate existing locoregional disease. The primary role of systemic therapy in HNCSCC is for palliative treatment of patients with incurable locoregional or distant disease.[1,28] Systemic therapy also has been considered in both the adjuvant and neoadjuvant settings; however, a definitive role in these settings has not yet been established. Available guidelines for the application of systemic therapy in HNCSCC and commonly used systemic agents and their utility in HNCSCC are reviewed in the following sections.

National Comprehensive Cancer Network Guidelines

The National Comprehensive Cancer Network (NCCN) has published clinical guidelines commonly used to assist with decision making in the care of cancer patients. In operable patients with HNCSCC, the guidelines hold few definitive recommendations regarding the use of systemic therapy.[1,28] If systemic therapy is being considered, multidisciplinary team discussion is recommended, ideally in the setting of a tumor board. The guidelines also suggest consideration of concurrent chemotherapy if nodal disease is excised incompletely or if there is residual disease where further surgery is not feasible. Systemic therapy is not recommended for local disease amenable to surgery or in cases of fully resected regional disease. The NCCN guidelines do suggest consideration of concurrent chemoradiation therapy (CCRT) within the context of a clinical trial if extracapsular nodal extension (ENE) is identified on pathology after neck dissection.[1] This recommendation is under scrutiny, however, due to recent data. The recently published multi-institutional randomized phase III Trans-Tasman Radiation Oncology Group (TROG) 05.01 Trial compared RT versus carboplatin in addition to RT in the adjuvant setting for high-risk CSCC, and there was no significant improvement observed in the carboplatin/RT arm.[29] Thus, the benefit of adding chemotherapy in this setting has not been established (discussed in more detail later).

　　For inoperable patients, systemic therapy alone can be used if curative treatment is not feasible. For concurrent use with RT, cisplatin, cisplatin plus 5-FU, EGFR inhibitors, or carboplatin is suggested. If concurrent curative RT is not feasible, the guidelines suggest the PD-1 inhibitor cemiplimab as the preferred option. If immunotherapy is not possible, platinum-based regimens or EGF receptor (EGFR) inhibitors are suggested. The guidelines also recommend clinical trial enrollment in this setting. When cemiplimab is being considered, other anti–PD-1 inhibitors could be effective in this setting based on the recently reported clinical experiences and preliminary data from ongoing trials. In cases of regional recurrence or distant metastatic disease, the preference of NCCN is cemiplimab.[1] Clinical trial platinum-based regimens or EGFR inhibitors are alternatives.

LOCALLY ADVANCED UNRESECTABLE DISEASE AND METASTATIC DISEASE

Regimens that have been examined and have shown some success in the unresectable and recurrent/metastatic setting include platinum-based chemotherapy, targeted agents, and immunotherapy.

The response rate with platinum-based regimens is reasonably high in CSCC.[5,6,30,31] In a small cohort of unresectable patients, combined treatment with cisplatin plus 5-FU plus bleomycin resulted in 31% complete response (CR) rate, and a 54% partial response rate. Most patients went on to definitive treatment.[6] The experience of systemic therapies at Roswell Park Comprehensive Cancer Center was published in 2016. They found that platinum-based regimens were superior to taxanes and EGFR therapies.[32] Dereure and colleagues[9] studied carboplatin in combination with cetuximab with disappointing results, including a 21% response rate, with no CRs, and a 2.6-month survival rate. In a prospective phase II study, concurrent radiation and platinum-based therapy was administered to locally or regionally advanced unresectable CSCC patients.[33] Of 19 patients, an impressive 10 (53%) achieved a CR with 2 others salvaged by surgery. The overall CR was 63%.[33] These regimens tend to be toxic, especially compared with potential targeted agents and immune checkpoint inhibitors as alternatives. Toxicity is important, particularly for a majority of patients who suffer from advanced CSCC, who often are elderly and/or immunosuppressed persons.[6] Responses to platinum agents tend to not be highly durable.[20,32]

EGFR targeted antibodies and tyrosine kinase inhibitors have been examined in recurrent/metastatic CSCC based on the principle that many tumors overexpress EGFR.[34] Erlotinib[11] and gefitinib[21] both have been studied in phase II trials in this context. The response rate to gefitinib was impressive, at 45%, when administered before definitive treatment in locally advanced patients.[21] CR was seen in 18%. Patients with unresectable/incurable disease, however, had a much lower response rate (11%).[21] Erlotinib, a similar agent, was studied in locally advanced unresectable or metastatic patients, and the results were disappointing.[11] Of the 29 patients who completed the treatment course, only 3 patients (10%) had a confirmed partial response. The remainder exhibited stable disease or progressed. Median progression-free survival was 4.7 months. Patients with chronic lymphocytic leukemia were excluded from the study.[11] Panitumumab, the humanized EGFR monoclonal antibody, also was studied as a single agent in incurable CSCC.[10] In 16 patients, the overall response rate was 31%, with 2 CRs.[10] Cetuximab similarly has been studied as first-line therapy in this population. In a phase II trial, the combined complete and partial response rate was 28%.[16] For unresectable locally advanced HNCSCC, concurrent RT with cetuximab or platinum-based regimens has been compared retrospectively adjuvant and definitive settings.[15,35] An analysis of 12 patients treated with concurrent cetuximab and radiation demonstrated CR of 36% and partial response of 27%, but toxicities were high.[35] In a comparative study, the clinical outcomes between the 2 regimens were improved slightly with cetuximab versus platinum regimens, but the flawed methodology of this study inhibits the ability draw any definitive conclusions.[15]

Immune checkpoint inhibitors have been studied in advanced unresectable locoregional disease and recurrent/metastatic CSCC, and cemiplimab and pembrolizumab (both PD-1 inhibitors), have been approved by the FDA for this indication. Cemiplimab is well tolerated and effective. A phase I/II study by Migden and colleagues[2] reported an objective response rate of approximately 50% of patients with locally advanced unresectable or metastatic CSCC. These responses generally were durable, with a duration of response exceeding 6 months in 57% of patients. Toxicities occurred in the minority of patients and were consistent with those typical of checkpoint inhibitors.[2] In another phase II trial, cemiplimab also showed excellent results among 78 patients with locally advanced disease deemed unresectable and ineligible for radiation, with a CR rate of 13% and partial response rate of 31%.[36] In the KEYNOTE-629 trial published in 2020, investigators administered single-agent pembrolizumab to 105 patients with recurrent or metastatic disease not amenable to surgery or radiation. The response rate was 34.4% with a median progression-free survival of 6.9 months. The 6-month progression-free survival rate was 50.4%. There were grades 3 to 5 toxicities in 5.7% of patients, including 1 death, but generally side effects were mild. They also reported response regardless of PD-L1 combined positive score.[27] Based on this study, the FDA approved pembrolizumab for the treatment-recurrent/metastatic CSCC. Patients with chronic lymphocytic leukemia or immunosuppressed states, including solid organ transplant patients, usually are excluded from immunotherapy trials. The transplant rejection rate is unacceptably high with immunotherapy, reportedly 52% for nivolumab, 27% for pembrolizumab, and 25% for ipilimumab.[37] Studies are emerging to examine markers that will identify which patients would respond to particular immune checkpoint therapies.

In summary, systemic therapy for CSCC has relied on cytotoxic agents, such as cisplatin and EGFR targeted therapy, based on limited reports. More recently, PD-1 checkpoint inhibitors have emerged as the preferred systemic treatment modality. **Fig. 2** provides examples of patients with both advanced local and metastatic disease who have responded exquisitely to PD-1 immune checkpoint inhibition.

Adjuvant Chemotherapy and Chemoradiation

As discussed previously, the seminal study guiding current decision making in the postoperative setting for advanced CSCC is the randomized phase III TROG 05.01 Trial, published in 2018.[29] Prior to this trial, rationale for adjuvant cytotoxic platinum-based chemoradiation regimens for patients with high-risk disease (ie, with positive surgical margins and/or ENE of lymph node disease) was extrapolated from studies that established benefit from concurrent cisplatin with radiation among high-risk head and neck aerodigestive squamous cell carcinoma patients.[38,39] In the TROG 05.01 Trial, carboplatin was the agent of choice for the concurrent chemoradiation therapy (CCRT) treatment arm. This was compared with adjuvant radiation (RT) alone. For both study arms, the rate of freedom from local relapse (FFLR) at 5-years was 83% in the RT arm and 87% in the CCRT arm, which were not significantly different. There also was no significant difference in overall survival. Locoregional failure rate was 7% in both arms. They included an analysis among patients with ENE, which was present in approximately equal proportions in each arm and found no significant difference in FFLR between arms among this subcohort.[29] Other studies have confirmed that there is no survival advantage for radiation alone versus chemoradiation in the postoperative setting for patients with regionally metastatic HNCSCC.[40,41] Tanvetyanon and colleagues[42] reported a decreased risk of recurrence or death with

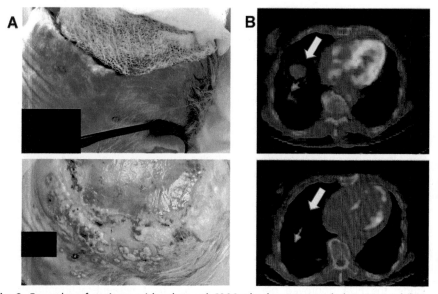

Fig. 2. Examples of patients with advanced CSCC who have responded to PD-1 inhibitor treatment. (A) Patient who developed extensive dermal metastases that rapidly developed 6 weeks after wide resection of a large, advanced scalp squamous cancer (arrows). The patient reduced his immunosuppressive medication for a renal transplant allograft and was given 2 cycles of cemiplimab, with an outstanding response (lower panel). (B). Example PET-computed tomography imaging from a patient with advanced scalp CSCC who developed pulmonary metastases (upper panel [arrow]). Durable CR after 1 year of ongoing cempilimab treatment (lower panel [arrow]).

CRT rather than RT alone in a retrospective study, but they did not find a difference in overall survival. ENE certainly is a poor prognosticator in CSCC.[40,43] Unlike mucosal squamous cell carcinoma, however, it is not clear that there is a benefit from adding chemotherapy for positive margins or ENE.[29,41]

Data regarding postoperative adjuvant therapy with other agents are limited. At least 1 small retrospective study has compared postoperative cetuximab with radiation to concurrent cisplatin and radiation,[15] with both exhibiting similar outcomes. Currently, immune checkpoint inhibitors are being evaluated as adjuvant agents combined with radiation in the postoperative setting. At the time this article was written, there is 1 active trial examining cemiplimab in this setting (NCT03969004), a second trial examining cemiplimab both before and after surgery (NCT04428671), and a trial examining concurrent pembrolizumab and radiation in the postoperative setting (NCT03833167).

For patients who are unresectable and receiving radiation as primary treatment, data supporting concurrent systemic therapy are limited to small case series and retrospective reports. Platinum-based agents commonly are used, but the most effective agents, which include the agents discussed in this review, are not known. In most cases, primary CRT is considered for patients with very advanced local disease (unresectable) or for patients with extensive comorbidities who would not tolerate surgery. It is likely that immune checkpoint therapy will play a major role in these settings, either as a single agent or perhaps given concurrently with radiation.

Table 2
Summary of key completed systemic therapy trials for patients with cutaneous squamous cell carcinoma

Trial, Year	Study Design	N	Outcome
Maubec et al,[16] 2011	Phase II, single arm, cetuximab, unresectable	36	DCR 69% at 6 wk; overall RR 28%; CR 6%
TROG 05.01,[29] 2018	Postoperative CCRT (carboplatin) vs RT	157 (RT) vs 153 (CRT)	FFLRR 83% (RT) vs 87% (CRT) at 5 y. DM 7% both arms
Migden et al,[2] 2018	Phase I/II, cemiplimab, locally advanced/metastatic	26 (phase I) 59 (phase II)	RR 47%–50%; duration of response >6 mo in 57%
KEYNOTE-629,[27] 2020	Phase II, pembrolizumab, recurrent/metastatic	105	DCR 52%; objective RR 34%

Abbreviations: DCR, disease control rate; DM, distant metastasis; RR, response rate.

Neoadjuvant and Induction Systemic Therapy

Limited studies exist evaluating neoadjuvant or induction systemic therapy prior to definitive treatment of advanced CSCC. Neoadjuvant cetuximab alone or cetuximab plus platinum plus 5-FU was examined in a trial of 34 patients who were mostly elderly; 92% of patients who initially had unresectable tumors became operable, and a pathologic CR was identified in 65% of those patients. The 2 patients who did not proceed to surgery still did well and were alive at greater than 21 months of follow-up.[17] Immune checkpoint inhibitors currently are the agents of choice for emerging neoadjuvant treatment strategies, with several planned or recently opened trials.[22] Several clinical trials are under way to examine this promising strategy. The preliminary results of a phase II trial of neoadjuvant cemiplimab in advanced HNCSCC (NCT03565783) were presented at the American Society of Clinical Oncology annual

Table 3
List of several[a] current clinical trials examining programmed cell death protein 1 receptor inhibitor therapy for new indications for patients with cutaneous squamous cell carcinoma

Agent	Setting	National Clinical Trial (NCT) Number
Cemiplimab	Recurrent stage III or IV, prior to surgery	NCT03565783
	Recurrent, intralesional injection prior to surgery	NCT03889912
	Adjuvant, after surgery and radiation	NCT03969004
	Stages II–IV, neoadjuvant	NCT04154943
Pembrolizumab	High-risk locally advanced, adjuvant after surgery and RT	NCT03833167
	With postoperative RT	NCT03057613
	Combination with cetuximab	NCT03082534
Nivolumab	Metastatic in immunosuppressed patients, alone or with ipilimumab	NCT 03816332

Each agent also is being studied in the unresectable/metastatic setting, and in combination strategies with novel agents.

Please visit ClinicalTrials.gov to find a comprehensive and updated list of clinical trials active for CSCC.

[a] Note this list is not a comprehensive list of all active trials studying immune checkpoint inhibitors.

meeting in 2019.[44] Of 20 patients included, there were no surgical delays. Overall response was 30% and a pathologic CR was observed in 55%. Despite planned post-operative radiation, 55% did not received this. No recurrences were observed at the median follow-up of 3.8 months.[44] There otherwise are few data regarding induction and neoadjuvant therapy with chemotherapy or targeted agents in CSCC.

SUMMARY

The role of systemic therapy for advanced CSCC traditionally has been understudied and limited. Cisplatin-based regimens and agents targeting the EGFR pathway have been utilized most. Recent advances are helping to clarify precise applications for systemic regimens and are leading to strategies using new agents. Specifically, adjuvant cisplatin-based CRT for advanced resectable CSCC has been called into question based on the results of the TROG 05.01 Trial,[29] and the PD-1 inhibitors cemiplimab and pembrolizumab now are FDA approved for the treatment of unresectable/metastatic CSCC. A selection of key clinical trials that help guide current application of systemic agents is presented in **Table 2**. New trials likely will lead to more wide indications for immune checkpoint inhibitors and molecularly targeted agents. **Table 3** highlights several active clinical trials studying new applications of immune checkpoint inhibitors in CSCC.

CLINICS CARE POINTS

- Advanced HNCSCC should undergo careful pathologic and imaging review by a multidisciplinary team that specializes in this disease in order to determine the appropriate role for systemic therapy.

- Because many patients with advanced and recurrent HNCSCC are elderly and/or immunocompromised, cases where systemic therapy may be considered often are challenging. This emphasizes the need for multidisciplinary decision making based on the best available data in a field that is progressing rapidly.

- Based on recent level I evidence (TROG 05.01), adjuvant platinum-based chemoradiation in the postoperative setting is not superior to radiation alone for patients with advanced resectable HNCSCC.

- PD-1 inhibitors now play an important role in the management of patients with unresectable and/or metastatic HNCSCC.

DISCLOSURE

Dr C.P. McMullen and Dr T.J. Ow have no commercial or financial conflicts of interest to disclose related to this article.

REFERENCES

1. National comprehensive cancer network. Squamous cell skin cancer (Version 2.2020). Available at: https://www.nccn.org/professionals/physician_gls/pdf/squamous.pdf. Accessed September 28, 2020.
2. Migden MR, Rischin D, Schmults CD, et al. PD-1 blockade with cemiplimab in advanced cutaneous squamous-cell carcinoma. N Engl J Med 2018;379(4):341–51.

3. Stratigos A, Garbe C, Lebbe C, et al. Diagnosis and treatment of invasive squamous cell carcinoma of the skin: European consensus-based interdisciplinary guideline. Eur J Cancer 2015;51(14):1989–2007.

4. Guthrie TH Jr, Porubsky ES, Luxenberg MN, et al. Cisplatin-based chemotherapy in advanced basal and squamous cell carcinomas of the skin: results in 28 patients including 13 patients receiving multimodality therapy. J Clin Oncol 1990; 8(2):342–6.

5. Khansur T, Kennedy A. Cisplatin and 5-fluorouracil for advanced locoregional and metastatic squamous cell carcinoma of the skin. Cancer 1991;67(8):2030–2.

6. Sadek H, Azli N, Wendling JL, et al. Treatment of advanced squamous cell carcinoma of the skin with cisplatin, 5-fluorouracil, and bleomycin. Cancer 1990; 66(8):1692–6.

7. Wieduwilt MJ, Moasser MM. The epidermal growth factor receptor family: biology driving targeted therapeutics. Cell Mol Life Sci 2008;65(10):1566–84.

8. Cañueto J, Cardeñoso E, García JL, et al. Epidermal growth factor receptor expression is associated with poor outcome in cutaneous squamous cell carcinoma. Br J Dermatol 2017;176(5):1279–87.

9. Dereure O, Missan H, Girard C, et al. Efficacy and tolerance of cetuximab alone or combined with chemotherapy in locally advanced or metastatic cutaneous squamous cell carcinoma: an open study of 14 patients. Dermatology 2016; 232(6):721–30.

10. Foote MC, McGrath M, Guminski A, et al. Phase II study of single-agent panitumumab in patients with incurable cutaneous squamous cell carcinoma. Ann Oncol 2014;25(10):2047–52.

11. Gold KA, Kies MS, William WN Jr, et al. Erlotinib in the treatment of recurrent or metastatic cutaneous squamous cell carcinoma: a single-arm phase 2 clinical trial. Cancer 2018;124(10):2169–73.

12. Heath CH, Deep NL, Nabell L, et al. Phase 1 study of erlotinib plus radiation therapy in patients with advanced cutaneous squamous cell carcinoma. Int J Radiat Oncol Biol Phys 2013;85(5):1275–81.

13. Jenni D, Karpova MB, Mühleisen B, et al. A prospective clinical trial to assess lapatinib effects on cutaneous squamous cell carcinoma and actinic keratosis. ESMO Open 2016;1(1):e000003.

14. Lewis CM, Glisson BS, Feng L, et al. A phase II study of gefitinib for aggressive cutaneous squamous cell carcinoma of the head and neck. Clin Cancer Res 2012;18(5):1435–46.

15. Lu SM, Lien WW. Concurrent radiotherapy with cetuximab or platinum-based chemotherapy for locally advanced cutaneous squamous cell carcinoma of the head and neck. Am J Clin Oncol 2018;41(1):95–9.

16. Maubec E, Petrow P, Scheer-Senyarich I, et al. Phase II study of cetuximab as first-line single-drug therapy in patients with unresectable squamous cell carcinoma of the skin. J Clin Oncol 2011;29(25):3419–26.

17. Reigneau M, Robert C, Routier E, et al. Efficacy of neoadjuvant cetuximab alone or with platinum salt for the treatment of unresectable advanced nonmetastatic cutaneous squamous cell carcinomas. Br J Dermatol 2015;173(2):527–34.

18. Stinchcombe TE, Socinski MA. Gefitinib in advanced non-small cell lung cancer: does it deserve a second chance? Oncologist 2008;13(9):933–44.

19. Thatcher N, Chang A, Parikh P, et al. Gefitinib plus best supportive care in previously treated patients with refractory advanced non-small-cell lung cancer: results from a randomised, placebo-controlled, multicentre study (Iressa Survival Evaluation in Lung Cancer). Lancet 2005;366(9496):1527–37.

20. Trodello C, Pepper JP, Wong M, et al. Cisplatin and cetuximab treatment for metastatic cutaneous squamous cell carcinoma: a systematic review. Dermatol Surg 2017;43(1):40–9.

21. William WN Jr, Feng L, Ferrarotto R, et al. Gefitinib for patients with incurable cutaneous squamous cell carcinoma: a single-arm phase II clinical trial. J Am Acad Dermatol 2017;77(6):1110–1113 e1112.

22. Corchado-Cobos R, García-Sancha N, González-Sarmiento R, et al. Cutaneous squamous cell carcinoma: from biology to therapy. Int J Mol Sci 2020;21(8).

23. Euvrard S, Morelon E, Rostaing L, et al. Sirolimus and secondary skin-cancer prevention in kidney transplantation. N Engl J Med 2012;367(4):329–39.

24. Campbell SB, Walker R, Tai SS, et al. Randomized controlled trial of sirolimus for renal transplant recipients at high risk for nonmelanoma skin cancer. Am J Transplant 2012;12(5):1146–56.

25. Pickering CR, Zhou JH, Lee JJ, et al. Mutational landscape of aggressive cutaneous squamous cell carcinoma. Clin Cancer Res 2014;20(24):6582–92.

26. Ding L, Chen F. Predicting tumor response to PD-1 Blockade. N Engl J Med 2019; 381(5):477–9.

27. Grob JJ, Gonzalez R, Basset-Seguin N, et al. Pembrolizumab monotherapy for recurrent or metastatic cutaneous squamous cell carcinoma: a single-arm phase II Trial (KEYNOTE-629). J Clin Oncol 2020;38(25):2916–25.

28. Ow TJ, Wang HR, McLellan B, et al. AHNS series - Do you know your guidelines? Diagnosis and management of cutaneous squamous cell carcinoma. Head Neck 2016;38(11):1589–95.

29. Porceddu SV, Bressel M, Poulsen MG, et al. Postoperative concurrent chemoradiotherapy versus postoperative radiotherapy in high-risk cutaneous squamous cell carcinoma of the head and neck: the randomized phase III TROG 05.01 Trial. J Clin Oncol 2018;36(13):1275–83.

30. Denic S. Preoperative treatment of advanced skin carcinoma with cisplatin and bleomycin. Am J Clin Oncol 1999;22(1):32–4.

31. Guthrie TH Jr, McElveen LJ, Porubsky ES, et al. Cisplatin and doxorubicin. An effective chemotherapy combination in the treatment of advanced basal cell and squamous carcinoma of the skin. Cancer 1985;55(8):1629–32.

32. Jarkowski A 3rd, Hare R, Loud P, et al. Systemic therapy in advanced cutaneous squamous cell carcinoma (CSCC): the roswell park experience and a review of the literature. Am J Clin Oncol 2016;39(6):545–8.

33. Nottage MK, Lin C, Hughes BG, et al. Prospective study of definitive chemoradiation in locally or regionally advanced squamous cell carcinoma of the skin. Head Neck 2017;39(4):679–83.

34. Maubec E, Duvillard P, Velasco V, et al. Immunohistochemical analysis of EGFR and HER-2 in patients with metastatic squamous cell carcinoma of the skin. Anticancer Res 2005;25(2B):1205–10.

35. Samstein RM, Ho AL, Lee NY, et al. Locally advanced and unresectable cutaneous squamous cell carcinoma: outcomes of concurrent cetuximab and radiotherapy. J Skin Cancer 2014;2014:284582.

36. Migden MR, Khushalani NI, Chang ALS, et al. Cemiplimab in locally advanced cutaneous squamous cell carcinoma: results from an open-label, phase 2, single-arm trial. Lancet Oncol 2020;21(2):294–305.

37. Fisher J, Zeitouni N, Fan W, et al. Immune checkpoint inhibitor therapy in solid organ transplant recipients: a patient-centered systematic review. J Am Acad Dermatol 2020;82(6):1490–500.

38. Bernier J, Domenge C, Ozsahin M, et al. Postoperative irradiation with or without concomitant chemotherapy for locally advanced head and neck cancer. N Engl J Med 2004;350(19):1945–52.

39. Cooper JS, Pajak TF, Forastiere AA, et al. Postoperative concurrent radiotherapy and chemotherapy for high-risk squamous-cell carcinoma of the head and neck. N Engl J Med 2004;350(19):1937–44.

40. Amoils M, Lee CS, Sunwoo J, et al. Node-positive cutaneous squamous cell carcinoma of the head and neck: Survival, high-risk features, and adjuvant chemoradiotherapy outcomes. Head & neck 2017;39(5):881–5.

41. Trosman SJ, Zhu A, Nicolli EA, et al. High-risk cutaneous squamous cell cancer of the head and neck: risk factors for recurrence and impact of adjuvant treatment. Laryngoscope 2020. https://doi.org/10.1002/lary.28564.

42. Tanvetyanon T, Padhya T, McCaffrey J, et al. Postoperative concurrent chemotherapy and radiotherapy for high-risk cutaneous squamous cell carcinoma of the head and neck. Head Neck 2015;37(6):840–5.

43. Hasmat S, Mooney C, Gao K, et al. Regional metastasis in head and neck cutaneous squamous cell carcinoma: an update on the significance of extra-nodal extension and soft tissue metastasis. Ann Surg Oncol 2020;27(8):2840–5.

44. Gross NFR, Nagarajan P, Bell D, et al. LBA74 Phase II study of neoadjuvant cemiplimab prior to surgery in patients with stage II/IV (M0) cutaneous squamous cell carcinoma of the head and neck (CSCC-HN). Ann Oncol 2019; 30(Supplement 5).

Surgical Management of Merkel Cell Carcinoma

Miriam Lango, MD[a],*, Yelizaveta Shnayder, MD[b]

KEYWORDS

- Merkel cell carcinoma surgery • Sentinel lymph node biopsy
- Lymph node metastases • Adjuvant radiation

KEY POINTS

- Merkel cell carcinoma is a rare aggressive cutaneous malignancy occurring most commonly in the head and neck region.
- Risk factors for development of Merkel cell carcinoma include sun exposure, age older than 65 years, immunosuppression, and infection with Merkel cell polyomavirus.
- Prognosis depends on factors, such as stage at presentation, tumor thickness, polyoma viral status, presence of tumor infiltrating lymphocytes, and lymphovascular invasion.
- Treatment of stage I and II Merkel cell carcinoma includes surgical resection and sentinel lymph node biopsy followed by the selective use adjuvant radiation.
- Treatment of stage III Merkel cell carcinoma requires multimodality treatment, including surgical resection of the primary site, lymphadenectomy, and adjuvant radiation or chemoradiation.

INTRODUCTION

Merkel cell carcinoma (MCC) is a rare aggressive neuroendocrine cutaneous malignancy that occurs most commonly in the head and neck region. Annual incidence of MCC is 0.6 cases per 100,000 persons and has been increasing.[1] The incidence of MCC in the United States, approximately 1600 cases per year, is expected to reach 3000 cases annually by 2025.[2] When analyzing characteristics of 4376 patients with MCC from the Surveillance, Epidemiology, and End Results database diagnosed between 1980 and 2008, Smith and colleagues[3] reported that most MCC tumors (48.1%) were located in the head and neck, followed by upper extremity (24.6%).

---

[a] Department of Head and Neck Surgery, University of Texas MD Anderson Cancer Center, 1515 Holcombe Boulevard, Houston, TX 77030, USA; [b] Department of Otolaryngology–Head and Neck Surgery, University of Kansas School of Medicine, 3901 Rainbow Boulevard, Kansas City, KS 66160, USA
* Corresponding author.
E-mail address: MNLango@mdanderson.org

Otolaryngol Clin N Am 54 (2021) 357–368
https://doi.org/10.1016/j.otc.2020.11.008
0030-6665/21/© 2020 Elsevier Inc. All rights reserved.

ETIOLOGY AND RISK FACTORS

Risk factors for MCC include age greater than 65 years, sun exposure, immunosuppression, and infection with Merkel cell polyomavirus; 80% of MCCs have evidence of viral genome, whereas the rest exhibit UV-related DNA damage[2]; 98% of MCCs occur in whites; and 81% of cases occur in sun-exposed skin. MCC presents as an erythematous or violaceous dermal papule (**Figs. 1** and **2**). Up to 30% of patients present with clinical evidence of cervical or intraparotid lymph node metastases.[4]

DIAGNOSIS, STAGING, PROGNOSIS

A punch biopsy or an excisional biopsy of a suspicious skin lesion with narrow margins is preferred to shave biopsy, in order to accurately diagnose depth of invasion of the lesion. In addition to standard hematoxylin-eosin histopathologic evaluation, immunohistochemical staining plays an important role in the diagnosis of MCC. Positive immunostaining for cytokeratin 20 (CK20) in the presence of negative thyroid transcription factor 1 (TTF-1) staining suggests the diagnosis.[5] Poorly differentiated MCCs may lose the CK20 marker. Positive stains for chromogranin A, synaptophysin, or CD 56 (neural cell adhesion molecule) and the negativity for TTF-1 distinguish MCCs from small cell carcinomas.[5]

A thorough history and complete head and neck examination, including palpation of the parotid, occipital, and cervical lymph node regions, should be performed. Imaging

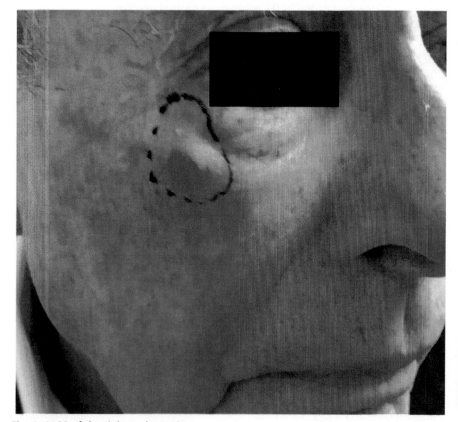

Fig. 1. MCC of the right malar region.

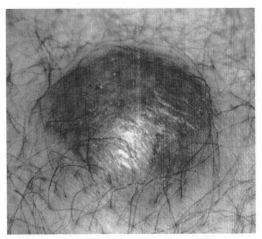

Fig. 2. MCC appears as an erythematous or violaceous dermal papule.

of the neck is a helpful adjunct to clinical staging. Lymphoscintigraphy with sentinel lymph node biopsy (SLNB) plays a critical role in staging MCCs and facilitates treatment planning. Up to one-half of patients with early-stage disease are reclassified as having late-stage disease following SLN biopsy. According to the National Comprehensive Cancer Network (NCCN) guidelines, SLNB is recommended for all patients with clinically node-negative disease who are fit for surgery.

Staging

The American Joint Committee on Cancer staging system incorporates well-established prognostic factors in MCC. In TNM staging, T classification is determined primarily by tumor diameter (**Table 1**). N classification is determined by the presence of lymph node metastases as well as dermal lymphatic metastases. Staging for MCC distinguishes lymph node metastases, which are identified clinically or radiographically versus those identified pathologically. Similar to melanoma, MCC is upstaged from stage I–II to stage IIIA, if clinically occult lymph nodes yield pathologic evidence of nodal metastases. Clinically positive nodal disease is considered at least stage IIIB, except T0/unknown primary (UP) MCCs, which are considered IIIA despite the presence of clinical nodal disease.

Dermal lymphatic metastases, or in-transit metastases, are features of MCCs and other cutaneous malignancies, which can complicate treatment. At a minimum, the presence of in-transit disease increases overall stage to III. In-transit disease located at a site distant from the primary tumor alters overall staging to M1a or stage IV.

Other, less well established clinicopathologic or immunologic factors have been investigated as independent predictors of prognosis, including tumor site,[3] tumor thickness,[6–9] growth pattern,[7,8] MCC viral status,[10,11] tumor-infiltrating lymphocytes,[7,12,13] and lymphovascular invasion (LVI).[7,14–16]

Prognostic Factors

The rates of metastatic spread of MCCs are far higher than those of most other cutaneous malignancies and upstage patients with clinical stage I–II to pathologic stage IIIA disease.[3,17,18] MCCs arising in head and neck sites have been linked to higher rates of occult nodal disease. In analyzing characteristics of 4376 patients with MCC, male sex, location of the primary tumor in the lip, intermediate tumor size

Table 1
Merkel cell carcinoma staging

Clinical Primary Tumor (T)	
TX	Primary tumor cannot be assessed (eg, curetted)
T0	No evidence of primary tumor
Tis	In situ primary tumor
T1	Maximum clinical tumor diameter, ≤2 cm
T2	Maximum clinical tumor diameter >2 but ≤5 cm
T3	Maximum clinical tumor diameter >5 cm
T4	Primary tumor invades fascia, muscle, cartilage, or bone
Clinical lymph node metastases (N)	
NX	Regional lymph nodes cannot be clinically assessed (eg, previously removed for another reason, or because of body habitus)
N0	No regional lymph node metastasis detected on clinical and/or radiologic examination
N1	Metastasis in regional lymph node(s)
N2	In-transit metastasis (discontinuous from primary tumor; located between primary tumor and draining regional nodal basin, or distal to the primary tumor) without lymph node metastasis
N3	In-transit metastasis (discontinuous from primary tumor; located between primary tumor and draining regional nodal basin, or distal to the primary tumor) with lymph node metastasis
Pathologic regional metastases (pN)	
pNX	Regional lymph nodes cannot be accessed (eg, previously removed for another reason or not removed for pathologic evaluation)
pN0	No regional lymph node metastasis detected on pathologic evaluation
pN1	Metastasis in regional lymph node(s)
pN1a(sn)	Clinically occult regional lymph node metastasis identified only by sentinel lymph node biopsy
pN1a	Clinically occult regional lymph node metastasis following lymph node dissection
pN1b	Clinically and/or radiologically detected regional lymph node metastasis, microscopically confirmed
pN2	In-transit metastasis (discontinuous from primary tumor, located between primary tumor and draining regional nodal basin, or distal to the primary tumor) without lymph node metastasis
pN3	In-transit metastasis (discontinuous from primary tumor, located between primary tumor and draining regional nodal basin, or distal to the primary tumor) with lymph node metastasis

Overall stage: clinical TNM	T classification	N classification	M classification
Stage 0	Tis	N0	M0
Stage I	T1	N0	M0
Stage IIA	T2–T3	N0	M0
Stage IIB	T4	N0	M0
Stage III	T0–T4	N1–3	M0
Stage IV	T0–T4	Any N	M1

Overall stage: pathologic TNM	T classification	N classification	M classification
Stage 0	Tis	N0	M0
Stage I	T1	N0	M0
Stage IIA	T2–T3	N0	M0
Stage IIB	T4	N0	M0
Stage IIIA	T1–T4	N1a(sn) or N1a	M0
	T0	N1b	M0
Stage IIIB	T1–T4	N1b–3	M0
Stage IV	T0–T4	Any N	M1

Data from NCCN Clinical Practice Guidelines in Oncology. Merkel Cell Carcinoma. Version 1.2020. October 2, 2019, 1-66.

2 cm to 5 cm, increasing tumor extension beyond the dermis, nodal metastasis, and distant metastasis each were independently associated with an increased risk of death from MCC.[3] The investigators found high frequency of lymph node metastases, 30.6% in non–head and neck MCC and 43.6% in head and neck MCC, even in small tumors less than 2 cm in size, indicating aggressiveness of MCC located in the head and neck region.

LVI, believed to be an early event in MCC pathogenesis,[19] has been associated with even higher rates of microscopic nodal disease and worse survival, independent of other factors.[7,15,16] LVI in the primary tumor has been associated with a 65% rate of occult metastases.[16]

Immunologic markers also have been investigated as prognostic biomarkers, based on observations of greater susceptibility and worse survival in immunosuppressed groups. Intratumoral CD8[+] lymphocyte infiltration has been shown to provide independent prognostic information.[12] Studies of predictive biomarkers of response to immunotherapy are ongoing.[20,21] For example, patients with an absence of Merkel cell polyomavirus oncoprotein (MCPyV) antibodies to a virus-related MCCs may be subject to higher recurrence rates. Currently, MCPyV serology may be included in the initial work-up as well as post-treatment surveillance of MCC patients.[22]

Imaging in Merkel Cell Carcinoma

Imaging plays an important role in the initial staging of MCC, due to MCC's propensity for early metastasis. Anatomic imaging, such as computerized tomography (CT) scan or magnetic resonance imaging and/or whole-body PET with fused axial imaging, may be useful to identify regional and distant metastases.[23] PET-CT scan is most useful for advanced disease. Imaging is less reliable for identifying occult metastatic disease in clinically stage I–II cases than is SLNB.[24] SLNB frequently has been utilized in the staging of MCC,[16,17,25] but there is no absolute consensus on the independent survival benefit of SLNB.[15] It facilitates, however, tailoring of the radiotherapy (RT) treatment to the disease[16] and provides a rationale for systemic therapy use, off or on protocol.

SURGICAL MANAGEMENT: EARLY-STAGE DISEASE (STAGES I AND II)

Wide local excision (WLE) of the primary MCC tumor with 1-cm to 2-cm margins, or to the level of investing fascia or periosteum, is the mainstay of treatment.[22] For early-stage T1 and T2 primary MCC tumors of the head and neck region, Mohs micrographic surgery (MMS) also has been utilized successfully, with overall survival outcomes comparable to those of WLE.[25] Although used infrequently overall, MMS is more likely to be utilized for small MCCs in head and neck sites, followed by adjuvant radiation[25,26] and performed less often in conjunction with an SLNB.[26] If MMS is chosen as a treatment, then SLNB should be performed prior to MMS, in order not to cause alteration in lymphatic drainage of the primary MCC. SLNB ideally should be performed at the time of the WLE of the primary tumor.[22,26]

Absence of SLNB precludes complete pathologic staging and impedes targeted adjuvant radiation planning.[16] Synoptic reporting of pathologic findings after MMS is underutilized, which also may affect staging and additional treatment. According to the NCCN guidelines, the following elements have to be included in the pathology report: largest tumor diameter (centimeters); peripheral and deep margin status; LVI; and extracutaneous extension to bone, muscle, fascia, or cartilage.[22] Additional clinically relevant factors to be included are Breslow depth (millimeters), tumor-infiltrating lymphocytes (not identified, brisk, nonbrisk), tumor growth pattern (nodular or infiltrative), and presence of secondary cutaneous malignancy in the specimen, such as squamous cell or basal cell carcinoma.[22]

SURGICAL MANAGEMENT: STAGE III
Stage IIIA

The surgical management of stage III is distinguished based on the presence of microscopic (stage IIIA) or clinically positive lymph node metastases (stage IIIB). Stage I–II MCCs without clinically or radiographically apparent nodal metastases that are found to have lymph node metastases postoperatively are reclassified as pathologic stage IIIA. A positive SLNB prompts additional treatment. The NCCN guidelines recommend nodal dissection and/or RT to the nodal basin, based on 2 small single-institution studies that suggested equivalent nodal control and survival after RT or completion lymph node dissection (CLND).[27,28] A larger study of more than 400 SLN-positive MCC patients from the National Cancer Database (NCDB) showed that patients treated with RT with or without CLND conferred a survival benefit compared with completion nodal dissection alone. The investigators recommended a personalized approach to adding CLND to adjuvant RT based on age, comorbidities, lymph node basin, and burden of disease.[29]

Stage IIIB

Early studies suggested aggressive treatment that included WLE, lymph node dissection, and adjuvant RT improved the survival of MCC patients.[30–32] Surgery and radiation have remained the mainstay in the treatment of MCCs with clinically apparent lymph node metastases without evidence of distant metastatic spread.[33] Chemotherapy (etoposide, and cisplatin or carboplatin) frequently is added, although the survival benefit of cytotoxic chemotherapy has not been demonstrated. Multimodality treatment has yielded 5-year overall survival rates of 30% to 40%.[34,35] RT to the primary site and nodal basin improved locoregional control[36–38] and disease-free[39] and overall survival.[40,41] Although primary RT in the setting of clinically positive nodal disease has been reported, locoregional control appears to be better with combined lymphadenectomy and postoperative RT.[42] The number of clinically involved lymph nodes[43] and immune-suppressed status[44] influence recurrence-free and disease-specific survival rates.

The use of immunotherapy, in particular, programmed cell death-1 inhibitors, as neoadjuvant treatment prior to surgical management of advanced resectable MCC is promising. The CheckMate 358 trial, which recently was published, showed notable antitumor efficacy in patients with advanced MCC. Administration of nivolumab prior to surgery in 39 MCC patients with predominantly stage IIIB disease resulted in pathologic complete responses (pCRs) in 47%, with at least a major pathologic response in 61.5% of patients. Recurrence-free survival rates at 12 months and 24 months postoperatively were 77.5% (95% CI, 58.4% to 88.7%) and 68.5% (95% CI, 47.5% to 82.6%), respectively, comparing favorably with historical controls. The 12-month and 24-month recurrence-free survival rates of patients with pCRs were 100% and 89%, respectively.[45] The investigators suggested that patients with pCRs may not require adjuvant RT. Response to therapy was determined more reliably with surgery, using pathologic review rather than radiographic restaging. Given these impressive results, it seems likely that immunotherapy will be incorporated into the standard treatment of locoregionally advanced MCC. Moreover, these responses appear to be durable in nature. Historically, overall survival for all patients with MCC of the head and neck was reported as low as 54% at 5 years and 37% at 10 years,[46] due to high rates of local recurrence as well as regional lymph node metastases.

SURGICAL MANAGEMENT OF UNKNOWN PRIMARY MERKEL CELL CARCINOMA

In 5% to 20% of MCCs, the primary cutaneous origin of metastatic MCC in the lymph nodes never is identified.[47,48] A full-body dermatologic survey and whole-body PET-CT scan are helpful in staging and work-up (**Fig. 3**).

UP MCC is characterized by infrequent intradermal metastases and portends a more favorable survival than other MCCs with similar nodal disease burden levels.[49] UP MCC has a lower association with MCC polyomavirus than with cutaneous MCC.[50] Other clinically distinctive characteristics have been identified, including decreased frequency of preexisting immunosuppression and higher tumor mutational burdens with UV-specific genetic signatures. Stronger underlying immune response against MCC is believed to contribute to regression of the primary lesion and improved survival associated with UP MCC.[51,52] Despite these distinctive features, there is no evidence that these represent a separate entity, such as primary lymph node MCC.[51,53]

The NCCN guidelines recommend that after multidisciplinary consultation, patients with MCC lymph node metastases undergo lymphadenectomy and adjuvant RT. Primary RT may be considered in some cases.[48] Surgery for UP MCC in the head and neck frequently involves parotidectomy and neck dissection. The lymphadenectomies approximate those performed for other cutaneous malignancies that include removal of external jugulodigastric, suboccipital, and/or postauricular lymphatics, due to the presumed cutaneous origin of these cancers.[51,53]

ROLE OF ADJUVANT RADIOTHERAPY

Surgical treatment of MCC often is followed by adjuvant radiation to the primary tumor bed with or without regional radiation to the lymph node basin.

For localized MCC (stages I and II), surgery followed by adjuvant RT has been shown to improve locoregional control[38,40] and overall survival[40,54] over surgery alone. Many studies do not distinguish between the utilization of local RT and regional RT, making it more difficult to assess the impact of the treatment on outcomes. Adjuvant local RT is employed far more commonly than elective nodal RT, particularly in the setting of a negative SLNB.[16] Indications for adjuvant local RT with or without regional RT include close or positive margins but other factors may be considered, such as larger primary tumor size and the presence of LVI or immunosuppression, at the discretion of the multidisciplinary treatment team. The NCCN recommends timely initiation of postoperative RT.[22] An NCDB review of 5952 patients with stage I–II MCC

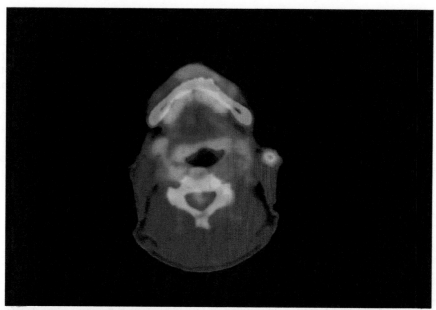

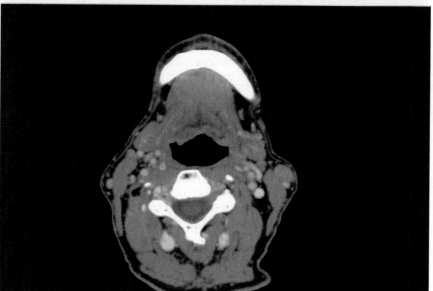

Fig. 3. PET-CT (*upper*) and CT with contrast (*lower*) both reveal a single metastatic lymph node within the left external jugular/parotid tail region, in a patient with MCC of UP. Complete skin examination failed to identify the primary tumor source. The patient underwent left parotidectomy with facial nerve preservation and selective neck dissection followed by adjuvant RT. He has no evidence of disease 3 years later.

revealed no detrimental effect of delays from completion of surgical treatment to initiation of adjuvant RT on overall survival, ranging from 4 weeks to 24 weeks. In this study, however, predictors of worse overall survival included advanced age, greater comorbidities, male sex, lower regional income, earlier year of diagnosis, more advanced tumor and nodal staging, positive margins, head and neck location, and treatment at community facilities.[55]

In patients with regional nodal metastases (stage III), adjuvant RT improves locoregional control but may not improve overall survival.[54] Patients are subject to rapid recurrences at locoregional and distant sites. High-risk patients should be considered for participation in clinical trials.

ROLE OF SYSTEMIC THERAPY

In the primary treatment of nondisseminated MCC, adjuvant cisplatin or carboplatin with or without etoposide may be considered in patients with regional disease. According to the NCCN guidelines, adjuvant chemotherapy should not be recommended routinely, because no overall survival benefit has been demonstrated in retrospective studies; it may be considered in select cases. A retrospective analysis of 2065 stage III MCC patients from the NCDB failed to show statistically significant improvement in overall survival with addition of adjuvant chemotherapy.[54] Cytotoxic chemotherapies no longer are recommended first-line treatments of disseminated disease. They largely have been replaced by immune checkpoint inhibitors (avelumab, pembrolizumab, and nivolumab) but may be considered second-line treatment. The NCCN recommends enrolling high-risk patients in clinical trials.

ACKNOWLEDGMENTS

Research support: None.

DISCLOSURES

None.

REFERENCES

1. Hughes MP, Hardee ME, Cornelius LA, et al. Merkel cell carcinoma: epidemiology, target, and therapy. Curr Dermatol Rep 2014;3(1):46–53.
2. Villani A, Fabbrocini G, Costa C, et al. Merkel cell carcinoma: therapeutic updates and emerging therapies. Dermatol Ther 2019;9:209–22.
3. Smith V, Ramsay Camp E, Lentsch E. Merkel cell carcinoma: identification of prognostic factors unique to tumors in the head and neck based on analysis of SEER Data. Laryngoscope 2012;122:1283–90.
4. Raju S, Vazirnia A, Totri C, et al. Treatment of merkel cell carcinoma of the head and neck: a systematic review. Dermatol Surg 2014;40:1273–83.
5. Leech SN, Kolar AJ, Barrett PD, et al. Merkel cell carcinoma can be distinguished from metastatic small cell carcinoma using antibodies to cytokeratin 20 and thyroid transcription factor 1. J Clin Pathol 2001;54(9):727–9.
6. Sandel HD, Day T, Richardson MS, et al. Merkel cell carcinoma: does tumor size or depth of invasion correlate with recurrence, metastasis, or patient survival? Laryngoscope 2006;116(5):791–5.
7. Andea AA, Coit DG, Amin B, et al. (2008). Merkel cell carcinoma: histologic features and prognosis. Cancer 2008;113(9):2549–58.

8. Schwartz JL, Griffith KA, Lowe L, et al. Features predicting sentinel lymph node positivity in Merkel cell carcinoma. J Clin Oncol 2011;29(8):1036–41.

9. Smith FO, Yue B, Marzban SS, et al. Both tumor depth and diameter are predictive of sentinel lymph node status and survival in Merkel cell carcinoma. Cancer 2015;121(18):3252–60.

10. Moshiri AS, Nghiem P. Milestones in the staging, classification, and biology of Merkel cell carcinoma. J Natl Compr Canc Netw 2014;12(9):1255–62.

11. Moshiri AS, Doumani R, Yelistratova L, et al. Polyomavirus-negative Merkel cell carcinoma: a more aggressive subtype based on analysis of 282 cases using multimodal tumor virus detection. J Invest Dermatol 2017;137(4):819–27.

12. Paulson KG, Iyer JG, Tegeder AR, et al. Transcriptome-wide studies of Merkel Cell Carcinoma and validation of intratumoral CD8+ lymphocyte invasion as an independent predictor of survival. J Clin Oncol 2011;29(12):1539–46.

13. Paulson KG, Iyer JG, Simonson WT, et al. CD8+ lymphocyte intratumoral infiltration as a stage-independent predictor of Merkel cell carcinoma survival: a population-based study. Am J Clin Pathol 2014;142(4):452–8.

14. Fields RC, Busam KJ, Chou JF, et al. Five hundred patients with Merkel cell carcinoma evaluated at a single institution. Ann Surg 2011;254(3):465–73 [discussion 473–65].

15. Fields RC, Busam KJ, Chou JF, et al. Recurrence and survival in patients undergoing sentinel lymph node biopsy for merkel cell carcinoma: analysis of 153 patients from a single institution. Ann Surg Oncol 2011;18(9):2529–37.

16. Harounian JA, Molin N, Galloway TJ, et al. Effect of sentinel lymph node biopsy and LVI on merkel cell carcinoma prognosis and treatment. Laryngoscope 2020. https://doi.org/10.1002/lary.28866.

17. Gupta SG, Wang LC, Peñas PF, et al. Sentinel lymph node biopsy for evaluation and treatment of patients with Merkel cell carcinoma: the Dana-Farber experience and meta-analysis of the literature. Arch Dermatol 2006;142(6):685–90.

18. Becker JC, Stang A, DeCaprio JA, et al. Merkel cell carcinoma. Nat Rev Dis Primers 2017;3:170–7.

19. Kukko HM, Koljonen VS, Tukiainen EJ, et al. Vascular invasion is an early event in pathogenesis of Merkel cell carcinoma. Mod Pathol 2010;23(8):1151–6.

20. Knepper TC, Montesion M, Russell JS, et al. The Genomic Landscape of Merkel Cell Carcinoma and Clinicogenomic Biomarkers of Response ot Immune Checkpoint Inhibitor Therapy. Clin Cancer Res 2019;25(19):5961-71.

21. Miller NJ, Church CD, Fling SP, et al. Merkel cell polyomavirus-specific immune responses in patients with Merkel cell carcinoma receiving anti-PD-1 therapy. J Immunother Cancer 2018;6(1):131–9.

22. National Comprehensive Cancer Network. Merkel Cell Carcinoma (Version 1.2020). https://www.nccn.org/professionals/physician_gls/pdf/mcc_blocks.pdf. Accessed June 28, 2020.

23. Poulsen M, Macfarlane D, Veness M, et al. Prospective analysis of the utility of 18-FDG PET in Merkel cell carcinoma of the skin: A trans tasman radiation oncology group study, TROG 09:03. J Med Imaging Radiat Oncol 2018;62(3):412–9.

24. Liu J, Larcos G, Howle J, et al. Lack of clinical impact of (18) F-fluorodeoxyglucose positron emission tomography with simultaneous computed tomography for stage I and II Merkel cell carcinoma with concurrent sentinel lymph node biopsy staging: a single institutional experience from Westmead Hospital, Sydney. Australas J Dermatol 2017;58(2):99–105.

25. Singh B, Qureshi MM, Truong MT, et al. Demographics and outcomes of stage I and II Merkel cell carcinoma treated with Mohs' micrographic surgery compared

to wide local excision in the national cancer database. J Am Acad Dermatol 2018; 79(1):126–34.

26. Shaikh WR, Sobanko JF, Etzkorn JR, et al. Utilization patterns and survival outcomes after wide local excision or Mohs' micrographic surgery for Merkel cell carcinoma in the United States 2004-2009. J Am Acad Dermatol 2018;78(1): 175–7.

27. Jenkins LN, Howle JR, Veness MJ. Sentinel lymph node biopsy in clinically node-negative Merkel cell carcinoma: the Westmead Hospital experience. ANZ J Surg 2019;89(5):520–3.

28. Lee JS, Durham AB, Bichakjian CK, et al. Completion lymph node dissection or radiation therapy for sentinel node metastasis in Merkel cell carcinoma. Ann Surg Oncol 2019;26(2):386–94.

29. Cramer JD, Suresh K, Sridharan S. Completion lymph node dissection for merkel cell carcinoma. Am J Surg 2020. https://doi.org/10.1016/j.amjsurg.2020.02.018.

30. Kokoska ER, Kokoska MS, Collins BT, et al. Early aggressive treatment for Merkel cell carcinoma improves outcome. Am J Surg 1997;174(6):688–93.

31. Lawenda BD, Thiringer JK, Foss RD, et al. Merkel cell carcinoma arising in the head and neck: optimizing therapy. Am J Clin Oncol 2001;24(1):35–42.

32. Brissett AE, Olsen KD, Kasperbauer JL, et al. Merkel cell carcinoma of the head and neck: a retrospective case series. Head Neck 2002;24(11):982–8.

33. Miles BA, Goldenberg D, Education Committee of the American H, Neck S. Merkel cell carcinoma: do you know your guidelines? Head Neck 2016;38(5):647–52.

34. Sridharan V, Muralidhar V, Margalit DN, et al. Merkel cell carcinoma: a population analysis on survival. J Natl Compr Canc Netw 2016;14(10):1247–57.

35. Steuten L, Garmo V, Phatak H, et al. Treatment patterns, overall survival, and total healthcare costs of advanced Merkel cell carcinoma in the USA. Appl Health Econ Health Policy 2019;17(5):733–40.

36. Eich HT, Eich D, Staar S, et al. Role of postoperative radiotherapy in the management of Merkel cell carcinoma. Am J Clin Oncol 2002;25(1):50–6.

37. Eng TY, Boersma MG, Fuller CD, et al. Treatment of merkel cell carcinoma. Am J Clin Oncol 2004;27(5):510–5.

38. Strom T, Naghavi AO, Messina JL, et al. Improved local and regional control with radiotherapy for Merkel cell carcinoma of the head and neck. Head Neck 2017; 39(1):48–55.

39. Veness MJ, Morgan GJ, Palme CE, et al. Surgery and adjuvant radiotherapy in patients with cutaneous head and neck squamous cell carcinoma metastatic to lymph nodes: combined treatment should be considered best practice. Laryngoscope 2005;115(5):870–5.

40. Mojica P, Smith D, Ellenhorn JD. Adjuvant radiation therapy is associated with improved survival in Merkel cell carcinoma of the skin. J Clin Oncol 2007;25(9): 1043–7.

41. Kim JA, Choi AH. Effect of radiation therapy on survival in patients with resected Merkel cell carcinoma: a propensity score surveillance, epidemiology, and end results database analysis. JAMA Dermatol 2013;149(7):831–8.

42. Fang LC, Lemos B, Douglas J, et al. Radiation monotherapy as regional treatment for lymph node-positive Merkel cell carcinoma. Cancer 2010;116(7):1783–90.

43. Iyer JG, Storer BE, Paulson KG, et al. Relationships among primary tumor size, number of involved nodes, and survival for 8044 cases of Merkel cell carcinoma. J Am Acad Dermatol 2014;70(4):637–43.

44. Bryant MK, Ward C, Gaber CE, et al. Decreased survival and increased recurrence in Merkel cell carcinoma significantly linked with immunosuppression. J Surg Oncol 2020. https://doi.org/10.1002/jso.26048.

45. Topalian SL, Bhatia S, Amin A, et al. Neoadjuvant nivolumab for patients with resectable Merkel Cell Carcinoma in the CheckMate 358 Trial. J Clin Oncol 2020;JCO2000201. https://doi.org/10.1200/JCO.20.00201.

46. Timmer FC, Klop WM, Relyveld GN, et al. Merkel cell carcinoma of the head and neck: emphasizing the risk of undertreatment. Eur Arch Otorhinolaryngol 2016; 273(5):1243–51.

47. Medina-Franco H, Urist MM, Fiveash J, et al. Multimodality treatment of Merkel cell carcinoma: case series and literature review of 1024 cases. Ann Surg Oncol 2001;8(3):204–8.

48. Deneve JL, Messina JL, Marzban SS, et al. Merkel cell carcinoma of unknown primary origin. Ann Surg Oncol 2012;19(7):2360–6.

49. Tarantola TI, Vallow LA, Halyard MY, et al. Unknown primary Merkel cell carcinoma: 23 new cases and a review. J Am Acad Dermatol 2013;68(3):433–40.

50. Pan Z, Chen YY, Wu X, et al. Merkel cell carcinoma of lymph node with unknown primary has a significantly lower association with Merkel cell polyomavirus than its cutaneous counterpart. Mod Pathol 2014;27(9):1182–92.

51. Vandeven N, Lewis CW, Makarov V, et al. Merkel cell carcinoma patients presenting without a primary lesion have elevated markers of immunity, higher tumor mutation burden, and improved survival. Clin Cancer Res 2018;24(4):963–71.

52. Chen KT, Papavasiliou P, Edwards K, et al. A better prognosis for Merkel cell carcinoma of unknown primary origin. Am J Surg 2013;206(5):752–7.

53. Lawrence LEB, Saleem A, Sahoo MK, et al. Is merkel cell carcinoma of lymph node actually metastatic cutaneous merkel cell carcinoma? Am J Clin Pathol 2020. https://doi.org/10.1093/ajcp/aqaa051.

54. Bhatia S, Storer BE, Iyer JG, et al. Adjuvant radiation therapy and chemotherapy in merkel cell carcinoma: survival analyses of 6908 cases from the national cancer dataBase. J Natl Cancer Inst 2016;108(9).

55. Shinde A, Verma V, Jones BL, et al. The effect of time to postoperative radiation therapy on survival in resected merkel cell carcinoma. Am J Clin Oncol 2019;42: 636–42.

Cutaneous Sarcomas

Brittny N. Tillman, MD[a],*, Jeffrey C. Liu, MD[b]

KEYWORDS

- Sarcoma • Cutaneous • Surgery for cutaneous sarcoma
- Dermatofibrosarcoma protuberans • Atypical fibroxanthoma
- Pleomorphic dermal sarcoma • Leiomyosarcoma • Angiosarcoma

KEY POINTS

- The various types of cutaneous sarcomas are discussed including presentation, diagnosis, and management.
- Adequate biopsy and a thorough pathologic analysis are critical to diagnosis.
- The mainstay of treatment is surgical resection with complete margin analysis given propensity for recurrence.

DERMATOFIBROSARCOMA PROTUBERANS

Dermatofibrosarcoma protuberans (DFSP) is a low-grade cutaneous sarcoma with an approximate yearly incidence of 4 cases per million in the United States (**Tables 1 and 2**).[1] It is among the most common of cutaneous sarcomas, accounting for 18% of the overall incidence with peaks in the third to fifth decades of life.[2] There is also an increased incidence in black patients and women.[3]

DFSP originates from dermal fibroblasts and possibly dermal dendrocytes. It is associated with a t(17;22) (q22:q13) translocation that results in the fusion of a beta-type platelet-derived growth factor receptor gene to the COL1A1 (collagen type 1 alpha 1) gene. Excessive activation of the beta-type platelet-derived growth factor receptor–dependent signaling pathway results in uncontrolled cell growth.[4]

DFSP usually presents as a slow growing asymptomatic plaque most commonly on the trunk followed by lower extremities and scalp. Untreated, DFSP can become very large, locally invasive, and destructive.[2] DFSP has a high reported recurrence rate of 50%; when excised with margins that are greater than 2 cm, the recurrence rate improves to 13%.[5] Although positive margins are more frequent with wide local excision than Mohs micrographic surgery (MMS), the local recurrence rates have been

[a] Department of Otolaryngology–Head and Neck Surgery, University of Texas Southwestern Medical School, 2001 Inwood Road, Dallas, TX 75390-8868, USA; [b] Department of Otolaryngology–Head and Neck Surgery, Lewis Katz School of Medicine at Temple University, Fox Chase Cancer Center, 3440 North Broad Street, Philadelphia, PA 19140, USA
* Corresponding author.
E-mail address: brittny.tillman@utsw.edu

Otolaryngol Clin N Am 54 (2021) 369–378
https://doi.org/10.1016/j.otc.2020.11.010
0030-6665/21/Published by Elsevier Inc.

oto.theclinics.com

Table 1
Characteristics of patient population and presentation by tumor type

Tumor	Population	Presentation
DFSP	Peak in third to fifth decades More common in women More common in black patients	Slow growing plaque with one or more nodules Erythematous, brown, or skin colored Often >3 cm at presentation
Atypical fibroxanthoma	Peak in seventh to eighth decades More common in men	Rapid growth of firm, nodular, exophytic tumor on sun damaged skin Erythematous or skin colored May become ulcerated
Pleomorphic dermal sarcoma	Peak in eighth decade More common in men	Rapid growth of exophytic, nodular, or plaque like tumor on sun damaged skin Brown or erythematous
Cutaneous leiomyosarcoma	Peak in sixth decade More common in men More common in white patients	Nodules or plaques which may be irregular or ulcerative Skin colored May be associated with pain, itching, and/or bleeding
Angiosarcoma	Average seventh Decade May present 2–30 y after radiation May present 10–15 y after lymphedema	Highly variable Red cutaneous lesion similar to hematoma May also seem to be similar to rosacea, eczema, plaque, nodule, cellulitis, or cutaneous edema

statistically similar.[6] One series of 204 retrospective patients with DFSP showed a recurrence rate of 1% using wide excision as a standardized approach, emphasizing the importance of margin control.[7]

The overall prognosis of DFSP is excellent with a 10-year survival rate of 99.1%.[1] Classic DFSP has a rare metastasis rate of 1% to 4%, with the lungs being the most common site.[5] Negative prognostic factors include advanced patient age at the time of diagnosis, large tumor size, and male sex.[8] Histologic variants include Bednar, myxoid, giant cell fibroblastoma, sclerosing, atrophic, and fibrosarcomatous. The fibrosarcomatous variant exhibits the highest rate of metastasis (14%) and poorest prognosis.[2,9,10]

On pathologic analysis, DFSP is characterized by storiform, monomorphic spindle cells, and minimal atypia. The infiltration of adipose tissue by tumor is characterized by a honeycomb appearance. Tumors stain positively for CD34 and negatively for factor XIIIa with rare exceptions. CD34 is an important immunohistochemical marker that may be absent in less differentiated cases. In these cases reverse transcriptase polymerase chain reaction or fluorescence in situ hybridization may be diagnostically useful in identifying the characteristic t(17;22) (q22;q13) translocation.[2]

MRI should be considered if extracutaneous extension is suspected.[11] In advanced tumors and more aggressive subtypes such as fibrosarcomatous, a metastatic workup including lung imaging with a chest computed tomography scan should also be considered.[2,12]

Table 2
Pathogenesis, histologic findings, and treatment strategy by tumor type

Tumor	Pathogenesis	Histology	Treatment
DFSP	Dermal fibroblasts and dendrocytes t (17;22) (q22:q13) translocation	Monomorphic spindle cells with minimal atypia (+) CD34 and (−) factor XIIIa	Wide excision with 2–4 cm margins vs Mohs MRI for extensive disease Regional/distant imaging for fibrosarcomatous subtype Radiation therapy vs imatinib for select cases
Atypical fibroxanthoma	Myofibroblastic cells P53 and telomerase reverse transcriptase mutations	Dermal atypical spindle, pleomorphic, histiocytic, and multinucleated giant cells with occasional atypical mitosis Diagnosis of exclusion	Wide excision with at least 1–2 cm margins vs Mohs Consider imaging for advanced disease[a]
Pleomorphic dermal sarcoma	Possibly a deeper and more aggressive variant of AFX P53, HRAS, CDKN2A, PIK3CA mutations	Resembles AFX with a predilection for subcutaneous structure invasion, perineural invasion, and necrosis Diagnosis of exclusion	Wide excision with at least 1–2 cm margins vs Mohs Consider imaging given 10% risk of metastasis[a]
Cutaneous leiomyosarcoma	Erector pili muscles of hair follicles	Interlacing fascicles of spindle cells with mitotic figures (+) Vimentin and smooth muscle actin (+) Desmin, cytokeratin, S100 in some cases	Wide excision with 3–5 cm margins vs Mohs Consider imaging for advanced disease[a] Adjuvant radiation therapy for tumors >5 cm Multiple systemic regimens reported for advanced disease
Angiosarcoma	Vascular endothelial cells	Dilated disorganized vascular structures or high-grade epithelioid spindle cells without clear vessels High mitotic rates	Preoperative mapping biopsies Wide excision with at least 3 cm margins Consider imaging for advanced disease[a] Multiple systemic regimens reported for advanced and metastatic disease Poor prognosis

[a] No formal guidelines exist.

Once the diagnosis is confirmed, the treatment of choice includes both wide local excision with generous margins of 2 to 4 cm and MMS. Given its widely infiltrative nature, excision should extend to investing fascia of muscle or pericranium when feasible. Margin control may require hematoxylin and eosin sections supplemented by CD34 immunohistochemistory.[13] When MMS is used, a debulking specimen should be examined to identify the more aggressive fibrosarcomatous transformation.[11]

Any complex closure should be delayed until after the final margins are cleared histologically.[2,14] Elective nodal dissection is not advised secondary to infrequent regional nodal metastasis (1%).[5] Although DFSP is radiosensitive, radiation therapy is usually used in either adjuvant or palliative contexts.[2]

Imatinib is a proven systemic therapy to be considered for unresectable, recurrent or metastatic DFSP. It is a multikinase inhibitor in the PDGFRB signaling pathway dysregulated by the t(17;22) translocation often seen in DFSP.[15] It is important to note that tumors lacking the t(17;22) translocation may not respond to imatinib and therefore molecular analysis is recommended before the initiation of imatinib therapy.[13]

ATYPICAL FIBROXANTHOMA

Atypical fibroxanthoma (AFX) is a low-grade superficial sarcoma often considered a superficial variant of dermal pleomorphic sarcoma. The true overall prevalence of AFX is difficult to elucidate because it is a diagnosis of exclusion, which is fraught with misclassification. It is seen more often in the seventh and eighth decades of life and is more common in men.[2]

UV light is thought to contribute to malignant transformation of myofibroblastic cells leading to AFX. Additional studies show telomerase reverse transcriptase promotor mutations and dysregulation of the CCND1/CDK4/6/RB1 signaling pathway, allowing cells to escape apoptosis through telomerase activation as well as decouple the cell cycle with subsequent tumor cell proliferation.[16,17]

AFX typically arises in the head and neck of elderly patients and less commonly in sun-exposed extremities.[18] It typically presents as an exophytic tumor on sun-damaged skin with a tendency toward rapid growth (over weeks).[2] They may become large and ulcerated.[17] Histologically, AFX is predominantly confined to the dermis with atypical spindle or pleomorphic cells, histiocytic cells, and multinucleated giant cells in variable growth patterns with occasional atypical mitosis. There may be hemorrhagic areas and ample vasculature. It is a well-circumscribed pleomorphic neoplasm with increased proliferation, lacking tumor necrosis and infiltrative growth.[18]

Ultimately, AFX is a diagnosis of exclusion and should include a panel of immunostains to rule out other tumor types.[18] It is critical that amelanotic melanoma be ruled out with appropriate markers such as S100 and pancytokeratin.[17] Although vimentin and CD68 staining may be positive, there is no immunohistochemical marker that allows for unequivocal diagnosis.

AFX is thought to represent a less aggressive and superficial version of pleomorphic dermal sarcoma (PDS), the cutaneous variant of undifferentiated pleomorphic sarcoma. Prior research has failed to make the distinction between AFX and dedifferentiated sarcomas, leading clinicians to question the true metastatic potential of AFX.[17] There is ongoing debate on a definitive distinction between AFX and PDS.[19]

The initial workup should include a history and physical examination, complete skin and regional nodal examination, and biopsy. Punch, incisional, or core biopsies are preferred to decrease misdiagnosis associated with a superficial specimen. The role of clinical imaging is unclear, but regional nodal evaluation can be considered with an ultrasound examination or a computed tomography scan, particularly for advanced cases.[17]

Treatment of the primary includes wide local excision with at least 1- to 2-cm margins or MMS. The entire specimen should be evaluated for infiltration beyond the dermis.[17] Regional nodal dissection should be performed as clinically indicated, although there are no absolute guidelines for management. Although metastasis has been reported in 0.5% to 10.0% of all cases, in general, metastasis is rare and the prognosis is generally favorable.[17]

PLEOMORPHIC DERMAL SARCOMA

PDS is also referred to as cutaneous pleomorphic sarcoma and cutaneous undifferentiated pleomorphic sarcoma, which has led to confusion with regard to its true incidence. Furthermore, it is thought to be both a superficial variant of soft tissue undifferentiated pleomorphic sarcoma and a deep variant of AFX. It has also fallen under the term "malignant fibrous histiocytoma," which was previously used to classify most dedifferentiated sarcomas and is no longer used.[17] Because CUPS is a fairly new entity, there are currently no reliable reporting of overall incidence rates. It is diagnosed most often in the eighth decade of life and is more common in men.[2]

PDS typically presents as an exophytic, nodular, or plaque-like growth on sun-damaged skin with rapid growth in elderly patients.[2] PDS resembles a more aggressive form of AFX, although the histopathologic distinction between the 2 entities is not clearly defined. PDS has a predilection for subcutaneous structure invasion, perineural invasion, and necrosis.[17,20]

Like AFX, PDS is also a diagnosis of exclusion that should evaluated with an adequate biopsy and immuhistochemistry.[18] Amelanotic melanoma must be ruled out.[17] Regional metastasis has been described in up to 10% of cases; therefore, radiologic nodal evaluation should be considered.[17] The treatment of choice is excision with at least 1- to 2-cm margins.[19]

CUTANEOUS LEIOMYOSARCOMA

Cutaneous leiomyosarcoma (LMS) is a rare cutaneous sarcoma that presents later in life, with an average age of diagnosis at 62 years. It presents predominantly in white males (94% white and 78% male).[21] Cutaneous LMS is separated into 2 main groups: a cutaneous (dermal) malignancy that rarely metastases, and a subcutaneous variant with greater metastatic potential. LMS can also arise from visceral sites, like the uterus or retroperitoneum, with metastasis to other sites. This review focuses on the cutaneous types.

The presentation of LMS is evenly distributed across the body: 25.5% in the lower limb and hip, 24.0% in the upper limb and shoulder, and 22.5% in the trunk 27.9%, as reported in the Surveillance, Epidemiology, and End Results database.[21] The cutaneous LMS subtype presents more frequently in the head and neck, representing 48% of cutaneous LMS cases.[22,23] Cutaneous LMS is thought to arise from the erector pili muscles of the hair follicles, whereas subcutaneous LMS is thought to arise from smooth muscle in vessels, although this remains speculative. LMS lesions present as skin-colored or erythematous nodules or plaques. They can be irregular or ulcerative. Pain is sometimes associated with presentation, although itching, burning, and bleeding can also occur.[24] Most of these findings described are usually seen with cutaneous LMS, with subcutaneous LMS presenting with normal overlying skin.

Histologically, LMS shows interlacing fascicles of spindle cells, usually with mitotic figures. For cutaneous LMS, these are vimentin and smooth muscle actin positive.

Desmin is positive in approximately 60% of cases.[25] Cytokeratins and S100 stains may occasionally be positive.[26] Necrosis, sclerosis, hemorrhage, hyalinization, and myxoid changes may occasionally be seen.[27]

Cutaneous LMS have a different metastatic pattern compared with subcutaneous LMS, although the data are limited. Although metastasis with cutaneous LMS has been rarely reported, as many as 30% of metastasis were reported in subcutaneous LMS.[24] After an appropriate workup, for disease confined to the local site the mainstay of treatment is surgical resection. Like all sarcomas, negative histologic margins are important to achieve. Some studies have recommended a 3- to 5-cm margin, which is very difficult to achieve in the head and neck.[23] Adjuvant therapy with radiation therapy is generally recommended for lesions greater than 5 cm in size, as noted in the National Comprehensive Care Network guidelines.[13,28] MMS has been reported for LMS with good results and acceptable local control rates.[29]

Despite appropriate treatment, recurrence remains an issue. For cutaneous LMS, the recurrence rate is lower, with 1 series reporting a rate as low as 14%. For subcutaneous LMS, the recurrence rate is reported to be much higher, with as many as one-half of all patients having a recurrence.[23,27] Distant metastases with the subcutaneous variant are uncommon and present in approximately 15% of cases, most commonly to the lungs.[27] For advanced disease, multiple chemotherapy regimens have been reported, which include the use of doxorubicin, ifosfamide, dacarbazine, and gemcitabine.[27] Additional treatment with tyrosine kinase inhibitors in LMS have been reported in clinical trials on sarcoma.[30]

ANGIOSARCOMA

Angiosarcomas (AS) are rare tumors that arise from vascular endothelial cells. They are aggressive tumors, with difficult rates of local control and a high rate of metastasis. The most common type is spontaneous formation in the head neck, known as the Wilson–Jones type. The tumor is rare, and represents about 10% of head and neck sarcomas.[31] AS can also present as a radiation-induced cancer, or develop after chronic lymphedema.[32,33] For the purpose of this review, we focus on cutaneous AS that present spontaneously in the head and neck.

The presentation of AS is varied and its diagnosis is difficult. It can present as a red lesion like a cutaneous hematoma, but may also have a similar presentation to rosacea, eczema, plaque, nodule, cellulitis, or cutaneous edema.[34] Histologically, the AS is variable as well. The cancer can have dilated disorganized vascular structures, with similarities to a hemangioma, but may also present as high-grade epithelioid spindle cells without clear vessels. The malignant endothelium may appear pleomorphic with varied growth patterns. Mitotic rates are usually very high.[35] The presence of an epithelioid morphology and necrosis are both associated with a worse prognosis.[36] For head and neck AS, the most common presentation site is the scalp and neck (61%) and the face (34%).[37]

In evaluating the patient with AS, a workup for both local and regional disease is recommended. MRI may be a consideration for these lesions given the soft tissue nature of the disease. A Surveillance, Epidemiology, and End Results database analysis showed that although 51% of patients were reported as having only localized disease, an additional 23% presented with regional disease, supporting the need for regional evaluation.[38] Distant metastasis was rare (8%).

Surgery remains the mainstay of therapy for treatment, with adjuvant radiation common.[37] A significant challenge in this disease is difficulty in achieving negative histologic margins on the primary site. Only about 20% to 47% of AS resection margins are reported as histologically negative.[38] Recurrence rates of 63% have been reported.[39] Unfortunately, the outcomes of patients who undergo resection with residual positive margins are almost no different than patients who do not receive surgery at all.[37] Neoadjuvant chemotherapy has been advocated as a treatment concept and is under investigation.[40,41]

To help better establish the margin of resection, preoperative localization and mapping biopsies have been advocated. Biopsies at the planned resection margin are taken preoperatively, usually with a punch biopsy, to map out the resection. The recommended margin size varies, but margins of 3 cm or more have been advocated.[13] A distinct challenge is that grossly normal appearing skin will microscopically be positive for AS. Intraoperative frozen sections are not reliable, with 1 series reporting that 67% of patients with AS with a negative intraoperative frozen section had positive margins on permanent section.[42] Collectively, these data show the challenge of achieving R0 surgical resection in AS. Given the high frequency of positive margins, adjuvant radiation is often reported performed after surgical resection of AS.[42]

The outcomes of head and neck AS are poor. A meta-analysis/systemic review shows the 5-year overall survival rate for AS to be between 11% and 50%.[43] Age is a major determinate of outcomes, with the 5-year overall survival for those less than 70 years of age to be 50% to 80%, whereas for those older than 70 years of age, it is reported 0% to 51%. Both Surveillance, Epidemiology, and End Results database and National Cancer Data Base studies report similar 5-year overall survival rate outcomes.[37,38]

Given the poor survival, there has been a significant interest in identifying agents that may improve survival.[44] The first line of treatment for metastatic disease has been with paclitaxel, with multiple phase II trials showing response.[45,46] Multiple agents have been tested for AS, including bevacizumab.[47] The tyrosine kinase inhibitor pazopanib has been reported, as well as propranolol and other agents.[48–51] Immune checkpoint inhibitors are currently being explored for efficacy.[52] Clinicaltrials.gov identifies at least 11 actively recruiting trials for AS, with dozens more in development.[53]

SUMMARY

Although cutaneous sarcomas are rare, awareness of these diseases is important to otolaryngologist—head and neck surgeons. An appropriate biopsy technique with careful pathologic analysis is critical to establish an accurate diagnosis. Surgical resection with adequate margins and complete histologic analysis is the gold standard for the initial treatment of most of these malignancies, per the National Comprehensive Care Network guidelines. Adjuvant therapy depends on the tumor type and its stage. Detailed understanding of the biology and nature of these cancers is important to delivering the best care. Multidisciplinary discussion should be considered for these cases.

DISCLOSURE

The authors have no conflicts of interest to disclose.

REFERENCES

1. Rouhani P, Fletcher CDM, Devesa SS, et al. Cutaneous soft tissue sarcoma incidence patterns in the U.S.: an analysis of 12,114 cases. Cancer 2008;113: 616–27.

2. Bhatt MD, Nambudiri VE. Cutaneous sarcomas. Hematol Oncol Clin North Am 2019;33:87–101.

3. Kreicher KL, Kurlander DE, Gittleman HR, et al. Incidence and survival of primary dermatofibrosarcoma protuberans in the United States. Dermatol Surg 2016;42: S24–31.

4. Patel KU, Sara SS, Vivian SH, et al. Dermatofibrosarcoma protuberans COL1A1-PDGFB fusion is identified in virtually all dermatofibrosarcoma protuberans cases when investigated by newly developed multiplex reverse transcription polymerase chain reaction and fluorescence in situ hybridization assays. Hum Pathol 2008;39:184–93.

5. Rutgers Th, E J, Kroon BBR, et al. Dermatofibrosarcoma protuberans: treatment and prognosis. Eur J Surg Oncol 1992;18:241–8.

6. Meguerditchian AN, Jiping W, Bethany L, et al. Wide excision or Mohs micrographic surgery for the treatment of primary dermatofibrosarcoma protuberans. Am J Clin Oncol 2010;33:300–3.

7. Farma JM, John BA, Jonathan SZ, et al. Dermatofibrosarcoma protuberans: how wide should WE resect? Ann Surg Oncol 2010;17:2112–8.

8. Criscito MC, Martires KJ, Stein JA. Prognostic factors, treatment, and survival in dermatofibrosarcoma protuberans. JAMA Dermatol 2016;152:1365–71.

9. Bogucki B, Neuhaus I, Hurst EA. Dermatofibrosarcoma protuberans: a review of the literature. Dermatol Surg 2012;38:537–51.

10. Mentzel T, Beham A, Katenkamp D, et al. Fibrosarcomatous ('high-grade') dermatofibrosarcoma protuberans: clinicopathologic and immunohistochemical study of a series of 41 cases with emphasis on prognostic significance. Am J Surg Pathol 1998;22:576–87.

11. Bichakjian CK, Thomas O, Murad A, et al. Dermatofibrosarcoma protuberans, version 1.2014. J Natl Compr Canc Netw 2014;12:863–8.

12. Acosta AE, Vélez CS. Dermatofibrosarcoma Protuberans. Curr Treat Options Oncol 2017;18:56.

13. NCCN, N. National Comprehensive Care Network (NCCN). Available at: https://www.nccn.org/. Accessed May 15, 2020.

14. Reha J, Katz SC. Dermatofibrosarcoma Protuberans. Surg Clin North Am 2016; 96:1031–46.

15. Johnson-Jahangir H, Sherman W, Ratner D. Using imatinib as neoadjuvant therapy in dermatofibrosarcoma protuberans: potential pluses and minuses. J Natl Compr Canc Netw 2010;8:881–5.

16. Griewank KG, Bastian S, Rajmohan M, et al. TERT promoter mutations are frequent in atypical fibroxanthomas and pleomorphic dermal sarcomas. Mod Pathol 2014;27:502–8.

17. Kohlmeyer J, Steimle-Grauer SA, Hein R. Cutaneous sarcomas. J Dtsch Dermatol Ges 2017;15:630–48.

18. Mentzel T, Requena L, Brenn T. Atypical Fibroxanthoma Revisited. Surg Pathol Clin 2017;10:319–35.

19. Soleymani T, Tyler Hollmig S. Conception and management of a poorly understood spectrum of dermatologic neoplasms: atypical fibroxanthoma, pleomorphic dermal sarcoma, and undifferentiated pleomorphic sarcoma. Curr Treat Options Oncol 2017;18:50.

20. Ziemer M. Atypical fibroxanthoma. J Dtsch Dermatol Ges 2012. https://doi.org/10.1111/j.1610-0387.2012.07980.x.

21. Sandhu N, Sauvageau AP, Groman A, et al. Cutaneous leiomyosarcoma: a SEER database analysis. Dermatol Surg 2020;46:159–64.

22. Annest NM, Grekin SJ, Stone MS, et al. Cutaneous leiomyosarcoma: a tumor of the head and neck. Dermatol Surg 2007;33:628–33.
23. Bernstein SC, Roenigk RK. Leiomyosarcoma of the skin. Treatment of 34 cases. Dermatol Surg 1996;22:631–5.
24. Fields JP, Helwig EB. Leiomyosarcoma of the skin and subcutaneous tissue. Cancer 1981;47:156–69.
25. Kaddu S, Beham A, Cerroni L, et al. Cutaneous leiomyosarcoma. Am J Surg Pathol 1997;21:979–87.
26. Jensen ML, Jensen OM, Michalski W, et al. Intradermal and subcutaneous leiomyosarcoma: a clinicopathological and immunohistochemical study of 41 cases. J Cutan Pathol 1996;23:458–63.
27. Zacher M, Markus VH, Titus JB, et al. Primary leiomyosarcoma of the skin: a comprehensive review on diagnosis and treatment. Med Oncol 2018;35:135.
28. Pisters PWT, Raphael EP, Valerae OL, et al. Long-term results of prospective trial of surgery alone with selective use of radiation for patients with T1 extremity and trunk soft tissue sarcomas. Ann Surg 2007;246:675–81.
29. Starling J, Coldiron BM. Mohs micrographic surgery for the treatment of cutaneous leiomyosarcoma. J Am Acad Dermatol 2011;64:1119–22.
30. Von Mehren M, Cathryn R, John RG, et al. Phase 2 Southwest Oncology Group-directed intergroup trial (S0505) of sorafenib in advanced soft tissue sarcomas. Cancer 2012;118:770–6.
31. Peng KA, Grogan T, Wang MB. Head and neck sarcomas: analysis of the SEER database. Otolaryngol Head Neck Surg 2014;151:627–33.
32. Lindford A, Böhling T, Vaalavirta L, et al. Surgical management of radiation-associated cutaneous breast angiosarcoma. J Plast Reconstr Aesthet Surg. 2011;64:1036–42.
33. Farzaliyev F, Hamacher R, Steinau Professor HU, et al. Secondary angiosarcoma: a fatal complication of chronic lymphedema. J Surg Oncol 2020;121:85–90.
34. Shustef E, Kazlouskaya V, Prieto VG, et al. Cutaneous angiosarcoma: a current update. J Clin Pathol 2017;70:917–25.
35. Antonescu C. Malignant vascular tumors-an update. Mod Pathol 2014;27:S30–8.
36. Deyrup AT, McKenney JK, Tighiouart M, et al. Sporadic cutaneous angiosarcomas: a proposal for risk stratification based on 69 cases. Am J Surg Pathol 2008;32:72–7.
37. Chang C, Peter Wu S, Kenneth H, et al. Patterns of care and survival of cutaneous angiosarcoma of the head and neck. Otolaryngol Head Neck Surg 2020;162:881–7.
38. Conic RRZ, Giovanni D, Alice F, et al. Incidence and outcomes of cutaneous angiosarcoma: a SEER population-based study. J Am Acad Dermatol 2020. https://doi.org/10.1016/j.jaad.2019.07.024. 1–8.
39. Guadagnolo BA, Gunar KZ, Dejka A, et al. Outcomes after definitive treatment for cutaneous angiosarcoma of the face and scalp. Head Neck 2011;33:661–7.
40. Constantinidou A, Nicolas S, Silvia S, et al. Evaluation of the use and efficacy of (neo)adjuvant chemotherapy in angiosarcoma: a multicentre study. ESMO Open 2020;5:e000787.
41. Schlemmer M, Reichardt P, Verweij J, et al. Paclitaxel in patients with advanced angiosarcomas of soft tissue: a retrospective study of the EORTC soft tissue and bone sarcoma group. Eur J Cancer 2008;44:2433–6.
42. Pawlik TM, Augusto FP, Cornelius JM, et al. Cutaneous angiosarcoma of the scalp: a multidisciplinary approach. Cancer 2003;98:1716–26.

43. Shin JY, Roh SG, Lee NH, et al. Predisposing factors for poor prognosis of angiosarcoma of the scalp and face: systematic review and meta-analysis. Head Neck 2017;39:380–6.

44. Ishida Y, Otsuka A, Kabashima K. Cutaneous angiosarcoma: update on biology and latest treatment. Curr Opin Oncol 2018;30:107–12.

45. Penel N, Binh NB, Jacques-Olivier B, et al. Phase II trial of weekly paclitaxel for unresectable angiosarcoma: the ANGIOTAX study. J Clin Oncol 2008;26: 5269–74.

46. Sikov WM, Donald AB, Charles MP, et al. Impact of the addition of carboplatin and/or bevacizumab to neoadjuvant once-per-week paclitaxel followed by dose-dense doxorubicin and cyclophosphamide on pathologic complete response rates in stage II to III triple-negative breast cancer: CALGB 40603 (Alliance). J Clin Oncol 2015;33:13–21.

47. Agulnik M, Yarber JL, Okuno SH, et al. An open-label, multicenter, phase II study of bevacizumab for the treatment of angiosarcoma and epithelioid hemangioendotheliomas. Ann Oncol 2013;24:257–63. Available at: https://pubmed.ncbi.nlm.nih.gov/22910841/.

48. Kollár A, Jones RL, Stacchiotti S, et al. Pazopanib in advanced vascular sarcomas: an EORTC soft tissue and bone sarcoma group (STBSG) retrospective analysis. Acta Oncol (Madr) 2017;56:88–92.

49. Patienten S, Therapie N. PAKT inhibitor may promote better responses to abiraterone in mCRPC. Onclive 2020;7:1–7.

50. Pasquier E, Nicolas A, Janine S, et al. Effective management of advanced angiosarcoma by the synergistic combination of propranolol and vinblastine-based metronomic chemotherapy: a bench to bedside study. EBioMedicine 2016;6: 87–95.

51. Chow W, et al. Growth attenuation of cutaneous angiosarcoma with propranolol-mediated β-blockade. JAMA Dermatol 2015;151:1226–9.

52. Florou V, Wilky BA. Current and future directions for angiosarcoma therapy. Curr Treat Options Oncol 2018;19:14.

53. Available at: clinicaltrials.gov; www.clinicaltrials.gov. Accessed May 15, 2020.

Reconstruction of Cutaneous Cancer Defects of the Head and Neck

Issam N. Eid, MD[a], Oneida A. Arosarena, MD[a,b],*

KEYWORDS

- Head and neck reconstruction • Mohs • Local flaps • Cutaneous malignancy
- Microvascular free tissue transfer

KEY POINTS

- The goal of cutaneous malignancy reconstruction is to restore the best functional and aesthetic outcome.
- Reconstruction should aim to restore all layers of the defect.
- The range of reconstructive options varies from healing by secondary intention to microvascular free tissue transfer for the different head and neck subsites.
- Local flaps are the mainstay of head and neck Mohs reconstruction.

INTRODUCTION

Mohs defect reconstruction in the head and neck requires functional and aesthetic restoration.[1] Well-established principles include replacing losses in kind.[2] Factors to consider when planning Mohs reconstruction include aesthetic subunits, relaxed skin tension lines (RSTLs), available tissue recruitment areas, structures that should not be distorted, and the patient's ability to participate in postoperative care.[3–6] It is best to place scars along aesthetic subunit borders or in RSTLs in order to camouflage them. Structures that should not be distorted include the anterior hairline, brows, eyelids, and auricular lobules.[3]

Reconstructive surgeons have often approached head and neck defects with the reconstructive ladder concept. This advocates a graduated approach from the simplest reconstruction method to more advanced methods.[7] However, the decision

[a] Department of Otolaryngology–Head and Neck Surgery, Lewis Katz School of Medicine at Temple University, 3440 North Broad Street, Suite 300, Philadelphia, PA 19140, USA; [b] Office of Health Equity, Diversity and Inclusion, Lewis Katz School of Medicine at Temple University, 3500 North Broad Street, Room 324E, Philadelphia, PA 19140, USA
* Corresponding author. Office of Health Equity, Diversity and Inclusion, Lewis Katz School of Medicine at Temple University, 3500 North Broad Street, Room 324E, Philadelphia, PA 19140, USA.
E-mail address: Oneida.Arosarena@tuhs.temple.edu

Otolaryngol Clin N Am 54 (2021) 379–395
https://doi.org/10.1016/j.otc.2020.11.011
0030-6665/21/© 2020 Elsevier Inc. All rights reserved.

oto.theclinics.com

on which reconstructive method to use should depend on defect characteristics and the patient's and surgeon's preferences in order to achieve the best outcome.

HEALING BY SECONDARY INTENTION

Healing by secondary intention is a useful reconstructive method in patients with multiple comorbidities that make a general anesthetic less desirable.[2] This approach's advantages include ease of cancer surveillance, procedural cost avoidance, and lower risk of complications.[2,8] The disadvantages include length of time and extent of wound care needed. The wound should be kept moist with an occlusive dressing. Healing by secondary intention is useful in scalp and forehead defects, even in cases of defects down to or with missing periosteum. It can be particularly advantageous in areas with absence of surrounding skin laxity from prior resections.[9] It can also be used for small defects of the cheek, medial canthal area, temple, and concave surfaces of the ear and nose.[2,4,8,9]

SKIN AND COMPOSITE GRAFT PHYSIOLOGY

Optimizing the wound bed by removing nonvital tissue promotes graft survival. Full-thickness skin grafts (FTSGs) offer better color match, and decreased contraction and depression compared with split-thickness skin grafts (STSGs). STSGs are commonly indicated for large scalp defects, for coverage of a wound bed being monitored for cancer recurrence, or for muscle free flap coverage. Delay of grafting by 12 to 14 days with wound care allows granulation tissue in-growth, which in turn decreases graft loss, depression, and contracture.[5,10] Composite graft cooling for 7 to 14 days reduces metabolic requirements and has been shown to improve survival.[5]

SKIN FLAP PHYSIOLOGY

Local flaps have several advantages over healing by secondary intention and skin grafting, including better color and texture match and decreased wound contraction.[11–13] The arterial blood supply to the skin can be categorized as musculocutaneous, direct cutaneous, and septocutaneous. Direct cutaneous arteries include the superficial temporal, posterior auricular, occipital, supratrochlear, and supraorbital arteries. Within the skin, at least 5 different vascular plexuses have been described: dermal, subdermal, subcutaneous, prefascial, and subfascial networks. These plexuses are interconnected via anastomosing (choke) vessels, creating collateral blood flow that allows cutaneous flap survival. Vascular delay enhances flap survival through loss of sympathetic tone, and axial reorientation and dilatation of choke vessels.[14]

Flaps may be categorized according to movement and/or blood supply. The basic flap movement types are advancement, rotation, and transposition. Advancement flaps are designed by moving tissue adjacent to the defect in 1 linear direction, while rotation flaps are curvilinear and rotate about a pivot point into the defect.[4,8,11,15] The simplest advancement flap is incisional closure with undermining. Advancement flaps can be subcategorized as unipedicle (eg, U-plasty), bipedicle (O→T, A→T), V→Y, Y→V, and H-plasty.[11] The ideal defect for a rotation flap is triangular in shape, with the triangle's height to width ratio being 2 to 1. The curve's radius should be 1 to 2 times the triangle's height. Transposition flaps are lifted over an incomplete skin bridge into the defect. Transposition flap examples include the rhombic, bilobe, and note flaps.[15]

Random pattern flaps rely on blood supply from surrounding reticular dermal vessels or perforating vessels from the subdermal plexus.[4,8] If the perfusion pressure at any portion of the flap falls below the arteriole closing pressure, the distal soft tissues will necrose.[14] Axial pattern flaps obtain their blood supply from a named artery.[4,8] Reconstruction within the major facial aesthetic subunits will be described in the rest of the article.

FOREHEAD AND SCALP

Considerations in scalp and forehead reconstruction include maintaining the hairline and avoiding hair-bearing skin loss (**Fig. 1**). Scalp skin is immobile, making reconstruction challenging.[16]

Primary closure is generally limited to defects that are less than 3 cm in diameter.[16] Healing by secondary intention is appropriate for large forehead defects that have first been reduced in size by advancement flaps. This may result in a better cosmetic result that skin grafting, and the resulting scar may be serially excised.[3]

Skin thickness of the scalp and forehead makes skin grafting a less desirable reconstructive option. Defects extending to the bone are better served by local advancement flaps. However, drilling the calvarium's outer cortex will increase STSG survivability.[16] Use of wound matrix material (Integra, Integra Life Sciences Corporation, Princeton, New Jersey) can aid grafting and has been used in full-thickness defects in patients who are not microvascular reconstruction candidates.[17]

Advancement flaps can be incised in forehead rhytids.[1,3,11] These are deal for eyebrow reconstruction.[11] Bilateral advancement flaps can be designed in H-plasty, A→T, and O→T/O→Z closures (**Figs. 2 and 3**).[3,8,11,15] Rotation flaps can be designed along the hairline.[1]

Healing by secondary intention or poor flap planning can lead to hairline and eyebrow position distortion in the forehead. Distortion can be minimized by securing the galea at the hairline or eyebrow to periosteum. Injury to the facial nerve's temporal branch can be avoided by dissection in a subcutaneous plane or at the deep temporal fascia level.[1]

OCULAR ADNEXA

Periocular reconstruction goals are to restore eyelid form and function, including globe protection.[1,18] Several techniques are available for eyelid reconstruction that depend

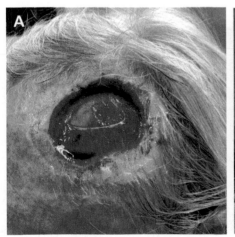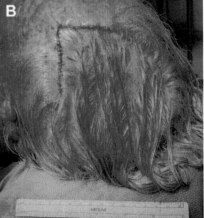

Fig. 1. (*A*) Scalp defect involving hairline. (*B*) Defect repaired with advancement/rotation flap.

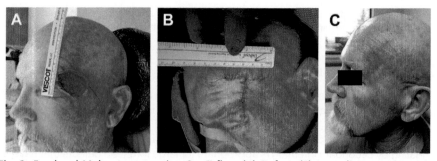

Fig. 2. Forehead Mohs reconstruction O→T flap. (A) Defect. (B) Immediate postoperative closure. (C) Several months postoperative result.

on defect size. Healing by secondary intention is appropriate for small (<1 cm), shallow, upper eyelid defects involving the concave medial canthal area.[8,12,18] Primary closure of small, nonmargin-involving, anterior lamella defects using an elliptical excision, M-plasty, O→-Z-plasty, or double-S ellipse also provides acceptable results.[8,12,13] Ellipses in the periorbital area should be oriented perpendicular to the RSTLs to avoid vertical tension on the eyelids.[13] For larger defects, local advancement and transposition (note, rhombic, V→Y, and bilobed flaps) can be designed from adjacent tissue.[12,13,18] FTSGs from the upper eyelid, pre- and postauricular area, supraclavicular area, and inner arm provide hairless skin with acceptable color matching for anterior lamellar defects.[8,12,13,18] Grafts should be oversized by up to 30% to prevent eyelid malposition.[8,18]

For larger defects involving the lower eyelid anterior lamella, a pedicled transposition flap from the upper eyelid can provide defect closure up to two-thirds the lower eyelid width.[8,12,13,19] Lower eyelid retraction can be prevented with lateral canthal tightening procedures and a suborbicularis fat lift.[13] Posterior lamellar defects can be repaired with nasal septal composite grafts, buccal mucosal grafts with cartilage support (eg, auricular cartilage), hard palate mucoperiosteum, or upper lid tarsoconjunctival grafts/flaps.[12,13,18]

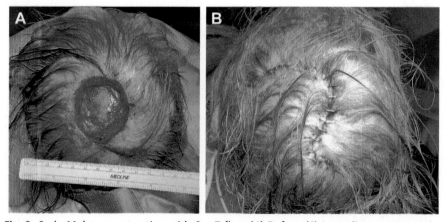

Fig. 3. Scalp Mohs reconstruction with O→Z flap. (A) Defect. (B) Immediate postoperative closure.

For full-thickness defects, end-to-end eyelid closure with wedge excision (with or without lateral canthotomy) is appropriate for defects less than 15 mm in length or less than 40% of the lid margin.[8,12,13,18,20] For defects up to two-thirds of the eyelid length, orbicularis flaps such as the Tenzel semicircular advancement flap, bolstered by cartilage grafts, may be used.[12,13,18] For larger, full-thickness defects, a cross-lid tarsoconjunctival flap may be used (Hughes procedure). When designing this flap, at least 4 mm of upper lid tarsus must be preserved to prevent eyelid malposition. The anterior lamella can be covered with a local flap, or a postauricular FTSG. The second-stage separation is performed after 4 to 6 weeks.[8,12,13,20] The Cutler-Beard flap is a cross-lid flap used to reconstruct the upper eyelid. This skin-muscle-conjunctival flap requires a cartilage graft between the lamellae to restore the upper eyelid tarsus.[12,18]

An alternative to the Hughes procedure is the cheek rotation (Mustardé) flap[8] with a nasal septal composite graft for posterior lamella reconstruction.[18] Drawbacks to this method's use include lower lid atonia and possible ectropion.[20] Frost sutures can prevent lower lid retraction.[8]

Defects involving the medial canthus are approached by securing the upper and lower lid remnants to the medial canthal tendon's posterior reflection or the lacrimal crest with permanent suture. The skin defect can then be replaced with an FTSG, or, if the defect extends to bone, with a paramedian forehead transposition flap (PFF).[8,12,18,20,21] Intubation of the remaining lacrimal canalicular system or conjunctivodacrocystorhinostomy can be performed at the time of reconstruction for defects involving the lacrimal system.[13,18] Lateral canthal reconstruction is directed toward the lateral orbital rim periosteum at Whitnall tubercle. If the periosteum is absent in this area, fixation may be performed with a drill hole placed at the Whitnall tubercle.[18]

Complications include epiphora, hypertrophic scarring, ectropion, edema, infection, exposure keratopathy, lagophthalmos, ptosis, corneal abrasion, trichiasis, and change in visual acuity.[1,13] Factors associated with complications are FTSG use and a defect more than one-half of the horizontal eyelid length repair. Webbing can complicate reconstruction in the medial canthal area and can be treated with Z-plasty.[1] When the medial canthus has been excised for margin control, superior or inferior canthal displacement and angle deformity can result.[20]

NOSE

Nasal reconstruction goals are to restore contour and maintain the airway.[1] Cartilaginous alar batten or sidewall support grafts are used to prevent airway compromise, minimize scar contracture and restore contour.[22-24]

Healing by secondary intention is limited to defects less than 5 mm on concave surfaces. Primary closure of defects less than 1 cm may be used for nasal dorsum and sidewall defects.[22,25,26] FTSG use is most successful in patients with Fitzpatrick 1 or 2 skin types and nasal skin that is not very sebaceous.[3,22] Skin grafting should be avoided when the perichondrium and periosteum are not intact. Conchal bowl composite grafts may be used for defects less than 1 cm (**Fig. 4**).[22]

Cheek advancement flaps can be used to reconstruct nasal sidewall defects.[4] The Lemmo flap is a laterally based bipedicle advancement flap that advances skin from the upper nasal dorsum to reconstruct lower nasal dorsal defects. The glabellar defect is closed in a V → Y fashion, avoiding long dorsal scars for a more favorable glabellar scar.[25]

Transposition flaps commonly used for nasal skin reconstruction include the nasolabial, bilobed, rhombic and note flaps. These flaps are based on facial and angular

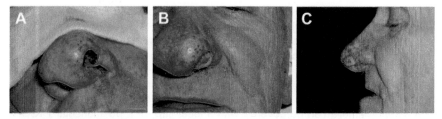

Fig. 4. (A) Defect of soft triangle. (B, C) early postoperative result of reconstruction with conchal composite graft.

artery branches that perforate the levator labii muscle,[3,4,23,27] or for medially-based bilobed flaps, on ophthalmic artery branches.[28] The bilobed flap is used for dorsum, sidewall, and nasal tip defects that are less than or equal to 1.5 to 2.0 cm.[3,15,22,25,26] It is designed so that the linear scar is situated at the dorsum-sidewall subunit boundary (**Fig. 5**).[3] The bilobed flap allows for greater tension dispersion than note or rhombic flaps.[15,22] The note flap is used for small-to-moderate sidewall defects. This triangular flap is drawn tangent to the defect above the alar groove and is 1.5 times the defect's diameter.[3,4,25–27]

Melolabial flaps may be used for defects involving the nasal sidewall, and partial- and full-thickness alar, columellar, and tip defects.[3,4,22,23,26,27] These include transposition and interpolated flaps.[4,23,26,29] Cheek interpolation flaps are advantageous for preserving the nasofacial junction, as they are transposed over the alar-facial sulcus.[22–24,26] The flap should be 1 mm larger than the defect in all dimensions to allow for contraction.[24] The pedicle is divided in a second stage 3 to 4 weeks after flap inset.[23,24] Melolabial flaps may be used to reconstruct full-thickness alar defects by folding the flaps on themselves to provide internal lining and external reconstruction.[23]

Glabellar rotation-advancement (Rieger) flaps may be used to reconstruct nasal defects up to 2.5 cm, with at least 5 mm of native tissue between the defect and free alar margin to prevent retraction.[22,25,26] The PFF is a workhorse flap for defect reconstruction ranging from a single subunit to total nasal reconstruction, and can provide both internal and external lining for through-and-through defects. Based on the supratrochlear artery, the PFF gives some of the most natural-appearing results. The flap can be performed in a 2- or 3-stage fashion with 3 to 5 weeks between each stage (**Fig. 6**).[21,26,30,31]

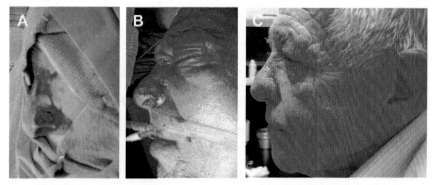

Fig. 5. (A) Defect involving nasal alar subunit. Bilobe flap design depicted. (B) Intraoperative repair. (C) Postoperative result.

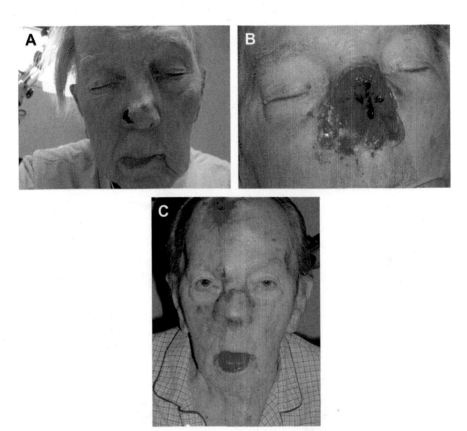

Fig. 6. (*A*) Advanced basal cell carcinoma in dementia patient. (*B*) Through-and-through defect following tumor excision. (*C*) Postoperative result following structural reconstruction with bilateral conchal cartilage grafts, and PFF used for cutaneous reconstruction and internal nasal lining.

Options for restoring the internal nasal lining include bipedicled vestibular skin advancement, septal mucosal or composite flaps (**Fig. 7**), conchal composite grafts, turbinate flaps, and microvascular free tissue transfer.[22,26] Costal cartilage or iliac crest bone can be used to restore the upper third of the nasal vault.[22] A forearm free flap with bone grafting is another option for reconstruction of the upper third in the setting of a large soft tissue defect.

Complications include nasal obstruction (from valve stenosis or synechiae), alar retraction, nasal deformity (eg, saddle deformity, asymmetry, pin-cushioning, or tip ptosis), and septal perforation.[1,29] Alar retraction, valve stenosis, tip ptosis, and saddle deformity can be prevented by use of cartilage grafting. Pin cushioning can be treated with steroid injections and dermabrasion postoperatively.[1] Cheek interpolation flap use can result in terminal hair transfer to the nose in men.[24] Superiorly based melolabial flaps are prone to nasofacial junction obliteration.[23]

CHEEK

Healing by secondary intention is reserved for small nasofacial, melolabial, preauricular, and alar-facial sulcus defects.[6] Cheek defects less than 1 to 2 cm can usually

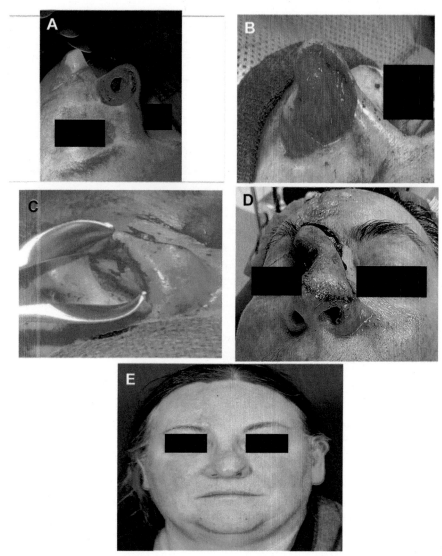

Fig. 7. Nose through-and-through defect reconstructed with composite graft and PFF. (*A*) Defect. (*B*) Composite graft inset. (*C*) Lining reconstructed with composite graft. (*D*) PFF inset. (*E*) Postoperative result.

be closed primarily, particularly if they abut subunit boundaries or are able to be closed parallel to RSTLs.[6,11] Cervicofacial advancement and rotation flaps are commonly used for upper medial cheek defects[1,3,6,8,32] (**Fig. 8**), although these defects can also be reconstructed with a PFF.[21] Defects that abut the nose and lip may be reconstructed with perialar crescentic advancement flaps.[32]

V→Y advancement flaps may be used for reconstruction of medial cheek defects that abut the melolabial crease,[3,32] or for lateral cheek defects.[6] Note transposition flaps may be used for medial cheek defects up to 3 cm in size.[6] Lateral and central cheek defects can be reconstructed with rhombic transposition flaps.[3,6] Similarly, defects of the

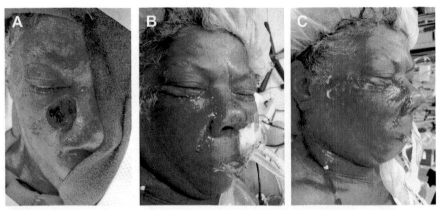

Fig. 8. (*A*) Medial cheek defect following excision of basal cell carcinoma. (*B, C*) Cervicofacial rotation flap repair.

perilabial cheek that abut the chin may be reconstructed with bilobed flaps.[6,32] O→T and A→T closures may be used for defects abutting the preauricular sulcus.

Microvascular free tissue transfer is indicated for combined cheek and eyelid defects with exposed bone, or when soft tissue bulk is required (**Figs. 9** and **10**). FTSGs may be used to reconstruct cheek defects in patients whose medical condition may not allow for local flap reconstruction. Limitations of free flaps and FTSG include inability to provide color-matched skin.[32]

PERIORAL RECONSTRUCTION

Perioral reconstruction goals are to maintain oral competence, motion, sensation, and cosmesis. Aesthetic subunits (ie, the vermillion border, philtral ridges, cupid's bow and

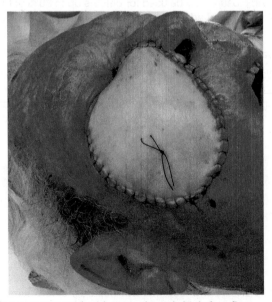

Fig. 9. Cheek defect reconstructed with anterolateral thigh free flap.

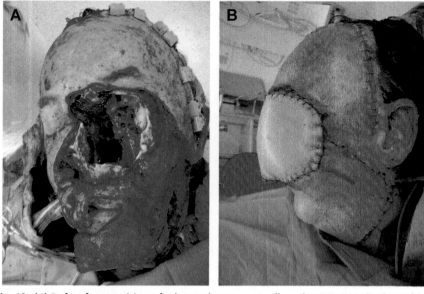

Fig. 10. (*A*) Defect from excision of advanced squamous cell carcinoma necessitating orbital exenteration, en-bloc ethmoidectomy and resection of cheek soft tissue; (*B*) reconstruction with rectus abdominus free flap.

labiomental crease) should be reconstructed while maintaining lip height and projection.

Primary Closure of Small Cutaneous Defects

Primary, V-shaped closure may be used for defects up to 30% of the lip.[2] This is done with wide undermining and advancement for tension-free closure (**Fig. 11**).

Bilateral Mucosal Advancement Flaps for Isolated Red Lip Defects

Advancement flaps such as the Burow wedge flap can be used for partial-thickness, lateral upper lip defects.[33] Rhombic flaps may be used for central and lateral upper lip defects, allowing incisions to fall at the philtral ridges, vermilion-cutaneous border, and nasolabial fold.[34] Central upper lip defects may also be reconstructed with a PFF.[21]

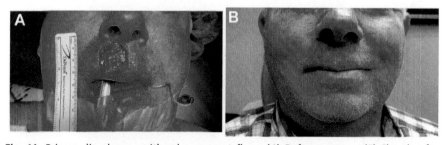

Fig. 11. Primary lip closure with advancement flaps. (*A*) Before surgery. (*B*) Shortly after surgery.

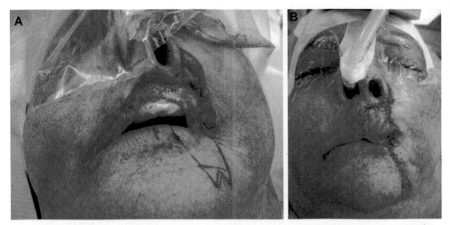

Fig. 12. (*A*) Defect resulting from excision of basal cell carcinoma of upper lip. Abbe flap marked with perialar crescentic excision for cheek advancement. (*B*) Abbe flap transposed with cheek advancement.

Lip Switch Flaps (Abbe or Estlander)

Lip switch flaps are based on the labial artery. These flaps involve a lip switch from the opposite lip with the same lip height taken but half the width to distribute the tissue deficit between the donor site and the recipient. The Abbe flap is used for central defects and requires the pedicle to remain attached for a delayed section and inset, usually after 3 weeks (**Figs. 12 and 13**). The Estlander flap involves the oral commissure and can be done in a single stage.[2]

Bilateral Advancement Flaps

The most common among these flaps are the Karapanzic, the Gillies fan flap, and Bernard-von Burrow closure. These flaps borrow tissue from the cheek and upper lip to restore the lower lip, and cause some degree of microstomia. The Karapanzic flap's advantage is neurovascular structure preservation that aids in maintaining oral competence.[2]

Microvascular Free Tissue Transfer

Complete lower lip defects require microvascular tissue transfer for optimal results. The radial forearm free flap with palmaris tendon suspension yields the best results in this case (**Fig. 14**).

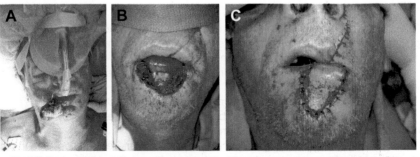

Fig. 13. (*A*) Lower lip squamous cell carcinoma with cutaneous horn. (*B*) Defect after excision and margin control. (*C*) Abbe flap transposed.

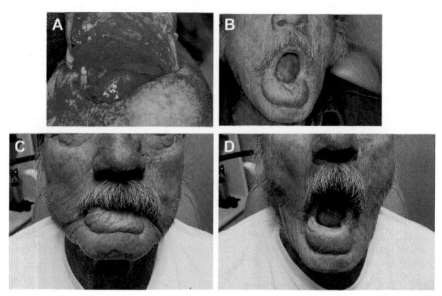

Fig. 14. Complete lower lip reconstruction. (*A*) Radial forearm flap inset with palmaris tendon sling. (*B*) 6-month follow-up (*C, D*) 2-year follow-up after debulking.

Complications

Upper lip reconstruction can lead to meliolabial fold distortion with the potential of bringing nonhair-bearing skin into the moustache area.[1,33] Other complications include microstomia; distortion of cupid's bow, the philtral ridges, and vermillion border; oral incompetence from lack of sensation; and oral commissure blunting.[1,33]

CHIN

Chin skin is the thickest skin in the face, leading to poorer scars, and is not very suitable for skin grafting.[35,36] Chin reconstruction is best accomplished by local advancement flaps. Primary vertical or horizonal closure is possible only for small defects.[36] H-plasty is a frequently used repair that employs bilateral advancement flaps with incisions hidden in the mentolabial crease. Other available options are the O → T closure and V → Y flap.[35]

EAR

Primary closure is advocated for small defects at the helix and antihelix skin.[37] A triangular wedge is taken with the triangle's apex extending to the concha around the helical root. This will inevitably lead to shortening of the ear.[36]

A wound that has intact perichondrium in a concave area is ideal for secondary intention healing.

FTSG use requires intact periosteum or a temporoparietal flap[24]

Helical rim advancement flaps can be used after wedge excision for defects up to one-fourth of the auricular circumference.[11,24]

Interpolated flaps from the retroauricular or preauricular areas can be used to reconstruct the helical rim, scaphoid fossa, and conchal bowl (**Fig. 15**).[24] The postauricular advancement flap is particularly useful for larger defects. It can be performed in 2

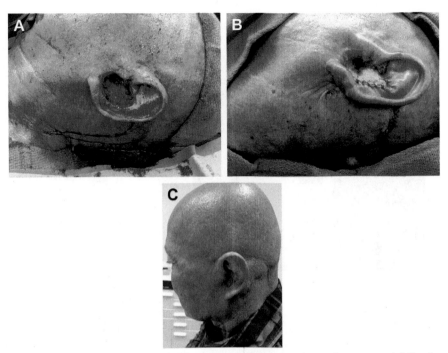

Fig. 15. (*A*) Through-and-through defect of conchal bowl and anterior ear canal following excision of basal cell carcinoma. V→Y advancement flap marked. (*B*) Folded advancement flap inset. (*C*) 4-month postoperative result.

stages with a possible cartilage harvest from the contralateral ear to give support and structure.[36]

Costochondral cartilage is the ideal framework for larger auricular defects and requires good soft tissue coverage with a local or regional skin flap.[37] Total auriculectomy defects can be addressed in several ways. Many patient factors come into play including patient aesthetic goals, while factoring in age and comorbidities. In older patients, an ear prosthetic is a viable option. Massive defects around the ear require flaps ranging from a supraclavicular flap to free tissue transfer such as a radial forearm or anterolateral thigh free flap for coverage. Reconstruction with alloplastic frameworks is prone to implant exposure.

Healing by secondary intention has a greater infection risk compared with other reconstructive methods. Healing by secondary intention and FTSG use are associated with wound depression. Wedge excision of defects greater than one-fourth of the auricular circumference can lead to distortion and auricular cupping. Postauricular tissue advancement can result in placing hair-bearing skin on the ear and postauricular sulcus blunting, which can make wearing glasses difficult. Reconstruction adjacent to or in the external auditory canal can result in stenosis.

SKIN EXPANSION

When defects are greater than half the cheek aesthetic unit, greater than one-third of the forehead, or over 6 cm in the scalp, expansion techniques are indicated (**Fig. 16**). Forehead skin expansion may be indicated for complete nasal reconstruction.

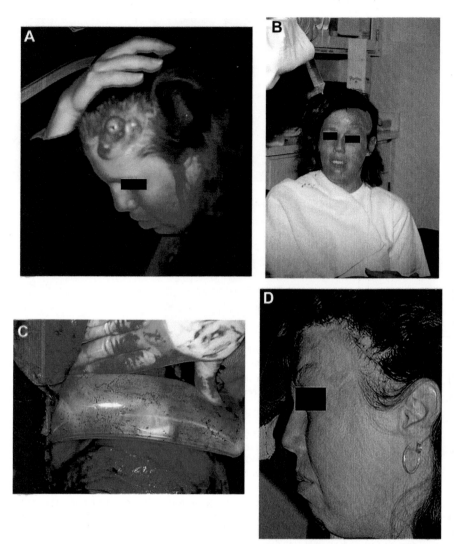

Fig. 16. (*A*) Patient with dermatofibrosarcoma protuberans of left scalp and forehead. (*B*) Defect initially covered with STSG at the time of expander placement. (*C*) Intraoperative implant removal after expansion complete. (*D*) Immediate postoperative result following advancement of expanded scalp skin.

Temporary cosmetic deformity and discomfort from expansion in the supraorbital region are this technique's disadvantages.[38] Tissue expander use includes risks of infection, implant extrusion, mechanical failure, tissue necrosis, bony changes, hematoma, and seroma formation.[1,38]

COMPLICATIONS

The incidence of complications following Mohs defect reconstruction varies from less than 0.5% in the glabella, jawline, and nasolabial folds, to greater than 45% in the nose. The complication rate also varies with the reconstructive method, ranging from less than 0.5% with primary closure and 27% with advancement flaps. Transposition and interpolated flaps, particularly if superiorly based, are prone to pincushioning.[1,21,23]

Complications increase in frequency with defect size. Excessive wound tension, vascular compromise, and infection can lead to complete or partial flap necrosis.[1,14] Smoking, uncontrolled hypertension, collagen disorders, diabetes mellitus, and previous radiation therapy can compromise flap and graft vascularity.[1,4,15,21,23,26] Other complications include persistent scar erythema, hypopigmented scar, sensory neuropathies, telangectasias,[1] incisional pain,[4] hematoma, bleeding,[4,21] and obscuring tumor recurrence.[4]

CLINICS CARE POINTS

- Healing by secondary intention is a useful reconstructive method in patients with comorbidities that preclude general anesthesia, or when surveillance for aggressive malignancies is necessary.
- When considering skin grafting, delay of skin grafting for 12-14 days to promote granulation tissue in-growth decreases the risk of graft loss, depression and contracture.
- Reconstruction with local flaps provide the best color and texture match, and decrease the risk of wound contracture.
- Smoking, uncontrolled hypertension, auto-immune disease, diabetes mellitus and previous radiation therapy can compromise flap and graft viability.

DISCLOSURE

The authors have no commercial or financial conflicts of interest, or any funding sources to disclose.

REFERENCES

1. Berens AM, Akkina SR, Patel SA. Complications in facial Mohs defect reconstruction. Curr Opin Otolaryngol Head Neck Surg 2017;25(4):258–64.
2. Becker GD, Adams LA, Levin BC. Secondary intention healing of exposed scalp and forehead bone after Mohs surgery. Otolaryngol Head Neck Surg 1999; 121(6):751–4.
3. Joseph AW, Joseph SS. Mohs reconstruction and scar revision. Otolaryngol Clin North Am 2019;52(3):461–71.
4. Chen EH, Johnson TM, Ratner D. Introduction to flap movement: reconstruction of five similar nasal defects using different flaps. Dermatol Surg 2005;31(8 Pt 2): 982–5.
5. Brenner MJ, Moyer JS. Skin and composite grafting techniques in facial reconstruction for skin cancer. Facial Plast Surg Clin North Am 2017;25(3):347–63.
6. Hanks JE, Moyer JS, Brenner MJ. Reconstruction of cheek defects secondary to mohs microsurgery or wide local excision. Facial Plast Surg Clin North Am 2017; 25(3):443–61.
7. Ge NN, McGuire JF, Dyson S, et al. Nonmelanoma skin cancer of the head and neck II: surgical treatment and reconstruction. Am J Otolaryngol 2009;30(3): 181–92.
8. Harvey DT, Taylor RS, Itani KM, et al. Mohs micrographic surgery of the eyelid: an overview of anatomy, pathophysiology, and reconstruction options. Dermatol Surg 2013;39(5):673–97.

9. Deutsch BD, Becker FF. Secondary healing of Mohs defects of the forehead, temple, and lower eyelid. Arch Otolaryngol Head Neck Surg 1997;123(5):529–34.

10. Robinson JK, Dillig G. The advantages of delayed nasal full-thickness skin grafting after Mohs micrographic surgery. Dermatol Surg 2002;28(9):845–51.

11. Shew M, Kriet JD, Humphrey CD. Flap basics II: advancement flaps. Facial Plast Surg Clin North Am 2017;25(3):323–35.

12. Huggins AB, Latting MW, Marx DP, et al. Ocular adnexal reconstruction for cutaneous periocular malignancies. Semin Plast Surg 2017;31(1):22–30.

13. Segal KL, Nelson CC. Periocular reconstruction. Facial Plast Surg Clin North Am 2019;27(1):105–18.

14. Lucas JB. The physiology and biomechanics of skin flaps. Facial Plast Surg Clin North Am 2017;25(3):303–11.

15. Starkman SJ, Williams CT, Sherris DA. Flap Basics I: rotation and transposition flaps. Facial Plast Surg Clin North Am 2017;25(3):313–21.

16. Olson MD, Hamilton GS 3rd. Scalp and forehead defects in the post-Mohs surgery patient. Facial Plast Surg Clin North Am 2017;25(3):365–75.

17. Richardson ML, Lange JP, Jordan JR. Reconstruction of full-thickness scalp defects using a dermal regeneration template. JAMA Facial Plast Surg 2016; 18(1):62–7.

18. Lu GN, Pelton RW, Humphrey CD, et al. Defect of the Eyelids. Facial Plast Surg Clin North Am 2017;25(3):377–92.

19. Perry MJ, Langtry J, Martin IC. Lower eyelid reconstruction using pedicled skin flap and palatal mucoperiosteum. Dermatol Surg 1997;23(5):395–7 [discussion: 397–8].

20. Moy RL, Ashjian AA. Periorbital reconstruction. J Dermatol Surg Oncol 1991; 17(2):153–9.

21. Reckley LK, Peck JJ, Roofe SB. Flap basics III: interpolated flaps. Facial Plast Surg Clin North Am 2017;25(3):337–46.

22. Dibelius GS, Toriumi DM. Reconstruction of cutaneous nasal defects. Facial Plast Surg Clin North Am 2017;25(3):409–26.

23. Carucci JA. Melolabial flap repair in nasal reconstruction. Dermatol Clin 2005; 23(1):65–71, vi.

24. Nguyen TH. Staged cheek-to-nose and auricular interpolation flaps. Dermatol Surg 2005;31(8 Pt 2):1034–45.

25. Lu GN, Kriet JD, Humphrey CD. Local cutaneous flaps in nasal reconstruction. Facial Plast Surg 2017;33(1):27–33.

26. Joseph AW, Truesdale C, Baker SR. Reconstruction of the nose. Facial Plast Surg Clin North Am 2019;27(1):43–54.

27. Alam M, Goldberg LH. Oblique advancement flap for defects of the lateral nasal supratip. Arch Dermatol 2003;139(8):1039–42.

28. Skaria AM. The medial based bi- or trilobed flap for repair of distal alar defects. Dermatology 2013;227(2):165–70.

29. Arden RL, Miguel GS. The subcutaneous melolabial island flap for nasal alar reconstruction: a clinical review with nuances in technique. Laryngoscope 2012;122(8):1685–9.

30. Menick FJ. Nasal reconstruction. Plast Reconstr Surg 2010;125(4):138e–50e.

31. Correa BJ, Weathers WM, Wolfswinkel EM, et al. The forehead flap: the gold standard of nasal soft tissue reconstruction. Semin Plast Surg 2013;27(02):096–103.

32. Rapstine ED, Knaus WJ 2nd, Thornton JF. Simplifying cheek reconstruction: a review of over 400 cases. Plast Reconstr Surg 2012;129(6):1291–9.

33. Oberemok S, Eliezri Y, Desciak E. Burow's wedge flap revisited. Dermatol Surg 2005;31(2):210–6 [discussion: 216].
34. Skaria AM. The transposition advancement flap for repair of postsurgical defects on the upper lip. Dermatology 2011;223(3):203–6.
35. Larrabee YC, Moyer JS. Reconstruction of Mohs defects of the lips and chin. Facial Plast Surg Clin North Am 2017;25(3):427–42.
36. Badash I, Shauly O, Lui CG, et al. Nonmelanoma facial skin cancer: a review of diagnostic strategies, surgical treatment, and reconstructive techniques. Clin Med Insights Ear Nose Throat 2019;12. 1179550619865278.
37. Smith RM, Byrne PJ. Reconstruction of the Ear. Facial Plast Surg Clin North Am 2019;27(1):95–104.
38. Hodgkinson DJ, Lam Q. Expansion techniques after Mohs' surgery on the face. Australas J Dermatol 2001;42(1):9–14.

Cutaneous Head and Neck Cancers in the High-Risk Immunosuppressed Population

Karen Y. Choi, MD[a,1], Cecelia E. Schmalbach, MD, MSc[b,*]

KEYWORDS

- Immunosuppression • Solid organ transplant • Cutaneous carcinoma
- Head and neck • Nonmelanoma skin cancer • Melanoma of the head and neck

KEY POINTS

- The immunosuppressed patient population is a uniquely high-risk group for aggressive cutaneous malignancies with worse outcomes.
- Rates of keratinocyte carcinomas, malignant melanoma, Merkel cell carcinoma, and Kaposi sarcoma are higher in the immunosuppressed patient cohort.
- The American Joint Committee on Cancer eighth edition cancer staging now acknowledges the poorer prognosis of cutaneous squamous cell carcinoma in the immunosuppressed population, but further studies are warranted to reconcile the heterogeneous data in order to fully delineate the impact of immune status on prognosis.
- Clinical trials for immunotherapy do not include the immunosuppressed population, and special considerations as well as close communication with the multidisciplinary transplant team is paramount when considering systemic therapy in this patient population.

INTRODUCTION

The immunosuppressed (IS) population encompasses a diverse cohort of patients to include iatrogenically immunocompromised organ transplant recipients (OTRs) as well as patients with chronic lymphoid malignancies, human immunodeficiency virus (HIV)/ acquired immunodeficiency syndrome (AIDS), and autoimmune disorders. Cutaneous cancers in this high-risk patient group are clinically distinct from the general immunocompetent population, showing aggressive behavior with associated poor outcomes.[1,2] This article reviews the pathogenesis, epidemiology, incidence,

[a] Department of Otolaryngology Head and Neck Surgery, The Pennsylvania State University, College of Medicine, Hershey, PA, USA; [b] Department of Otolaryngology Head and Neck Surgery, Lewis Katz School of Medicine, Temple University, 3440 North Broad Street, Kresge West 309, Philadelphia, PA 19140, USA
[1] Present address: 500 University Drive, MCHO91, Hershey, PA 17033.
* Corresponding author.
E-mail address: cecelia.schmalbach@tuhs.temple.edu

Otolaryngol Clin N Am 54 (2021) 397–413
https://doi.org/10.1016/j.otc.2020.11.012
0030-6665/21/© 2020 Elsevier Inc. All rights reserved.

prognosis, and special considerations required in managing cutaneous cancers in the IS patient population.

PATHOGENESIS

The skin serves as a mechanical barrier of protection. In addition it is widely accepted as a peripheral immunologic organ, housing many of the critical lymphoid organ cells to include dendritic antigen presenting cells and Langerhans cells commonly associated with the spleen, lymph nodes, and Waldeyer ring.[1,3,4] The dendritic cells housed in the epidermis and dermis are capable of inducing primary immune responses by presenting antigens encountered on the skin to T cells.[1,5]

The exact pathogenesis of cutaneous malignancies in the IS population is multifactorial. It is generally accepted that the major cause is the combination of ultraviolet (UV) radiation exposure with reduced immune surveillance secondary to the chronic immunosuppressive medications.[6–8] In addition, IS patients are more susceptible to oncogenic viruses such as Epstein-Barr virus, human papillomavirus (HPV),[8,9] Kaposi sarcoma herpesvirus or human herpesvirus 8 (HHV8), human T-cell leukemia virus type 1 (HTLV-1), and Merkel cell polyomavirus.[10,11]

INCIDENCE AND PROGNOSIS
Cutaneous Squamous Cell Carcinoma

Cutaneous squamous cell carcinoma (cSCC) is one of the most common malignancies following transplant.[12–14] As immunosuppressive regimens improve, patients are surviving longer.[6] This prolonged chronic immunosuppression increases the risk of de novo secondary cancers, the most common being cutaneous malignancies.[6,8,15] OTRs on chronic immunosuppression carry a 65-fold to 100-fold increase in cSCC compared with the general population; patients with chronic lymphoid malignancies carry an 8-fold to 13-fold increase in incidence.[2,6,16–22] Increased rates of cSCC are also found in other immunosuppressed patients, such as those with lymphoma and HIV.[23,24]

Overall, cSCC portends an excellent prognosis, with 5-year survival rates exceeding 90% in the general population. However, IS patients experience a more aggressive histology[12,25–27] and associated worse outcomes,[2,19,28,29] with recurrence rates reaching 7.2 times that of the general population.[25] Although cSCC metastasizes to regional lymph nodes or distant sites in 2% to 5% of the general population,[30,31] immunosuppression is recognized as an independent risk factor for regional metastasis,[31] with rates reaching 22.5%.[6,32–34] Similarly, locoregional recurrence (LRR) and distant metastasis are rare in the general population (13%–48% and 7%–19%, respectively).[2,22,35,36] However, immunosuppression is an independent prognostic factor for LRR as well, with increased risk ranging from 2.66 to 3.79 times higher than the general population.[37,38] Recurrence-free survival is significantly lower in the IS population, with rates of 47.3% versus 86.1% for immunocompetent patients, as well as lower locoregional progression-free survival rates at 38.7% versus 71.6% at 2 years.[2]

Ultimately, cSCC represents a significant cause of mortality in the IS population, with a decreased overall survival (OS) rate of 66% at 5 years and 43% at 10 years compared with the general population.[12,14,18,39–42] One retrospective cohort study found immunosuppressed patients had a significantly lower disease-specific survival (DSS) at 3 (75.8%), 5 (68.2%), and 10 years (62.4%) compared with the immunocompetent cohort (87.1%, 84.1%, 83.2%, respectively).[43]

Basal Cell Carcinoma

Basal cell carcinoma (BCC) is the most common cutaneous cancer overall and, similar to cSCC, has an increased incidence among OTRs. Together, BCC and cSCC develop in 40% of OTRs within 20 years after transplant, with 75% of patients diagnosed within 1 year.[16,44,45] The incidence ratio of BCC to cSCC among the general population is roughly 4:1, but this ratio is reversed in the IS population,[8,46,47] with OTRs 20 times more likely to develop cSCC than BCC.[8,15,20,48] However, the incidence of BCC in the IS population remains increased with respect to the general population, with a 10-fold higher risk.[12–14,49,50] Note that BCCs in the OTR population often develop in sun-protected areas and other unusual locations not typical of the general population, such as the external auditory canal, genitalia, hand, wrist, and axilla.[44]

Cutaneous Melanoma

Similar to cutaneous squamous cell carcinoma (SCC), IS patients are at higher risk of developing malignant melanoma, with rates 2-fold to 4-fold higher in OTRs compared with the general population.[20,51–57] Similarly, patients with HIV/AIDS are noted to have 2.6-fold increased risk of developing melanoma,[50,58,59] and patients with chronic lymphocytic leukemia (CLL) have an increased risk between 2.8-fold and 6.2-fold.[50,60–64]

Given the strong immunogenicity of melanoma biology, it is not surprising that melanoma in the setting of immunosuppression has a more aggressive course and worse prognoses.[65–67] OTRs have been shown to have a 3-fold higher risk of melanoma-specific mortality.[51,65,68,69] OS for OTRs with melanoma is significantly lower than that of the general population, with 2-year, 5-year, and 10-year rates reported to be 77%, 54.2%, and 40.6% respectively, compared with the general population rates of 95.6%, 82.1%, and 75.2%.[67] As expected, melanomas thicker than 2 mm had significantly worse OS, with a hazard ratio of 11.49 compared with the general population.[67,70,71] However, thinner melanomas (<1 mm) were also still noted to have an increased risk of mortality, with an HR 4.74 compared with the general population.[51] Differences in survival were not noted based on donor organ.[65]

Merkel Cell Carcinoma

Merkel cell carcinoma (MCC) is a rare cutaneous neuroendocrine malignancy associated with the Merkel cell polyomavirus.[10] Overall, IS patients who develop MCC tend to be younger and have a more aggressive behavior pattern leading to lower MCC-specific survival and OS in this population.[10,66,72–74] OTRs are at greater risk (10-fold to 24-fold) of developing MCC compared with the general population.[10,75–77] The incidence of MCC in the OTR population is associated with increased age at time of transplant, with more than 70% of cases occurring in patients more than 50 years old at time of transplant, and with increased duration of immunosuppression.[75] Increased incidences have also been shown in other immunodeficient states, including UV-induced immunosuppression, hematologic malignancies, HIV/AIDS, and autoimmune diseases.[10,78–81]

MCCs in the IS population is associated with a 12-fold increased risk of MCC-specific death in the OTR population.[10,73] Higher levels of intratumoral infiltrating lymphocytes were found to be an independent predictor of improved outcomes, showing the importance of an intact immune response in MCC.[82,83]

Kaposi Sarcoma

Kaposi sarcoma (KS) is an endothelial tumor caused by human herpesvirus 8 (HHV-8) infection and closely associated with immunosuppression, especially in HIV/AIDS, where it is often the first presentation of this disease.[20,52,84,85] Before the AIDS epidemic of the 1980s, rates of KS were extremely low, with an incidence in the United States of 0.2 per 100,000 person years.[86] This incidence increased to 200,000 among patients with AIDS compared with the general population.[87] KS also occurs at higher rates among OTRs, where it is diagnosed 200 times more often than the general population.[88] It develops quickly after transplant, with a mean time to diagnosis of 13 months.[6] Nonwhite men receiving lung transplants are at greater risk, as are patients of Mediterranean, Jewish, Arabic, Caribbean, or African descent.[6,84]

RISK FACTORS UNIQUE TO THE IMMUNOSUPPRESSED POPULATION

A host of risk factors in the IS population place them at greater risk of developing cutaneous malignancies. Similar to the general population, exposure to UV radiation remains an important factor, as does a prior history of skin cancer.[6] In addition, patient demographics play a role in developing posttransplant cSCC. Multiple studies have shown that white transplant recipients with Fitzpatrick scale of 1 to 3 were at highest risk of skin cancer.[46,89–99] Men were 3 times more likely to develop posttransplant skin cancer compared with women.[99]

Numerous studies found that patients with a history of pretransplant cSCC carry a high risk of developing cSCC posttransplant, and multiple multivariate models showed this to be the single strongest predictor of skin cancer risk.[100] The presence of actinic keratoses and viral warts around the time of transplant was also associated with increased risk of skin cancer.[101] Several observational studies suggested that lung, heart, and combined pancreas-kidney transplant patients were at higher risk than kidney and liver transplant recipients.[56,102,103] Patients who underwent transplant at an older age were also found to be at increased risk of developing cSCC sooner after transplant, with a median time from transplant to first cSCC of 3 years for patients more than 60 years old compared with 13 years for patients 18 to 40 years of age.[97,104]

Several risk factors have been associated with development of melanoma after OTR, including male gender and increased age at time of transplant.[51,105] In a comparison of the different types of solid organ transplants, patients who underwent liver or lung transplants were noted to have lower risk of developing melanoma compared with patients who received kidney transplants.[51] Vajdic and colleagues[52] also found that the intensity and duration of immunosuppression were further important determinations in the development of melanoma in OTR. Cases of transmission of melanoma from organ donors to recipients have been reported. In a study analyzing 104 donor-transmitted malignancies, melanoma was found to be the second most frequently transmitted malignancy, following renal cancer.[106] The exact mechanism of how this occurs is unknown, but it is hypothesized to be intricately involved with the tumor biology of melanoma.[50,107]

The connection between immunosuppressive medications and MCC was first reported by Penn and First[72] in 1999 after noting the increased aggressiveness of MCC compared with the general population and the appearance in younger patients (mean age of 53 years).[72,78] Clarke and colleagues[75] reviewed the US Scientific Registry of Transplant Recipients and noted that the risk of developing MCC was highest in older patients, with more than 70% of cases occurring in patients more than 50 years old at the time of transplant, and was more common in men (70% higher incidence), with 5 times higher risk in white compared with nonwhite recipients.

The role of HPV infection in the development of cSCC has been hypothesized.[8,108] Several studies showed increased frequency of HPV DNA in cSCC tumors compared with nonmalignant, normal skin of IS patients (90% vs 11%–32%).[9] One study showed this link to be unique to cSCC and found no similar association between HPV and BCC.[108] It remains unclear whether the high-risk alpha-HPV types versus the low-risk beta-HPV types play a more prevalent role in the carcinogenesis of these skin tumors,[109–111] and further study is required.

STAGING
American Joint Committee on Cancer

At present the American Joint Committee on Cancer (AJCC) provides cancer staging for cutaneous melanoma,[112] MCC,[113] BCC, and cSCC.[114] cSCC warrants special comment given the recent implementation of the eighth edition of AJCC staging, which specifically mentions the IS patient population.

The overall excellent prognosis of cSCC coupled with the lack of a dedicated, national registry makes accurate staging more challenging compared with cutaneous melanoma. Given these challenges and the propensity for cSCC to develop in the sun-exposed region of the head and neck (HN), the latest staging iteration was developed by a panel of HN experts and applies to this specific anatomic region.[114]

The new system remains founded on the traditional tumor-nodal-metastasis categories. Specifically, the tumor stage is based on the cancer diameter as well as invasion into surrounding structures, to include perineural and bone. Similar to other HN cancers, the nodal stage is based on number of metastatic nodes, nodal size, and the presence of extranodal extension. The metastatic stage is defined by the presence (M1) or absence (M0) of distant disease.

The designers of the staging system acknowledge that immunocompromised OTRs are more prone to cSCC and have a worse prognosis with respect to recurrence and survival.[114] Although strong consideration was given to incorporating immune status into this latest staging system, the literature was deemed conflicting and limited to small cohort studies. The panel identified only 1 supporting multivariate study comprising 31 IS patients, to include HN, trunk, and extremity. Therefore, immune status was not formally incorporated into the system but centers collecting data for prospective study are encouraged to denote immune status.

In order to address the heterogeneous nature of prior studies and the small cohort sizes, Elghouche and colleagues[12] recently conducted a systematic review of the literature with meta-analysis to specifically investigate the impact of immunosuppression on HN cSCC. The investigators identified 317 IS HN patients in 17 studies. Immunosuppression was found to have a statistically significant worse prognosis with respect to LRR (HR 2.20), DFS (HR 2.69), DSS (HR 3.61), and OS (HR 2.09).

Sentinel Node Biopsy

Because immunosuppression has been found to be an independent risk factor for developing metastatic disease,[31] with regional metastasis rate ranging between 2.2% and 21%,[32,115–117] increased consideration may be warranted for use of sentinel lymph node biopsy (SLNB) for nodal staging in the high-risk IS patient population.

SLNB provides a minimally invasive means for pathologic staging.[118] HN SLNB has been shown to be safe and reliable, with a false rate of omission (failure in a previously mapped regional nodal basin deemed negative for metastatic disease) of 4.7%, which mirrors that of cutaneous melanoma, where the technique is accepted as standard of care.[119] Current cSCC NCCN guidelines recommend consideration of SLNB for high-risk, localized tumors, which includes the IS population.[120] At present, SLNB remains only as a staging modality for cSCC, and the impact on survival remains unknown.

CUTANEOUS CANCER TREATMENT OF IMMUNOSUPPRESSED PATIENTS

Treatment recommendations for cutaneous malignancies in the IS population are based on tumor stage and mirror those of the general population.[120–125] However, some unique considerations do warrant further discussion.

Reduction in Immunosuppression

Treatment of cutaneous malignancies in the iatrogenically IS patient population should include close partnership with the multidisciplinary transplant team to safely reduce immunosuppression when possible. When considering reduction or modulation of immunosuppressive therapy, discussion with the patient's transplant team is paramount to ensure a safe balance between potential organ rejection, risk of development of skin cancers, as well as the psychological impact to the patient. Although specific guidelines have not been established, 1 expert consensus survey made recommendations on the level of immunosuppression based on type of solid organ transplant and skin cancer history.[126] Reduction should be considered in patients who have developed numerous cutaneous malignancies or those who develop recurrent or metastatic disease.[6,93,126,127]

One study of 231 transplant patients identified increased acute rejection rates in the setting of lower-dose immunosuppressive therapy (cyclosporine and azathioprine); however, overall graft survival rates were similar and patients experienced fewer cSCCs and BCCs (14.7% vs 22.6%).[128] In addition, numerous studies have shown decreased incidence of cutaneous malignancies with the use of mycophenolate mofetil (MMF) compared with azathioprine,[129,130] and mammalian target of rapamycin (mTOR) inhibitor use such as sirolimus or everolimus rather than calcineurin inhibitors.[131–135]

Although reduction of immunosuppression has been shown to decrease incidences of melanoma,[51] reduction may not be feasible for lifesaving organ transplants. As such, there has been much discussion surrounding safe use of systemic agents in this population. There are no specific guidelines for treatment of MCC in the IS population, and surgical excision with adjuvant radiation as indicated remains the standard of care in this cohort.[136] Some reports support temporary or partial regression of MCC in patients who had reduction of their immunosuppressive regimens; however, because of the overall rarity of this disease, generalized recommendations based on these data are limited.[137,138] If feasible, reducing immunosuppression to the lowest level possible without risking graft rejection is recommended.[126]

Targeted Immunotherapy

Surgical management with adjuvant therapy based on final pathology remains the standard of care for cutaneous malignancies in the IS population.[120–123] However, special consideration is required in the use of systemic immunotherapy. Ideally the treatment plan is formalized in the setting of a multidisciplinary tumor board well versed in the treatment of advanced cutaneous cancers.

Cemiplimab is a monoclonal antibody against programmed death 1 (PD-1). It was approved by the US Food and Drug Administration (FDA) for use in advanced and metastatic cSCC following results from a phase I/II trial published in 2018 showing response rates of 47% to 50% and durable disease control rates of 61% to 65%.[139] More recently, pembrolizumab received similar FDA approval.[140] Note that these trials did not include the IS population.[15] The PD-1 signaling pathway is thought to play an important role in pathogenesis of organ rejection[141]; thus, the use of anti–PD-1 inhibitors must be considered with extreme caution in OTRs and they are traditionally considered contraindicated in this high-risk patient population. One retrospective review at a US cancer center reported their experience treating 39 OTRs with checkpoint blockade, showing a 41% rate of allograft rejection with median time to rejection of 21 days and a total graft loss in 81% despite aggressive treatment with high-dose corticosteroids and/or sirolimus, tacrolimus, MMF, or intravenous immunoglobulin.[142] Furthermore, they showed a mortality of 46% in patients, related to allograft rejection or rejection complications.[142] Similarly, 1 case series reported increased mortality associated with cetuximab (anti–epidermal growth factor antibody) use in 2 lung transplant recipients secondary to diffuse alveolar hemorrhage, suggesting caution with use in this population.[143]

Ipilimumab is a CTLA-4 (cytotoxic T-lymphocyte-associated protein 4) checkpoint inhibitor that may be better tolerated than PD-1 inhibition. However, graft rejection has been reported with both medications.[144–146] Although several case reports have been published showing tolerance of ipilimumab in transplant patients, including 2 kidney transplants and 1 liver transplant,[146,147] further investigation is required.

Multiple clinical trials are underway to specifically explore the efficacy and safety of checkpoint blockade in OTRs, including an Australian trial evaluating nivolumab in the renal transplant population for treatment of cSCC (ACTRN12617000741381) and a US trial evaluating the effect of tacrolimus and prednisolone immunosuppression with nivolumab and ipilimumab in renal transplant recipients (NCT03816332).[141] Results from these studies will be extremely important in showing the objective clinical response in this vulnerable patient population and true rates of organ rejection.

It is worth noting that patients with CLL and autoimmune disorders are also often excluded from most clinical trial investigations using checkpoint blockade.[141] At present, knowledge surrounding the feasibility of checkpoint blockade in these populations is limited to small cohort studies. One retrospective study involving 3 with CLL treated with PD-L1 reported a 62% rate of objective response at median follow-up time of 16.5 months, and a 12-month progression-free survival of 68.4%.[148] Another case-control study evaluating response rates of checkpoint blockade in the setting of melanoma and CLL showed promising results similar to the Keynote 629 trial,[149] and further studies are investigating outcomes of checkpoint blockade with CLL in combination with other agents.[141] In patients with autoimmune diseases, off-label treatment with checkpoint inhibitors has suggested these patients may be treated; however, only under close and strict supervision because rates of exacerbation requiring immunosuppression are documented to be 2 to 3 times higher than in the general population. A higher rate of significant autoimmune toxicities has also been observed.[150]

Kaposi Sarcoma

The primary treatment of KS is to reduce the level of immunosuppression[93,151] or to bolster the immune system by initiating medications such as antiretroviral therapy (ART) in the case of AIDS-induced KS.[85] KS regression has been documented after altering immunosuppressive medications from cyclosporine as well as tacrolimus to sirolimus in renal transplant patients.[152–158] The introduction of ART dramatically decreased the incidence of AIDS-related KS[157] and treatment of HIV with ART may cause regression of some tumors, with up to 80% of early-stage disease managed by initiation of ART.[158]

PREVENTION

Mitigating risks is extremely important for high-risk IS patients. They should be counseled on sun avoidance, use of sunscreen, and the importance of sun-protective clothing. Before proceeding with organ transplant, dermatology consultation is strongly recommended for screening and treatment of any cutaneous malignancies or precursor lesions.[159,160] Depending on cancer type and stage, patients with a history of skin cancer may be advised to undergo a period of observation before proceeding with transplant.[160] For low-risk keratinocyte carcinomas, melanoma in situ, or lentigo melanoma, it is acceptable to proceed with transplant with frequent whole-body skin examinations. However, for patients with high-risk cSCC, MCC, or malignant melanoma, the general recommendation is to wait 2 to 5 years before transplant.[160]

It is imperative that IS patients undergo routine whole-body skin examination to evaluate for development of new cutaneous malignancies. One Canadian study followed more than 10,000 OTRs for more than 5 years and found that routine skin examination was associated with a 34% decrease in the development of advanced nonmelanoma skin cancers.[161] As noted earlier, partnership with the multidisciplinary transplant team is also imperative in reducing immunosuppressive therapy as safely as possible to avoid both recurrence and new cutaneous cancers.

SUMMARY

Immunosuppressed patients carry an increased risk of cutaneous malignancies, especially for cSCC among organ transplant patients. Although skin cancers traditionally portend an excellent prognosis, they are known to be aggressive with worse outcomes in this high-risk group. Diligent surveillance that includes patient education and early intervention is imperative to reduce the risk associated with skin cancer development. Treatment planning for patients with advanced cutaneous malignancies in the setting of immunosuppression ideally transpires in the setting of a multidisciplinary oncology team well versed in cutaneous cancers. In addition, treatment in the iatrogenically IS patient population necessitates close partnership with the multidisciplinary care team to safely reduce immunosuppression whenever possible.

DISCLOSURE

The authors have no related financial disclosures or conflicts of interest.

REFERENCES

1. Gerlini G, Romagnoli P, Pimpinelli N. Skin cancer and immunosuppression. Crit Rev Oncol Hematol 2005;56(1):127–36.
2. Manyam BV, Garsa AA, Chin RI, et al. A multi-institutional comparison of outcomes of immunosuppressed and immunocompetent patients treated with surgery and radiation therapy for cutaneous squamous cell carcinoma of the head and neck. Cancer 2017;123(11):2054–60.
3. Schwarz T. Skin immunity. Br J Dermatol 2003;149(Suppl 66):2–4.
4. Streilein JW, Alard P, Niizeki H. A new concept of skin-associated lymphoid tissue (SALT): UVB light impaired cutaneous immunity reveals a prominent role for cutaneous nerves. Keio J Med 1999;48(1):22–7.
5. Banchereau J, Steinman RM. Dendritic cells and the control of immunity. Nature 1998;392(6673):245–52.
6. Euvrard S, Kanitakis J, Claudy A. Skin cancers after organ transplantation. N Engl J Med 2003;348(17):1681–91.
7. Athar M, Walsh SB, Kopelovich L, et al. Pathogenesis of nonmelanoma skin cancers in organ transplant recipients. Arch Biochem Biophys 2011;508(2):159–63.

8. Mittal A, Colegio OR. Skin cancers in organ transplant recipients. Am J Transplant 2017;17(10):2509–30.
9. Nindl I, Gottschling M, Stockfleth E. Human papillomaviruses and non-melanoma skin cancer: basic virology and clinical manifestations. Dis Markers 2007;23(4):247–59.
10. Arron ST, Canavan T, Yu SS. Organ transplant recipients with Merkel cell carcinoma have reduced progression-free, overall, and disease-specific survival independent of stage at presentation. J Am Acad Dermatol 2014;71(4):684–90.
11. Gandhi RK, Rosenberg AS, Somach SC. Merkel cell polyomavirus: an update. J Cutan Pathol 2009;36(12):1327–9.
12. Elghouche AN, Pflum ZE, Schmalbach CE. Immunosuppression Impact on Head and Neck Cutaneous Squamous Cell Carcinoma: A Systematic Review with Meta-analysis. Otolaryngol Head Neck Surg 2019;160(3):439–46.
13. Marcen R, Pascual J, Tato AM, et al. Influence of immunosuppression on the prevalence of cancer after kidney transplantation. Transplant Proc 2003;35(5):1714–6.
14. Ritter A, Bachar G, Feinmesser R, et al. Nonmelanoma skin cancer of the head and neck region in solid organ transplant recipients. Head Neck 2019;41(2):374–80.
15. Greenberg JN, Zwald FO. Management of skin cancer in solid-organ transplant recipients: a multidisciplinary approach. Dermatol Clin 2011;29(2):231–41, ix.
16. Lindelof B, Sigurgeirsson B, Gabel H, et al. Incidence of skin cancer in 5356 patients following organ transplantation. Br J Dermatol 2000;143(3):513–9.
17. Adamson R, Obispo E, Dychter S, et al. High incidence and clinical course of aggressive skin cancer in heart transplant patients: a single-center study. Transplant Proc 1998;30(4):1124–6.
18. Garrett GL, Lowenstein SE, Singer JP, et al. Trends of skin cancer mortality after transplantation in the United States: 1987 to 2013. J Am Acad Dermatol 2016;75(1):106–12.
19. Kaplan AL, Cook JL. Cutaneous squamous cell carcinoma in patients with chronic lymphocytic leukemia. Skinmed 2005;4(5):300–4.
20. Moloney FJ, Comber H, O'Lorcain P, et al. A population-based study of skin cancer incidence and prevalence in renal transplant recipients. Br J Dermatol 2006;154(3):498–504.
21. Omland SH, Gniadecki R, Haedersdal M, et al. Skin cancer risk in hematopoietic stem-cell transplant recipients compared with background population and renal transplant recipients: a population-based cohort study. JAMA Dermatol 2016;152(2):177–83.
22. Zavos G, Karidis NP, Tsourouflis G, et al. Nonmelanoma skin cancer after renal transplantation: a single-center experience in 1736 transplantations. Int J Dermatol 2011;50(12):1496–500.
23. Wilkins K, Dolev JC, Turner R, et al. Approach to the treatment of cutaneous malignancy in HIV-infected patients. Dermatol Ther 2005;18(1):77–86.
24. Wilkins K, Turner R, Dolev JC, et al. Cutaneous malignancy and human immunodeficiency virus disease. J Am Acad Dermatol 2006;54(2):189–206 [quiz: 207–10].
25. Southwell KE, Chaplin JM, Eisenberg RL, et al. Effect of immunocompromise on metastatic cutaneous squamous cell carcinoma in the parotid and neck. Head Neck 2006;28(3):244–8.
26. Manyam BV, Gastman B, Zhang AY, et al. Inferior outcomes in immunosuppressed patients with high-risk cutaneous squamous cell carcinoma of the

head and neck treated with surgery and radiation therapy. J Am Acad Dermatol 2015;73(2):221–7.

27. Shao A, Wong DK, McIvor NP, et al. Parotid metastatic disease from cutaneous squamous cell carcinoma: prognostic role of facial nerve sacrifice, lateral temporal bone resection, immune status and P-stage. Head Neck 2014;36(4): 545–50.

28. Lott DG, Manz R, Koch C, et al. Aggressive behavior of nonmelanotic skin cancers in solid organ transplant recipients. Transplantation 2010;90(6):683–7.

29. Smith KJ, Hamza S, Skelton H. Histologic features in primary cutaneous squamous cell carcinomas in immunocompromised patients focusing on organ transplant patients. Dermatol Surg 2004;30(4 Pt 2):634–41.

30. Brougham ND, Dennett ER, Cameron R, et al. The incidence of metastasis from cutaneous squamous cell carcinoma and the impact of its risk factors. J Surg Oncol 2012;106(7):811–5.

31. Brantsch KD, Meisner C, Schonfisch B, et al. Analysis of risk factors determining prognosis of cutaneous squamous-cell carcinoma: a prospective study. Lancet Oncol 2008;9(8):713–20.

32. Rowe DE, Carroll RJ, Day CL Jr. Prognostic factors for local recurrence, metastasis, and survival rates in squamous cell carcinoma of the skin, ear, and lip. Implications for treatment modality selection. J Am Acad Dermatol 1992;26(6): 976–90.

33. McDowell L, Yom SS. Locally advanced non-melanomatous skin cancer: Contemporary radiotherapeutic management. Oral Oncol 2019;99:104443.

34. Sapir E, Tolpadi A, McHugh J, et al. Skin cancer of the head and neck with gross or microscopic perineural involvement: Patterns of failure. Radiother Oncol 2016;120(1):81–6.

35. Schmults CD, Karia PS, Carter JB, et al. Factors predictive of recurrence and death from cutaneous squamous cell carcinoma: a 10-year, single-institution cohort study. JAMA Dermatol 2013;149(5):541–7.

36. Velez NF, Karia PS, Vartanov AR, et al. Association of advanced leukemic stage and skin cancer tumor stage with poor skin cancer outcomes in patients with chronic lymphocytic leukemia. JAMA Dermatol 2014;150(3):280–7.

37. Xu MJ, Lazar AA, Garsa AA, et al. Major prognostic factors for recurrence and survival independent of the American Joint Committee on Cancer eighth edition staging system in patients with cutaneous squamous cell carcinoma treated with multimodality therapy. Head Neck 2018;40(7):1406–14.

38. Sahovaler A, Krishnan RJ, Yeh DH, et al. Outcomes of cutaneous squamous cell carcinoma in the head and neck region with regional lymph node metastasis: a systematic review and meta-analysis. JAMA Otolaryngol Head Neck Surg 2019; 145(4):352–60.

39. Ch'ng S, Clark JR, Brunner M, et al. Relevance of the primary lesion in the prognosis of metastatic cutaneous squamous cell carcinoma. Head Neck 2013; 35(2):190–4.

40. McLean T, Brunner M, Ebrahimi A, et al. Concurrent primary and metastatic cutaneous head and neck squamous cell carcinoma: Analysis of prognostic factors. Head Neck 2013;35(8):1144–8.

41. Palme CE, O'Brien CJ, Veness MJ, et al. Extent of parotid disease influences outcome in patients with metastatic cutaneous squamous cell carcinoma. Arch Otolaryngol Head Neck Surg 2003;129(7):750–3.

42. Berg D, Otley CC. Skin cancer in organ transplant recipients: Epidemiology, pathogenesis, and management. J Am Acad Dermatol 2002;47(1):1–17 [quiz: 18–20].

43. Tam S, Yao CMK, Amit M, et al. Association of immunosuppression with outcomes of patients with cutaneous squamous cell carcinoma of the head and neck. JAMA Otolaryngol Head Neck Surg 2019;05:05.

44. Kanitakis J, Alhaj-Ibrahim L, Euvrard S, et al. Basal cell carcinomas developing in solid organ transplant recipients: clinicopathologic study of 176 cases. Arch Dermatol 2003;139(9):1133–7.

45. Kempf W, Mertz KD, Hofbauer GF, et al. Skin cancer in organ transplant recipients. Pathobiology 2013;80(6):302–9.

46. Ramsay HM, Fryer AA, Hawley CM, et al. Non-melanoma skin cancer risk in the Queensland renal transplant population. Br J Dermatol 2002;147(5):950–6.

47. Hardie IR, Strong RW, Hartley LC, et al. Skin cancer in Caucasian renal allograft recipients living in a subtropical climate. Surgery 1980;87(2):177–83.

48. Krynitz B, Olsson H, Lundh Rozell B, et al. Risk of basal cell carcinoma in Swedish organ transplant recipients: a population-based study. Br J Dermatol 2016; 174(1):95–103.

49. Zamoiski RD, Yanik E, Gibson TM, et al. Risk of second malignancies in solid organ transplant recipients who develop keratinocyte cancers. Cancer Res 2017;77(15):4196–203.

50. Kubica AW, Brewer JD. Melanoma in immunosuppressed patients. Mayo Clin Proc 2012;87(10):991–1003.

51. Robbins HA, Clarke CA, Arron ST, et al. Melanoma risk and survival among organ transplant recipients. J Invest Dermatol 2015;135(11):2657–65.

52. Vajdic CM, van Leeuwen MT, Webster AC, et al. Cutaneous melanoma is related to immune suppression in kidney transplant recipients. Cancer Epidemiol Biomarkers Prev 2009;18(8):2297–303.

53. Vajdic CM, McDonald SP, McCredie MR, et al. Cancer incidence before and after kidney transplantation. JAMA 2006;296(23):2823–31.

54. Hollenbeak CS, Todd MM, Billingsley EM, et al. Increased incidence of melanoma in renal transplantation recipients. Cancer 2005;104(9):1962–7.

55. Kasiske BL, Snyder JJ, Gilbertson DT, et al. Cancer after kidney transplantation in the United States. Am J Transplant 2004;4(6):905–13.

56. Jensen P, Hansen S, Moller B, et al. Skin cancer in kidney and heart transplant recipients and different long-term immunosuppressive therapy regimens. J Am Acad Dermatol 1999;40(2 Pt 1):177–86.

57. Green AC, Olsen CM. Increased risk of melanoma in organ transplant recipients: systematic review and meta-analysis of cohort studies. Acta Derm Venereol 2015;95(8):923–7.

58. Burgi A, Brodine S, Wegner S, et al. Incidence and risk factors for the occurrence of non-AIDS-defining cancers among human immunodeficiency virus-infected individuals. Cancer 2005;104(7):1505–11.

59. Engels EA. Non-AIDS-defining malignancies in HIV-infected persons: etiologic puzzles, epidemiologic perils, prevention opportunities. AIDS 2009;23(8): 875–85.

60. Tsimberidou AM, Wen S, McLaughlin P, et al. Other malignancies in chronic lymphocytic leukemia/small lymphocytic lymphoma. J Clin Oncol 2009;27(6): 904–10.

61. McKenna DB, Stockton D, Brewster DH, et al. Evidence for an association between cutaneous malignant melanoma and lymphoid malignancy: a

population-based retrospective cohort study in Scotland. Br J Cancer 2003; 88(1):74–8.

62. Hisada M, Biggar RJ, Greene MH, et al. Solid tumors after chronic lymphocytic leukemia. Blood 2001;98(6):1979–81.

63. Adami J, Frisch M, Yuen J, et al. Evidence of an association between non-Hodgkin's lymphoma and skin cancer. BMJ 1995;310(6993):1491–5.

64. Travis LB, Curtis RE, Hankey BF, et al. Second cancers in patients with chronic lymphocytic leukemia. J Natl Cancer Inst 1992;84(18):1422–7.

65. Brewer JD, Christenson LJ, Weaver AL, et al. Malignant melanoma in solid transplant recipients: collection of database cases and comparison with surveillance, epidemiology, and end results data for outcome analysis. Arch Dermatol 2011; 147(7):790–6.

66. Brewer JD, Shanafelt TD, Otley CC, et al. Chronic lymphocytic leukemia is associated with decreased survival of patients with malignant melanoma and Merkel cell carcinoma in a SEER population-based study. J Clin Oncol 2012;30(8): 843–9.

67. Matin RN, Mesher D, Proby CM, et al. Melanoma in organ transplant recipients: clinicopathological features and outcome in 100 cases. Am J Transplant 2008; 8(9):1891–900.

68. Vajdic CM, Chong AH, Kelly PJ, et al. Survival after cutaneous melanoma in kidney transplant recipients: a population-based matched cohort study. Am J Transpl 2014;14(6):1368–75.

69. Krynitz B, Rozell BL, Lyth J, et al. Cutaneous malignant melanoma in the Swedish organ transplantation cohort: A study of clinicopathological characteristics and mortality. J Am Acad Dermatol 2015;73(1):106–113 e102.

70. Le Mire L, Hollowood K, Gray D, et al. Melanomas in renal transplant recipients. Br J Dermatol 2006;154(3):472–7.

71. Penn I. Malignant melanoma in organ allograft recipients. Transplantation 1996; 61(2):274–8.

72. Penn I, First MR. Merkel's cell carcinoma in organ recipients: report of 41 cases. Transplantation 1999;68(11):1717–21.

73. Paulson KG, Iyer JG, Blom A, et al. Systemic immune suppression predicts diminished Merkel cell carcinoma-specific survival independent of stage. J Invest Dermatol 2013;133(3):642–6.

74. Tarantola TI, Vallow LA, Halyard MY, et al. Prognostic factors in Merkel cell carcinoma: analysis of 240 cases. J Am Acad Dermatol 2013;68(3):425–32.

75. Clarke CA, Robbins HA, Tatalovich Z, et al. Risk of merkel cell carcinoma after solid organ transplantation. J Natl Cancer Inst 2015;107(2).

76. Koljonen V, Kukko H, Tukiainen E, et al. Incidence of Merkel cell carcinoma in renal transplant recipients. Nephrol Dial Transplant 2009;24(10):3231–5.

77. Keeling E, Murray SL, Williams Y, et al. Merkel cell carcinoma in kidney transplant recipients in Ireland 1964-2018. Br J Dermatol 2019;181(6):1314–5.

78. Koljonen V, Sahi H, Bohling T, et al. Post-transplant Merkel Cell Carcinoma. Acta Derm Venereol 2016;96(4):442–7.

79. Goes HFO, Lima CDS, Issa MCA, et al. Merkel cell carcinoma in an immunosuppressed patient. An Bras Dermatol 2017;92(3):386–8.

80. Tadmor T, Liphshitz I, Aviv A, et al. Increased incidence of chronic lymphocytic leukaemia and lymphomas in patients with Merkel cell carcinoma - a population based study of 335 cases with neuroendocrine skin tumour. Br J Haematol 2012; 157(4):457–62.

81. Engels EA, Frisch M, Goedert JJ, et al. Merkel cell carcinoma and HIV infection. Lancet 2002;359(9305):497–8.

82. Paulson KG, Iyer JG, Tegeder AR, et al. Transcriptome-wide studies of merkel cell carcinoma and validation of intratumoral CD8+ lymphocyte invasion as an independent predictor of survival. J Clin Oncol 2011;29(12):1539–46.

83. Sihto H, Bohling T, Kavola H, et al. Tumor infiltrating immune cells and outcome of Merkel cell carcinoma: a population-based study. Clin Cancer Res 2012; 18(10):2872–81.

84. Moosa MR. Kaposi's sarcoma in kidney transplant recipients: a 23-year experience. Qjm 2005;98(3):205–14.

85. Cesarman E, Damania B, Krown SE, et al. Kaposi sarcoma. Nat Rev Dis Primers 2019;5(1):9.

86. Cook-Mozaffari P, Newton R, Beral V, et al. The geographical distribution of Kaposi's sarcoma and of lymphomas in Africa before the AIDS epidemic. Br J Cancer 1998;78(11):1521–8.

87. Beral V, Peterman TA, Berkelman RL, et al. Kaposi's sarcoma among persons with AIDS: a sexually transmitted infection? Lancet 1990;335(8682):123–8.

88. Grulich AE, Vajdic CM. The epidemiology of cancers in human immunodeficiency virus infection and after organ transplantation. Semin Oncol 2015; 42(2):247–57.

89. Hiesse C, Rieu P, Kriaa F, et al. Malignancy after renal transplantation: analysis of incidence and risk factors in 1700 patients followed during a 25-year period. Transplant Proc 1997;29(1–2):831–3.

90. Ulrich C, Schmook T, Sachse MM, et al. Comparative epidemiology and pathogenic factors for nonmelanoma skin cancer in organ transplant patients. Dermatol Surg 2004;30(4 Pt 2):622–7.

91. Ulrich C, Kanitakis J, Stockfleth E, et al. Skin cancer in organ transplant recipients–where do we stand today? Am J Transplant 2008;8(11):2192–8.

92. Fortina AB, Caforio AL, Piaserico S, et al. Skin cancer in heart transplant recipients: frequency and risk factor analysis. J Heart Lung Transplant 2000;19(3): 249–55.

93. Otley CC, Cherikh WS, Salasche SJ, et al. Skin cancer in organ transplant recipients: effect of pretransplant end-organ disease. J Am Acad Dermatol 2005; 53(5):783–90.

94. Ramsay HM, Reece SM, Fryer AA, et al. Seven-year prospective study of nonmelanoma skin cancer incidence in U.K. renal transplant recipients. Transplantation 2007;84(3):437–9.

95. Bordea C, Wojnarowska F, Millard PR, et al. Skin cancers in renal-transplant recipients occur more frequently than previously recognized in a temperate climate. Transplantation 2004;77(4):574–9.

96. Espana A, Martinez-Gonzalez MA, Garcia-Granero M, et al. A prospective study of incident nonmelanoma skin cancer in heart transplant recipients. J Invest Dermatol 2000;115(6):1158–60.

97. Webb MC, Compton F, Andrews PA, et al. Skin tumours posttransplantation: a retrospective analysis of 28 years' experience at a single centre. Transplant Proc 1997;29(1–2):828–30.

98. Hartevelt MM, Bavinck JN, Kootte AM, et al. Incidence of skin cancer after renal transplantation in The Netherlands. Transplantation 1990;49(3):506–9.

99. Liddington M, Richardson AJ, Higgins RM, et al. Skin cancer in renal transplant recipients. Br J Surg 1989;76(10):1002–5.

100. Ramsay HM, Fryer AA, Hawley CM, et al. Factors associated with nonmelanoma skin cancer following renal transplantation in Queensland, Australia. J Am Acad Dermatol 2003;49(3):397–406.

101. Bouwes Bavinck JN, Euvrard S, Naldi L, et al. Keratotic skin lesions and other risk factors are associated with skin cancer in organ-transplant recipients: a case-control study in The Netherlands, United Kingdom, Germany, France, and Italy. J Invest Dermatol 2007;127(7):1647–56.

102. Wisgerhof HC, van der Boog PJ, de Fijter JW, et al. Increased risk of squamous-cell carcinoma in simultaneous pancreas kidney transplant recipients compared with kidney transplant recipients. J Invest Dermatol 2009;129(12):2886–94.

103. Rashtak S, Dierkhising RA, Kremers WK, et al. Incidence and risk factors for skin cancer following lung transplantation. J Am Acad Dermatol 2015;72(1):92–8.

104. Bouwes Bavinck JN, Hardie DR, Green A, et al. The risk of skin cancer in renal transplant recipients in Queensland, Australia. A follow-up study. Transplantation 1996;61(5):715–21.

105. Ascha M, Ascha MS, Tanenbaum J, et al. Risk Factors for Melanoma in Renal Transplant Recipients. JAMA Dermatol 2017;153(11):1130–6.

106. Xiao D, Craig JC, Chapman JR, et al. Donor cancer transmission in kidney transplantation: a systematic review. Am J Transplant 2013;13(10):2645–52.

107. Strauss DC, Thomas JM. Transmission of donor melanoma by organ transplantation. Lancet Oncol 2010;11(8):790–6.

108. Ally MS, Tang JY, Arron ST. Cutaneous human papillomavirus infection and Basal cell carcinoma of the skin. J Invest Dermatol 2013;133(6):1456–8.

109. Connolly K, Manders P, Earls P, et al. Papillomavirus-associated squamous skin cancers following transplant immunosuppression: one Notch closer to control. Cancer Treat Rev 2014;40(2):205–14.

110. Neale RE, Weissenborn S, Abeni D, et al. Human papillomavirus load in eyebrow hair follicles and risk of cutaneous squamous cell carcinoma. Cancer Epidemiol Biomarkers Prev 2013;22(4):719–27.

111. Reuschenbach M, Tran T, Faulstich F, et al. High-risk human papillomavirus in non-melanoma skin lesions from renal allograft recipients and immunocompetent patients. Br J Cancer 2011;104(8):1334–41.

112. Gershenwald JE, Scolyer RA, Hess KR, et al. Melanoma of the skin. In: Amin MB, Edge S, Green F, et al, editors. AJCC cancer staging manual. 8th edition. Springer International Publishing; 2017. p. 563–86.

113. Bichakjian CK, Nghiem P, Johnson T, et al. Merkel cell carcinoma. In: Amin MB, Edge S, Green F, et al, editors. AJCC cancer staging manual. 8th edition. Springer International Publishing; 2017. p. 549–62.

114. Califano J, Lydiatt WM, Nehal KS, et al. Cutaneous carcinoma of the head and neck. In: Amin MB, Edge S, Green F, et al, editors. AJCC cancer staging manual. 8th edition. Springer International Publishing; 2017. p. 171–81.

115. Moore BA, Weber RS, Prieto V, et al. Lymph node metastases from cutaneous squamous cell carcinoma of the head and neck. Laryngoscope 2005;115(9):1561–7.

116. Carroll RP, Ramsay HM, Fryer AA, et al. Incidence and prediction of nonmelanoma skin cancer post-renal transplantation: a prospective study in Queensland, Australia. Am J Kidney Dis 2003;41(3):676–83.

117. McLaughlin EJ, Miller L, Shin TM, et al. Rate of regional nodal metastases of cutaneous squamous cell carcinoma in the immunosuppressed patient. Am J Otolaryngol 2017;38(3):325–8.

118. Jackson RS, Schmalbach CE. New frontiers in surgical innovation. Otolaryngol Clin North Am 2017;50(4):733–46.

119. Ahmed MM, Moore BA, Schmalbach CE. Utility of head and neck cutaneous squamous cell carcinoma sentinel node biopsy: a systematic review. Otolaryngol Head Neck Surg 2014;150(2):180–7.

120. Network NCC. Squamous Cell Skin Cancer (Version 2.2020). Available at: https://www.nccn.org/professionals/physician_gls/pdf/squamous.pdf. Accessed August 6, 2020.

121. Network NCC. Basal Cell Skin Cancer (Version 1.2020). Available at: https://www.nccn.org/professionals/physician_gls/pdf/nmsc.pdf. Accessed June 8, 2020.

122. Network NCC. Merkel Cell Carcinoma (Version 1.2020). Available at: https://www.nccn.org/professionals/physician_gls/pdf/mcc.pdf. Accessed August 6, 2020.

123. Network NCC. Cutaneous Melanoma (Version 3.2020). Available at: https://www.nccn.org/professionals/physician_gls/pdf/cutaneous_melanoma.pdf. Accessed August 6, 2020.

124. Ow TJ, Wang HR, McLellan B, et al. AHNS series - Do you know your guidelines? Diagnosis and management of cutaneous squamous cell carcinoma. Head Neck 2016;38(11):1589–95.

125. Ow TJ, Grethlein SJ, Schmalbach CE. Do you know your guidelines? Diagnosis and management of cutaneous head and neck melanoma. Head Neck 2018;40(5):875–85.

126. Otley CC, Berg D, Ulrich C, et al. Reduction of immunosuppression for transplant-associated skin cancer: expert consensus survey. Br J Dermatol 2006;154(3):395–400.

127. Moloney FJ, Kelly PO, Kay EW, et al. Maintenance versus reduction of immunosuppression in renal transplant recipients with aggressive squamous cell carcinoma. Dermatol Surg 2004;30(4 Pt 2):674–8.

128. Dantal J, Hourmant M, Cantarovich D, et al. Effect of long-term immunosuppression in kidney-graft recipients on cancer incidence: randomised comparison of two cyclosporin regimens. Lancet 1998;351(9103):623–8.

129. Coghill AE, Johnson LG, Berg D, et al. Immunosuppressive medications and squamous cell skin carcinoma: nested case-control study within the skin cancer after organ transplant (SCOT) Cohort. Am J Transplant 2016;16(2):565–73.

130. Molina BD, Leiro MG, Pulpon LA, et al. Incidence and risk factors for nonmelanoma skin cancer after heart transplantation. Transplant Proc 2010;42(8):3001–5.

131. Euvrard S, Morelon E, Rostaing L, et al. Sirolimus and secondary skin-cancer prevention in kidney transplantation. N Engl J Med 2012;367(4):329–39.

132. Campbell SB, Walker R, Tai SS, et al. Randomized controlled trial of sirolimus for renal transplant recipients at high risk for nonmelanoma skin cancer. Am J Transpl 2012;12(5):1146–56.

133. Badve SV, Pascoe EM, Burke M, et al. Mammalian target of rapamycin inhibitors and clinical outcomes in adult kidney transplant recipients. Clin J Am Soc Nephrol 2016;11(10):1845–55.

134. Dantal J, Morelon E, Rostaing L, et al. Sirolimus for secondary prevention of skin cancer in kidney transplant recipients: 5-year results. J Clin Oncol 2018;36(25):2612–20.

135. Knoll GA, Kokolo MB, Mallick R, et al. Effect of sirolimus on malignancy and survival after kidney transplantation: systematic review and meta-analysis of individual patient data. BMJ 2014;349:g6679.

136. Zhan FQ, Packianathan VS, Zeitouni NC. Merkel cell carcinoma: a review of current advances. J Natl Compr Canc Netw 2009;7(3):333–9.

137. Muirhead R, Ritchie DM. Partial regression of Merkel cell carcinoma in response to withdrawal of azathioprine in an immunosuppression-induced case of metastatic Merkel cell carcinoma. Clin Oncol (R Coll Radiol) 2007;19(1):96.

138. Friedlaender MM, Rubinger D, Rosenbaum E, et al. Temporary regression of Merkel cell carcinoma metastases after cessation of cyclosporine. Transplantation 2002;73(11):1849–50.

139. Migden MR, Rischin D, Schmults CD, et al. PD-1 blockade with cemiplimab in advanced cutaneous squamous-cell carcinoma. N Engl J Med 2018;379(4):341–51.

140. Grob JJ, Gonzalez R, Basset-Seguin N, et al. Pembrolizumab monotherapy for recurrent or metastatic cutaneous squamous cell carcinoma: a single-arm phase II Trial (KEYNOTE-629). J Clin Oncol 2020;38(25):2916–25.

141. Guminski A, Stein B. Immunotherapy and other systemic therapies for cutaneous SCC. Oral Oncol 2019;99:104459.

142. Abdel-Wahab N, Safa H, Abudayyeh A, et al. Checkpoint inhibitor therapy for cancer in solid organ transplantation recipients: an institutional experience and a systematic review of the literature. J Immunother Cancer 2019;7(1):106.

143. Leard LE, Cho BK, Jones KD, et al. Fatal diffuse alveolar damage in two lung transplant patients treated with cetuximab. J Heart Lung Transplant 2007;26(12):1340–4.

144. Ranganath HA, Panella TJ. Administration of ipilimumab to a liver transplant recipient with unresectable metastatic melanoma. J Immunother 2015;38(5):211.

145. Spain L, Higgins R, Gopalakrishnan K, et al. Acute renal allograft rejection after immune checkpoint inhibitor therapy for metastatic melanoma. Ann Oncol 2016;27(6):1135–7.

146. Lipson EJ, Bodell MA, Kraus ES, et al. Successful administration of ipilimumab to two kidney transplantation patients with metastatic melanoma. J Clin Oncol 2014;32(19):e69–71.

147. Morales RE, Shoushtari AN, Walsh MM, et al. Safety and efficacy of ipilimumab to treat advanced melanoma in the setting of liver transplantation. J Immunother Cancer 2015;3:22.

148. Park MJ, Roh JL, Choi SH, et al. De novo head and neck cancer arising in solid organ transplantation recipients: The Asan Medical Center experience. Auris Nasus Larynx 2018;45(4):838–45.

149. Tobin JWD, Royle J, Mason R, et al. The effect of immune checkpoint inhibitors in patients with concomitant advanced melanoma and chronic lymphocytic leukaemia. Blood 2017;130(Supplement 1):5338.

150. Menzies AM, Johnson DB, Ramanujam S, et al. Anti-PD-1 therapy in patients with advanced melanoma and preexisting autoimmune disorders or major toxicity with ipilimumab. Ann Oncol 2017;28(2):368–76.

151. Zmonarski SC, Boratynska M, Rabczynski J, et al. Regression of Kaposi's sarcoma in renal graft recipients after conversion to sirolimus treatment. Transplant Proc 2005;37(2):964–6.

152. Johari Y, Nicholson ML. Complete resolution of oral Kaposi's sarcoma achieved by changing immunosuppression: a case report. Ann R Coll Surg Engl 2010; 92(5):W45–6.
153. Pranteda G, Feliziani G, Grimaldi M, et al. Sirolimus and regression of Kaposi's sarcoma in immunosuppressed transplant patient. J Eur Acad Dermatol Venereol 2008;22(8):1022–3.
154. Stallone G, Schena A, Infante B, et al. Sirolimus for Kaposi's sarcoma in renal-transplant recipients. N Engl J Med 2005;352(13):1317–23.
155. Campistol JM, Schena FP. Kaposi's sarcoma in renal transplant recipients–the impact of proliferation signal inhibitors. Nephrol Dial Transplant 2007;22(Suppl 1):i17–22.
156. Park YJ, Bae HJ, Chang JY, et al. Development of Kaposi sarcoma and hemophagocytic lymphohistiocytosis associated with human herpesvirus 8 in a renal transplant recipient. Korean J Intern Med 2017;32(4):750–2.
157. Roshan R, Labo N, Trivett M, et al. T-cell responses to KSHV infection: a systematic approach. Oncotarget 2017;8(65):109402–16.
158. Bower M, Dalla Pria A, Coyle C, et al. Prospective stage-stratified approach to AIDS-related Kaposi's sarcoma. J Clin Oncol 2014;32(5):409–14.
159. Kang W, Sampaio MS, Huang E, et al. Association of pretransplant skin cancer with posttransplant malignancy, graft failure and death in kidney transplant recipients. Transplantation 2017;101(6):1303–9.
160. Zwald F, Leitenberger J, Zeitouni N, et al. Recommendations for solid organ transplantation for transplant candidates with a pretransplant diagnosis of cutaneous squamous cell carcinoma, merkel cell carcinoma and melanoma: a consensus opinion from the international transplant skin cancer collaborative (ITSCC). Am J Transplant 2016;16(2):407–13.
161. Chan AW, Fung K, Austin PC, et al. Improved keratinocyte carcinoma outcomes with annual dermatology assessment after solid organ transplantation: Population-based cohort study. Am J Transplant 2019;19(2):522–31.

Ethical Considerations for Elderly Patients with Cutaneous Malignancy

Alyssa K. Ovaitt, MD[a], Brian B. Hughley, MD[b],
Susan McCammon, MFA, MD[c,d],*

KEYWORDS

- Cutaneous malignancy • Care of elderly • Medical decision-making capacity
- Shared decision making • Palliative care • Narrative • Ethics

KEY POINTS

- In elders, changes in ability and function affect the entire circle of caregiving—within the family and the social support system of nursing facilities and community-based services. Medical decision making needs to consider these repercussions.
- The traditional principles of medical ethics (beneficence, nonmaleficence, autonomy, and justice) may not be sufficient to account for the issues facing the elderly patient with advanced skin cancers and their care givers. The ethical framework of narrative ethics can offer additional understanding and guidance.

INTRODUCTION

Cutaneous malignancy, particularly in elderly patients, poses unique challenges to explanation, understanding, and decision making. Skin cancers, for many patients, elderly or not, have become a regular part of life with preventive skin screening examinations, proactive ablation of small lesions, and biopsy-proven cancers that are easily treated. Lay understanding of most nonmelanoma skin cancers is that they are a minor nuisance that can be easily dealt with, sometimes with just an ointment.

When faced with a skin cancer that has become life threatening, patients are challenged to recalibrate their thinking and expectations. This is particularly true if the

[a] Department of Otolaryngology–Head and Neck Surgery, University of Alabama at Birmingham, FOT 1155, 1720 2nd Avenue South, Birmingham, AL 35294-3412, USA; [b] Department of Otolaryngology–Head and Neck Surgery, University of Florida, 1345 Center Drive, Box #100264, Gainesville, FL 32610, USA; [c] Department of Otolaryngology—Head and Neck Surgery, The University of Alabama at Birmingham, Faculty Office Tower 1155, 1720 2nd Avenue South, Birmingham, AL 35294-3412, USA; [d] Department of Internal Medicine, Division of Gerontology, Geriatrics and Palliative Care, The University of Alabama at Birmingham, 1720 2nd Avenue South, Birmingham, AL 35294-3412, USA
* Corresponding author.
E-mail address: smccammon@uabmc.edu

Otolaryngol Clin N Am 54 (2021) 415–423
https://doi.org/10.1016/j.otc.2020.11.013

disease presents in an untreated nodal basin or recurs after well-tolerated treatment. Patients may have to come to terms with the fact that what has been previously treated in the office may now require general anesthesia, a hospital stay, or even life-changing surgery. For some, the introduction of a neck dissection or a parotidectomy seems like too much for a skin cancer. For patients facing more radical extirpations, such as a temporal bone resection or an orbital exenteration, it can be hard to make the mental transition that this is all necessary for a skin cancer. They may respond with denial or disproportionate fear, or they may be dealing with anger or decisional regret about prior treatments and decisions. Often the surgeon treating this patient and his or her care circle is coming into his or her skin cancer story, midway or more through, sometimes for the final and unwelcome chapters.[1,2]

Cutaneous malignancies of the head and neck, such as melanoma, Merkel cell carcinoma (MCC), and nonmelanoma skin cancer (NMSC) including basal cell carcinoma (BCC) and squamous cell carcinoma (SCC), have long plagued the aging population. Indeed, the incidence of invasive melanoma and MCC increases with age.[3–8] In addition to NMSC, more aggressive disease likely portends more intensive treatment, and discussions about the risks and benefits of management options become even more important.[6] In addition to an increased risk of skin cancer, elderly patients may have different goals and expectations for their remaining life, treatment, and symptom burden. Their medical decision-making capacity and autonomy may also be more limited in some cases.[6,9] Management of elderly patients requires frequent and in-depth discussions of options and goals, shared decision making, and thoughtful application of clinical ethics.

BACKGROUND

The most traditional and commonly taught ethical framework in medicine is principlism, which states that medical decisions should be made according to 4 core principles:[10]

- Beneficence: provide or maximize benefit to the patient
- Nonmaleficence: avoid or minimize harm to the patient
- Autonomy: respect the patient's right to make decisions
- Justice: promote fairness in distribution of scarce resources and acknowledge competing needs, rights, and obligations

Many individual and cultural factors challenge the application of these principles in situations with unclear solutions or competing principles.[11]

Elderly patients with cutaneous malignancies and those who care for them can find themselves in such situations. Although independence and medical decision-making capacity can be preserved into extreme old age, there is a greater incidence of dependent living and diminished capacity as people age.[12,13] Elderly patients may already be reliant on the care of loved ones or custodial care providers, or they may be only 1 episode away from becoming so. Thus, any decision that has the potential to affect their level of function or dependence necessarily affects their circle of care. This term, "circle of care," acknowledges the reality that some patients rely primarily on loved ones who may not be legally related family or may be family of choice. Other patients rely on paid provision of medical/custodial care, and medical decisions require recognition of their resources and how changes in their clinical and cognitive condition may affect their eligibility for services that they find acceptable.[14–17] The special characteristics of elderly patients with cutaneous malignancy offer an opportunity to explore shared decision making using the framework of narrative ethics.

Narrative ethics focus on the role that stories play in creating identity and ordering one's moral universe. Both the act of telling a story, and hearing a story, create a context for making sense of a situation. For narrative ethicists, such as Rita Charon and Arthur Frank, this applies to an individual and his or her particular circumstances, but it is also influential on a broader scale, guiding and shaping the decisions of others who use stories as generalizable moral guides—stories with morals. The use of literature to study narrative ethics in medicine has largely focused on the illness narratives that patients and their loved ones tell to make sense of their experience of pathology.[18]

Arthur Frank famously characterized 3 illness narratives: restitution (being restored to normal); quest (a journey to a new normal); and chaos (life interrupted, without trajectory.)[19] Qualitative researchers have identified similar narratives in cancer survivors and have correlated the choice of narrative to quality-of-life outcomes.[20] Beyond the patient's experience of telling a story, there is the practitioner's experience of hearing or witnessing the story.[18,21,22] Howard Brody in his book, The Healer's Power, illustrated the role of the physician in helping to repair a patient's "broken story." Physicians and patients thus benefit from training in empathic listening.[23]

Going a step further, physicians themselves are responsible for generating stories in how they explain diagnoses, treatment options, and possible outcomes to patients.[24,25] Every surgeon has had the experience of presenting information to a patient and having the patient lean toward a decision the physician does not think is in the patient's best interest, and feeling the need to explain it better, or differently. Whether physicians are aware of it or not, they have a long experience of developing narrative competence, or presenting information in a way that achieves a desired outcome. That outcome can be as generous as helping a patient achieve his or her own stated goals or as paternalistic as imposing what the physician thinks is the right decision.[26,27]

Describing options and their ramifications is an essential part of the decision-making and informed consent processes. These descriptions, however, are not value free, particularly when attempting to portray the natural progression of cancer. Palliative interventions are sometimes proposed to relieve a current symptom but can also be advocated to prevent predictable future suffering. Describing the possibility of imagined but not yet experienced suffering can be emotionally fraught for both patient and surgeon.[28,29]

The following cases will address some issues unique to elderly patients with cutaneous malignancy and the ethical resources that can be used to face them, focusing on eliciting goals and values and helping patients and their care circle make goal-concordant decisions.

CASE STUDIES
Case 1

An 87-year-old man underwent conservative excision of a 2 cm full-thickness cSCC of the scalp with rotational flap reconstruction 5 years ago, followed by radiation. Three years later, he returned with 2 full-thickness, ulcerative scalp defects with exposed calvarium (**Fig. 1**A, B) and biopsies returned with recurrent cSCC. He was denied treatment by his previous surgeon given his age and frailty. Since that time, he has experienced significant increases in pain with frequent bleeding from these sites, prompting him to stop his antiplatelet therapy that he takes for his mechanical valve replacement. He now presents to the clinic.

After much discussion, the patient elects to undergo excision of the scalp cSCC with free flap reconstruction. He has an uneventful postoperative hospitalization and

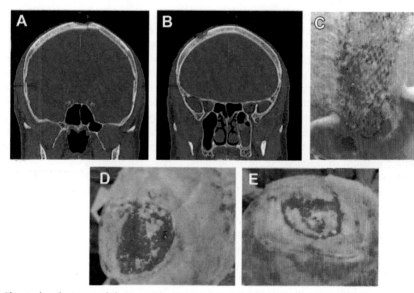

Fig. 1. (*A–E*): Case 1. (*A*): Coronal computed tomography (CT) scan showing midline soft tissue and bone defect resulting from chronic wound. (*B*): Coronal CT scan showing right lateral erosive soft tissue and bone lesion resulting from cutaneous squamous cell carcinoma. (*C*): 2-week postoperative photograph of well-healed right lateral scalp reconstruction with a latissimus dorsi free flap. (*D*): 2-week postoperative photograph of distal flap necrosis at scalp vertex. (*E*): 2-month postoperative photo of full-thickness distal tip flap necrosis with exposed calvarial bone.

is discharged to a skilled nursing facility to assist with wound care. At his 2-week postoperative visit, partial flap loss is noticed at the distal tip (**Fig. 1**C). He and his family are shown more complex wound management techniques that require dressing changes multiple times per day. After 2 months, he has full-thickness loss of the distal flap with exposed bone (**Fig. 1**D–E). Additional reconstructive surgery is offered, but the patient declines, stating that he prefers to "not go through that whole ordeal again" given his improved pain control and bleeding (see **Fig. 1**A–E).

Discussion

Elderly patients are often not treated aggressively for advanced cutaneous malignancies.[30] One can wonder if this patient was initially not offered guideline-based curative surgical treatment in an attempt to uphold the principle of nonmaleficence, despite it being well established that age alone is not a contraindication for curative treatment for cutaneous malignancies.[31] Because few elderly patients are included in studies and clinical trials because of age limitations within inclusion criteria, even fewer data exist to guide management algorithms in this age group.[32] In this instance, classic ethical thinking of nonmaleficence alone may not be sufficient.

After he did receive definitive treatment, the patient has what most physicians would consider a successful surgery, in that he developed no major or minor complications, and clear tumor margins were obtained. Additionally, he experienced relief of symptoms and had a relatively short convalescence for a major surgical procedure. He does, however, have a wound with exposed calvarium requiring chronic attention and long-term care. Although more reconstructive surgery has been offered, the patient refused; from his perspective, the original goals of stopping chronic bleeding and relieving pain have been met, and he wishes to avoid further surgery.

In such a case, the surgeon may be tempted to persuade the patient to complete the second reconstructive surgery. With such a recent, extensive surgery, it perhaps seems counterintuitive to leave such a chronic wound untreated, but this is where narrative ethics may be used as a guide. Listening to this patient's story is key to understanding and guiding medical decision making, perhaps at times against the physician's own goals or wishes. On further discussion with this patient, for example, he divulges that his wife of 65 years has an end-stage cancer diagnosis of her own, and he feels he cannot risk another hospitalization and stay at a nursing facility under these circumstances. In meeting patients within their narrative story and engaging in authentic discussion, one may allow both parties to understand more clearly what is at stake and reach decisions together.

Case 2

A 72-year-old woman presents to the clinic with a chief complaint of double vision for 2 months. She has a large, 12 × 15 cm fungating lesion of the forehead; biopsy confirms BCC. On further questioning, she states that the spot has been on her forehead for a few years and got a little bigger recently. She lives in a rural area and takes care of her 94-year-old father, who has Alzheimer disease; she has 1 estranged sister who lives across the country. The surgeon advises the patient that surgery would require removing her eye and a part of her face and replacing it with tissue from her leg. Even though it would be a big operation, it could potentially provide a durable cure. In counseling, she is shown photographs of an identical operation to help in understanding the process, and outcomes (**Fig. 2A–E**).

When asked to restate the goals for surgery in her own words, she states that, "I would like the bump removed so I can see better to take care of my father." She also insists that the surgery be performed as an outpatient with no general anesthesia because, "my dad had general anesthesia years ago for heart surgery and that's what gave him Alzheimer's." Given concerns about the patient's medical decision-making capacity, you call the patient's sister to discuss the next steps in management of both the patient, and her father.

Discussion

As discussed previously, a head and neck surgeon is often entering a pre-existing narrative for an elderly patient with an advanced cutaneous malignancy. The ability to hear and empathically respond to the patient's prior history and beliefs about current condition is important and helps frame the next steps in the discussion. In addition to eliciting the goals and values of the patient and his or her care circle, the physician then must consider how to craft his or her own story about what the immediate future may hold. For elderly patients, this story will need to include multiple possible outcomes and may utilize a scenario-planning decision tool such as the "Best Case-Worst Case" tool developed by vascular surgeon and bioethicist, Margaret Schwarze.[33,34]

In this case, multiple factors must be considered during care discussions, including the establishment of decision-making capacity and a surrogate decision maker (the sister), coordination of care for both the patient and her father, and management of disease at an advanced stage. For this patient, the best case scenario would be an uncomplicated surgery with a well healed flap. Although hedgehog inhibitors should be discussed as an option for eye preservation, this patient's desire for quick recovery and return to her father, as well as her prior delay in seeking care with concerns for

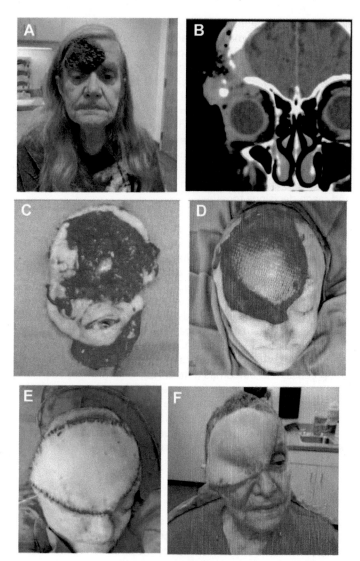

Fig. 2. (A–F): Case 2. (A): Image of a large, locally invasive basal cell carcinoma of the right forehead and brow. (B): Coronal image depicting the aggressive nature of the tumor. Bone destruction is noted, as well as intracranial and intraorbital invasion of tumor. (C): Surgical specimen clearly showing orbital exenteration as a component of the removed tumor. (D): Surgical reconstruction showing titanium mesh over the resected calvarial bone. (E): Soft tissue reconstruction with a large anterolateral thigh free flap. (F): 2-month postoperative photograph of the patient. (*Courtesy of* Peter Dziegielewski, MD, Gainesville, FL.)

medical decision-making capacity, may make definitive surgical management the better choice in this complicated case. Her father will likely require placement in a nursing facility during her hospitalization, and it is possible that both she and her father will require custodial care. Additionally, the failure of her sister to help with their father in the past may make the patient wary of relying on her for her own care or decision making, even if it is appropriate. By reframing the story of her acute problem to a more holistic view of the care needs of both her father and herself, she may be able to pursue what Arthur Frank would call a quest narrative to a new normal, where she and her father may be able to reside in the same facility with mutual assistance.

SUMMARY

Ethical considerations in a certain disease in the aging population begs the questions: How is this different from general medical ethics for all patients, with all diseases? And Is there something unique about elderly patients with cutaneous malignancy that requires specific ethical considerations? This article has argued that yes, this disease in these patients poses ethical challenges that are better met by a relational ethical framework such as narrative ethics, which can enrich traditional ethical principlism.

There are, of course, more universal, general ethical considerations that also apply. These are perhaps best summed up by the questions: What is too much?, What is too little?, and Who decides? Specifically, this article has looked at a case of a patient who made age-based decisions for conservative care and had to pay the price of progressive disease at a later more fragile state and have grappled with the social and cultural challenges surrounding the care of a partially capacitated patient.

Some cutaneous malignancies threaten to be life limiting even at the time of diagnosis, such as MCC, melanoma, and cancers in immunosuppressed patients. For many patients, however, skin cancer is not understood to be potentially fatal. When it is, or when it threatens to be so, it can shake one's understanding of life and health. An analogy may be a refractory decubitus ulcer at the end of life; physicians push nutrition and wound care, but, in truth, this is an organ failure as much as heart or kidney or lung failure. It is an unfixable problem that portends approaching death.[35] When skin cancers break their polite social boundaries and become invasive, disfiguring, or regionally or distantly metastatic, they too are announcing the failure of the body's largest organ. These 2 cases have illustrated the use of narrative to help guide the process of shared decision making.

CLINICS CARE POINTS

- Patients and their families make decisions based on the information physicians give them, and they understand that information in the context of their existing identity and narrative. Considerable care must be taken to be comprehensible, compassionate, and fair in descriptions of the outcomes of treatments ranging from extensive surgery to supportive care.

- A palliative approach to patient care attends to the whole caregiving circle that encompasses the patient. Decisions that will result in dependence or change in caregiving needs affect more than just an autonomous individual, and those considerations are ethically valid and morally essential.

DISCLOSURE

The authors have nothing to disclose.

REFERENCES

1. Nabozny MJ, Kruser JM, Steffens NM, et al. Patient-reported limitations to surgical buy-in: a qualitative study of patients facing high-risk surgery. Ann Surg 2016; 265(1):97–102.

2. Pecanac KE, Kehler JM, Brasel KJ, et al. It's big surgery: preoperative expressions of risk, responsibility, and commitment to treatment after high-risk operations. Ann Surg 2014;259(3):458–63.

3. Gandhi SA, Kampp J. Skin cancer epidemiology, detection, and management. Med Clin North Am 2015;99(6):1323–35.

4. Siegel RL, Miller KD, Jemal A. Cancer statistics, 2019. CA Cancer J Clin 2019; 69(1):7–34.

5. Ciocan D, Barbe C, Aubin F, et al. Distinctive features of melanoma and its management in elderly patients: a population-based study in France. JAMA Dermatol 2013;149(10):1150–7.

6. Renzi M Jr, Schimmel J, Decker A, et al. Management of skin cancer in the elderly. Dermatol Clin 2019;37(3):279–86.

7. Paulson KG, Park SY, Vandeven NA, et al. Merkel cell carcinoma: current US incidence and projected increases based on changing demographics. J Am Acad Dermatol 2018;78(3):457–463 e452.

8. Schadendorf D, Lebbe C, Zur Hausen A, et al. Merkel cell carcinoma: epidemiology, prognosis, therapy and unmet medical needs. Eur J Cancer 2017;71: 53–69.

9. Fontanella D, Grant-Kels JM, Patel T, et al. Ethical issues in geriatric dermatology. Clin Dermatol 2012;30(5):511–5.

10. Beauchamp TL, Childress JF. Principles of biomedical ethics. 8th edition. New York (NY): Oxford University Press; 2019.

11. Callahan D. Can the social sciences save bioethics? J Clin Ethics 2014; 25(1):32–5.

12. Moye J, Marson DC. Assessment of decision-making capacity in older adults: an emerging area of practice and research. J Gerontol B Psychol Sci Soc Sci 2007; 62(1):P3–11.

13. Brody H. Shared decision making and determining decision-making capacity. Prim Care 2005;32(3):645–658, vi.

14. Lucente FE. Ethical challenges in geriatric care. Otolaryngol Head Neck Surg 2009;140(6):809–11.

15. McKoy JM, Burhenn PS, Browner IS, et al. Assessing cognitive function and capacity in older adults with cancer. J Natl Compr Canc Netw 2014;12(1):138–44.

16. Rocque GB, Pisu M, Jackson BE, et al. Resource use and medicare costs during lay navigation for geriatric patients with cancer. JAMA Oncol 2017;3(6):817–25.

17. Szturz P, Vermorken JB. Treatment of elderly patients with squamous cell carcinoma of the head and neck. Front Oncol 2016;6:199.

18. Charon R. The patient-physician relationship. Narrative medicine: a model for empathy, reflection, profession, and trust. JAMA 2001;286(15):1897–902.

19. Frank AW. The wounded storyteller: body, illness, and ethics. Chicago (IL): University of Chicago Press; 1997.

20. Ratcliff C, Naik AD, Martin LA, et al. Examining cancer survivorship trajectories: exploring the intersection between qualitative illness narratives and quantitative screening instruments. Palliat Support Care 2018;16(6):712–8.

21. Frank AW. Truth telling, companionship, and witness: an agenda for narrative ethics. Hastings Cent Rep 2016;46(3):17–21.

22. Batt-Rawden SA, Chisolm MS, Anton B, et al. Teaching empathy to medical students: an updated, systematic review. Acad Med 2013;88(8):1171–7.

23. Brody H. The healer's power. New Haven (CT): Yale University Press; 1992.

24. Brody H. Transparency and self-censorship in shared decision-making. Am J Bioeth 2007;7(7):44–6.

25. Brody HA. New forces shaping the patient-physician relationship. Virtual Mentor 2009;11(3):253–6.

26. Putman MS, Yoon JD, Rasinski KA, et al. Directive counsel and morally controversial medical decision-making: findings from two national surveys of primary care physicians. J Gen Intern Med 2014;29(2):335–40.

27. Yoon JD, Rasinski KA, Curlin FA. Moral controversy, directive counsel, and the doctor's role: findings from a national survey of obstetrician-gynecologists. Acad Med 2010;85(9):1475–81.

28. Kleinman A. On illness meanings and clinical interpretation: not 'rational man', but a rational approach to man the sufferer/man the healer. Cult Med Psychiatry 1981; 5(4):373–7.

29. Kleinman A. Suffering, ethics, and the politics of moral life. Cult Med Psychiatry 1996;20(3):287–90.

30. Deilhes F, Boulinguez S, Pages C, et al. Advanced cutaneous squamous cell carcinoma is associated with suboptimal initial management in a cohort of 109 patients. Dermatology 2019;235(6):516–21.

31. Rogers EM, Connolly KL, Nehal KS, et al. Comorbidity scores associated with limited life expectancy in the very elderly with nonmelanoma skin cancer. J Am Acad Dermatol 2018;78(6):1119–24.

32. Hegde UP, Grant-Kels JM. Ethical issues in cutaneous melanoma. Clin Dermatol 2012;30(5):501–10.

33. Kruser JM, Nabozny MJ, Steffens NM, et al. Best Case/Worst Case": qualitative evaluation of a novel communication tool for difficult in-the-moment surgical decisions. J Am Geriatr Soc 2015;63(9):1805–11.

34. Schwarze ML, Kehler JM, Campbell TC. Navigating high risk procedures with more than just a street map. J Palliat Med 2013;16(10):1169–71.

35. Brody H, Hermer LD, Scott LD, et al. Artificial nutrition and hydration: the evolution of ethics, evidence, and policy. J Gen Intern Med 2011;26(9):1053–8.

Injectables in Head and Neck Cutaneous Melanoma Treatment

Brad Rumancik, PharmD, Lawrence Mark, MD, PhD*

KEYWORDS

- Otolaryngology • Cutaneous melanoma • Injectable • Talimogene laherparepvec
- Oncolytic virus

KEY POINTS

- Local injectables for cutaneous melanoma offer the benefit of local and possibly systemic antitumor effects with minimal adverse effects compared with other systemic therapies.
- Local injectables are particularly beneficial for unresectable melanomas, an occurrence often seen in otolaryngology.
- Talimogene laherparepvec, an attenuated type 1 herpes simplex virus, is the most clinically relevant local injectable for unresectable melanoma.
- In patients with unresectable stage IIIB to IV melanoma, talimogene laherparepvec showed a durable response rate of 19% and suggested overall survival advantages in phase III studies. Subanalyses showed strengthened durable response rates for lower-stage melanoma and treatment naivety. These findings were maintained in patients who had cutaneous head and neck melanoma.
- There are numerous ongoing trials for intratumoral injectables in melanoma, including talimogene laherparepvec combined with systemic immunotherapies, other oncolytic viruses, and a variety of nonviral agents.

INTRODUCTION: MELANOMA IN OTOLARYNGOLOGY

Up to 15% to 20% of cutaneous melanomas occur in the head and neck region, possibly because of increased sun exposure and melanocyte concentration in this region.[1–3] Several factors distinguish cutaneous head and neck melanomas from those occurring on other body parts. First, head and neck melanomas have lower survival and higher recurrence rates compared with other primary cutaneous melanomas.[1,3,4] There is a rich, complex, and superficial lymphatic system of the head and neck that is thought to play a role in facilitating metastases.[4] Importantly, surgical resection of

Department of Dermatology, Indiana University School of Medicine, 545 Barnhill Drive Emerson Hall 139, Indianapolis, IN 46202, USA
* Corresponding author.
E-mail address: lamark@iu.edu

Otolaryngol Clin N Am 54 (2021) 425–438
https://doi.org/10.1016/j.otc.2020.11.014
0030-6665/21/© 2020 Elsevier Inc. All rights reserved.

head and neck melanomas are often limited because of functional and cosmetic concerns. Although there have been many advances in melanoma therapy, management of head and neck melanoma has remained challenging.[5] Intratumoral injectables may aid in the management of head and neck melanomas where resection is difficult or impossible.

A Historical Perspective

The goal of intratumoral immunotherapies is to stimulate local and systemic immune responses through direct tumor injection. Theoretically, lysis of local tumor cells and release of tumor-derived antigens could evoke a systemic immune response, much like a vaccination. William Bradley Coley is often recognized as the father of cancer immunotherapy, because, in the 1890s, he refined previous reports of erysipelas-induced tumor regression by using heat-killed *Streptococcus pyogenes* and *Serratia marcescens* as a direct inoculum to manage recurrent sarcoma.[6] His contemporary, George Dock, reported the first viral-induced tumor regression in a patient with leukemia in 1904.[7]

In 1975, a metastatic melanoma case report described a remarkable response to direct tumor injection with bacillus Calmette-Guérin bacterium, an attenuated *Mycobacterium bovis* strain.[8] However, use of this technique in melanoma has been limited by serious adverse events (AEs) such as disseminated intravascular coagulation and death from hypersensitivity reactions.[9] Rose Bengal, an inflammatory dye, has been studied since the 1980s and is currently under investigation for melanoma, as described at the end of this article.[9] Other nonviral injectables, such as toll-like receptor agonists and immunomodulating cytokines (ie, interleukin-2 [IL-2]), have received continued attention since the 1990s.[9,10]

A large variety of viral species, predominately adenovirus, herpesvirus, vaccinia virus, and reovirus, have been studied for use as oncolytic viruses.[11] In 2005, the Chinese Food and Drug Administration provided the world's first approval of an oncolytic virus, H101 variant of adenovirus, for refractory nasopharyngeal carcinoma in combination with chemotherapy.[12] In 2015, talimogene laherparepvec (T-VEC), a modified herpes simplex virus, became the first, and currently the only, United States Food and Drug Administration (FDA)–approved oncolytic virus for use in melanoma.[13]

Talimogene Laherparepvec Background and Mechanism of Action

T-VEC is an FDA-approved oncolytic virus with the labeled indication for treating unresectable cutaneous, subcutaneous, and nodal melanoma lesions.[13] T-VEC is a second-generation, live attenuated, type 1 herpes simplex virus (HSV-1). First-generation oncolytic HSVs were developed through deletion of the *neurovirulence factor infected cell protein 34.5 (ICP 34.5)* gene. *ICP34.5* gene deletion attenuates HSV pathogenicity toward healthy cells while enhancing tumor-cell specificity.[14] In addition to maintaining deletion of the *ICP34.5* gene, T-VEC has further modifications summarized in **Table 1**.[15] Selective and rapid oncolysis causes release of tumor antigens and granulocyte-macrophage colony-stimulating factor (GM-CSF), thereby stimulating a local and sometimes systemic immune response against tumor cells (**Fig. 1**).[16,17]

Talimogene Laherparepvec Monotherapy: Clinical Trials

The phase III Oncovex[GM-CSF] Pivotal Trial in Melanoma (OPTiM) study is the largest randomized controlled trial studying oncolytic viruses for unresectable melanoma. In this multicenter study, patients with unresectable stage IIIB to IV melanoma were randomized in a 2:1 ratio to receive intralesional T-VEC versus subcutaneous GM-CSF. T-VEC was administered with an initial 10^6 plaque forming units (pfu)/mL dose, to

Table 1
Herpes simplex virus pathophysiology and talimogene laherparepvec modifications

Gene	Pathophysiologic Function	Modification
ICP34.5	Infection of neurons and other healthy cells	ICP34.5 deletion: tumor-selective virulence
ICP47	Inhibits HSV antigen presentation	ICP47 deletion: disinhibits antigen presentation and increases antigenicity of infected tumor cells
US11	Permits HSV-1 replication	US11 increased expression: increased viral replication and thus increased oncolytic potency
GM-CSF	Enhances dendritic cell recruitment (thereby increasing antigen presentation and T-cell activation)	GM-CSF gene insertion: release of GM-CSF on oncolysis thus strengthening local, and likely systemic, antitumor immune response

seroconvert HSV-seronegative patients. Three weeks later, 10^8 pfu/mL was then dosed once every 2 weeks thereafter. Injected volume per lesion varied from 0.1 mL to 4.0 mL based on the size of each lesion. Maximum total volume per treatment session was 4.0 mL. The GM-CSF regimen was 125 mg/m^2 subcutaneously once daily for 14 days in 28-day cycles. The primary end point was durable response rate (DRR), defined as the rate of complete response (CR) plus partial response (PR) lasting greater than or equal to 6 months and beginning within the first 12 months of therapy.[18]

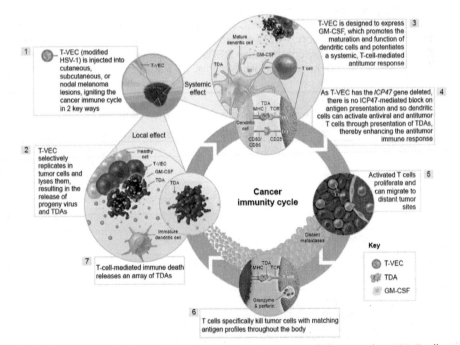

Fig. 1. Mechanism of action of T-VEC. MHC, major histocompatibility complex; TCR, T-cell receptor; TDA, tumor-derived antigen. (Used with permission of Amgen Inc.)

The OPTiM study included 436 patients in the intention-to-treat analysis, of which 57% of the patients had stage IIIB, IIIC, or IVM1a melanoma (considered lower stages in this trial). At time of final analysis, 3 years after the last patient was randomized, median duration of treatment was 23.1 weeks (range, 0.1–176.7 weeks) for T-VEC and 10 weeks (range, 0.6–120 weeks) for GM-CSF. Median follow-up time from randomization to analysis was 49 months. Regarding the primary end point, T-VEC had a favorable DRR compared with GM-CSF (**Table 2**). Exploratory analyses revealed improved T-VEC outcomes for lower melanoma stages compared with those with stage IVM1b or IVM1c disease. The following DRRs were calculated: stage IIIB/IIIC (T-VEC 33% vs GM-CSF 0%, $P<.0001$), IVM1a (24% vs 0%, $P = .0003$), IVM1b (6.3% vs 3.8%, $P = 1.0$), and IVM1c (9% vs 3.4%, $P = .67$). The primary OPTiM analysis also revealed patients had improved DRRs with T-VEC in treatment-naive disease (24% vs 0% with GM-CSF) compared with those receiving T-VEC as salvage therapy (10% vs 4% with GM-CSF).[18,19]

Systemic immune effects of local T-VEC injection were shown by responses seen in uninjected lesions, as described in **Table 3**. In addition, 5% of T-VEC patients developed vitiligo compared with 0.8% (n = 1) of GM-CSF patients, suggesting an immune response elicited against melanocyte proteins.[18]

Among responding patients, median time to response and median duration of response are summarized in **Table 2**. The final analysis of OPTiM further showed the durable response to T-VEC. Of the 17% of T-VEC–treated patients who obtained a CR, median duration of CR was not reached over a median follow-up period of 4 years.[19]

The final analysis of the OPTiM study in 2019 revealed no difference in median overall survival (OS) for T-VEC versus GM-CSF; however, in T-VEC–treated patients with CRs, the median OS was not reached, with an estimate of 90% living at 5 years[19]

A subanalysis was conducted on the OPTiM study patients who had cutaneous head and neck melanoma.[20] The T-VEC group consisted of 61 patients versus 26 patients in the GM-CSF group. T-VEC efficacy was maintained in the cutaneous head and neck melanoma subgroup because DRRs for T-VEC and GM-CSF were 36.1% versus 3.8% ($P = .001$), respectively. Notably, 29.5% of head and neck patients

Table 2
Oncovex[GM-CSF] pivotal trial in melanoma study: response rates and timing

	T-VEC n = 295	GM-CSF n = 141	Statistical Analysis
DRR (%)	19.0	1.4	Odds ratio (95% CI): 16.6 (4.0–69.2) $P<.0001$
ORR, % (95% CI)	31.5 (26.3–37.2)	6.4 (3.0–11.8)	$P<.0001$
CR, %	16.9	0.7	—
PR (%)	14.6	5.7	—
Median Time to Response, mo (Range)[a]	4.1 (1.2–16.7)	3.7 (1.9–9.1)	—
Median Duration of Response, mo (Range)[b]	Not reached	2.8 mo	—

Abbreviation: ORR, overall response rate.

[a] Values obtained from OPTiM 2015 primary analysis. In the 2019 final analysis, median time to CR in T-VEC–treated patients was 8.6 months (range, 2.1–42.3 months).

[b] Values obtained from OPTiM 2015 primary analysis. In the 2019 final analysis, duration of response was not reached over a median 4-year follow-up period for patients treated with T-VEC and who achieved a CR.

Table 3
2015 Oncovex^{GM-CSF} pivotal trial in melanoma study primary analysis: comparison of talimogene laherparepvec–treated general study population versus talimogene laherparepvec–treated patients with cutaneous head and neck melanoma

Parameter Measured	T-VEC OPTiM General Population n = 295	T-VEC OPTiM Head and Neck n = 61
Disease Stage		
IIIB (%)	8	15
IIIC (%)	22	28
IVM1a (%)	25	18
IVM1b (%)	22	25
IVM1c (%)	23	15
IIIB + IIIC (%)	30	43
DRR, % (95% CI)	16.3 (12.1–20.5)	36.1 (24.2–49.4)
ORR, % (95% CI)	26.4 (21.4–31.5)	47.5 (34.6–60.7)
CR (%)	10.8	29.5
PR (%)	15.6	18
Injected Lesions Response	64% of injected lesions decreased ≥50% in size	Responses were identified in 63.8% of injected lesions
Uninjected Lesions Response	34% of nonvisceral and 15% of visceral lesions decreased ≥50% in size	Responses were identified in 7.9% of uninjected lesions and 10.8% of visceral lesions

Abbreviations: CR, complete response; DRR, durable response rate; ORR, overall response rate; PR, partial response; T-VEC, talimogene laherparepvec.

had a CR with T-VEC compared with 0% with GM-CSF. T-VEC also produced an effect on uninjected lesions, as summarized in **Table 3**. Median OS for GM-CSF was 25.2 months but was not reached for the T-VEC group; additionally, a multivariate sensitivity analysis to adjust for baseline characteristics calculated that T-VEC had an improved OS (hazard ratio [HR], 0.38; 95% confidence interval [CI], 0.20–0.72; P = .003). Compared with the original OPTiM study T-VEC group, the T-VEC–treated patients with cutaneous head and neck melanoma had a higher DRR, overall response rate (ORR), CR, and PR (see **Table 3**). Importantly, these more favorable response rates were seen in the context of a higher proportion of stage IIIB and IIIC patients in the T-VEC–treated head and neck melanoma group (43%) compared with the T-VEC–treated original study population (30%).[18,20]

In summary, the phase III OPTiM study showed that T-VEC treatment leads to improved DRR and suggested OS advantages compared with GM-CSF. Improved DRR and OS in T-VEC–treated patients were most notable for stages IIIB to IVM1a and treatment-naive patients. Local T-VEC injections also showed clinically meaningfully effects on uninjected tumors. The beneficial effects of T-VEC were maintained in the head and neck population.

Talimogene Laherparepvec Combination Therapy: Clinical Trials

Immune checkpoint inhibitors, including ipilimumab, a cytotoxic T lymphocyte–associated antigen-4 (CLTA-4) inhibitor, and pembrolizumab, an anti–programmed death-1 (PD-1) receptor antibody, have led to improved survival responses with tolerable side effect profiles in patients with melanoma.[21] Data are maturing regarding T-VEC therapy combined with immune checkpoint inhibitors such as ipilimumab and pembrolizumab (discussed later).[10,22,23] Overall, T-VEC plus checkpoint inhibitors show promise; however, further studies and longer follow-up times are required to further elucidate the utility of T-VEC combination therapy.

Talimogene Laherparepvec Adverse Events

The OPTiM study found T-VEC to be well tolerated. The most common AEs were fatigue (50.3%), chills (48.6%), pyrexia (42.8%), nausea (35.6%), and influenzalike symptoms (30.5%). Within the T-VEC group, 11.3% of patients experienced grade 3 or grade 4 AEs versus 4.7% in the GM-CSF group. Immune-related AEs occurred in 8.1% of the T-VEC–treated patients, of which 4 events were grade 3 and there were no grade 4 immune-related AEs. Vitiligo, the presence of which suggests systemic immune response to melanocytes, was the most common immune-related AE seen in 6.2% of the T-VEC patients.[18] Overall, the incidence of grade 3 or grade 4 AEs was similar to reports for PD-1 inhibitors and lower than for CTLA-4, and T-VEC lacked the common AEs seen in immune checkpoint inhibitors, such as autoimmune thyroiditis, adrenalitis, hypophysitis, and hepatitis.[21,24,25]

Implications of Herpes Simplex Virus Oncolytic Virus and Talimogene Laherparepvec Administration

Using HSV as the oncolytic virus has several implications. First, during the phase I study of T-VEC, the initial dose of 10^8 pfu/mL had to be reduced to 10^6 pfu/mL for all HSV-seronegative patients because of pronounced AEs.[26] This dosing strategy, 10^6 pfu/mL for the first dosing session, was adopted for the subsequent phase III OPTiM study and is now the recommended strategy for all patients (**Tables 4** and **5**).[13] Baseline serology to assess HSV serostatus is not a requirement for starting

Table 4			
Talimogene laherparepvec dosing schedule			
Treatment Visit	**Treatment Interval**	**Concentration (PFU/mL)**	**Prioritization of Lesions to be Injected**
Initial	—	10^6	Inject largest lesions first. Prioritize injection of remaining lesions based on lesion size until maximum injection volume is reached or until all injectable lesions have been treated
Second	3 wk after initial treatment	10^8	Inject any new lesions (lesions that have developed since initial treatment) first Prioritize injection of remaining lesions based on lesion size until maximum injection volume is reached or until all injectable lesions have been treated
All subsequent treatments	2 wk after previous treatment	10^8	Inject any new lesions (lesions that have developed since previous treatment) first Prioritize injection of remaining lesions based on lesion size until maximum injection volume is reached or until all injectable lesions have been treated

Adapted from Imlygic® (talimogene laherparepvec) package insert. Used with permission of Amgen Inc.

Table 5
Recommended dosing ratio: injection volume to lesions size

Lesion Size (Longest Dimension) (cm)	Injection Volume[a] (mL)
>5	Up to 4
>2.5–5	Up to 2
>1.5–2.5 cm	Up to 1
>0.5–1.5 cm	Up to 0.5
≤0.5	Up to 0.1

[a] Maximum injection volume per treatment visit (eg, all lesions combined) is 4 mL.
Adapted from Imlygic® (talimogene laherparepvec) package insert. Used with permission of Amgen Inc.

T-VEC. There has been no statistically significant association between HSV serostatus and efficacy outcomes.[19,22]

The phase III OPTiM study had 16 subjects (5.5%) in the T-VEC group who developed HSV-related AEs (15 subjects developed oral herpes and 1 subject, with a past history of herpetic keratitis, had recurrence of herpetic keratitis).[18,27] Polymerase chain reaction testing was not performed to determine wild-type status, so the herpetic reactions may have been activation of dormant native HSV. T-VEC is contraindicated in immunocompromised patients because it is a live, attenuated HSV, which could lead to a life-threatening infection. Avoidance of T-VEC should also be considered on a case-by-case basis during pregnancy because of theoretic fetal risks.[28] Viral shedding risk is low and close contacts are at low risk of contracting HSV; however, patients should still be educated on viral shedding and advised to engage in safe practices, as elaborated on by Harrington and colleagues.[13,15,27,29]

T-VEC is stored at −90°C to −70°C and should be thawed at room temperature immediately before injection. T-VEC is to be injected directly into cutaneous, subcutaneous, and nodal lesions that are visible, palpable, or detectable by ultrasonography guidance using a single insertion point to create multiple tracts covering the radial distance of the needle (**Fig. 2**). Before rotating the needle to create a new tract, the needle should be withdrawn until the tip is just deep to the puncture site. This method prevents the possibility of a needle fracture from undue torque within fibrotic lesions. T-VEC does not have approval for visceral lesion injections. Lesion prioritization, T-VEC dosing, and injection frequency are summarized in **Tables 4** and **5**. Multiple injection sites, using a separate needle for each injection, may be used if the lesion is larger than the needle radial distance. If necrosis is present, injecting the border of

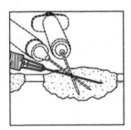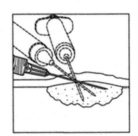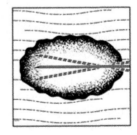

Fig. 2. Radial injection of (*left*) cutaneous, (*middle*) subcutaneous, and (*right*) nodal lesions. (Used with permission of Amgen Inc.)

the lesion theoretically increases chances of injecting viable tumor cells. Topical or local anesthesia may be used, but do not directly inject the lesion with anesthetic or mix anesthetic with T-VEC. The authors recommend using needles of 26 to 30 gauge for patient comfort. Small unit syringes (eg, 0.5-mL insulin syringes) enhance injection control. Needle withdrawal should be slow to prevent leakage from injection sites. After withdrawal, apply pressure with sterile gauze for 30 seconds, sterilize injection site and surrounding area with alcohol, change gloves or remove the top glove of 2 gloves, then apply an absorbent pad and dry occlusive dressing. Maintain dressing for 1 week, or longer if injection site oozing is present. Used dressings should be placed in a sealed plastic bag and discarded in the garbage.[13]

T-VEC has a biosafety level 1 classification and the risk for transmission to a healthy, adult health care worker using appropriate personal protective equipment (gowns, face shields, and gloves) is low.[15,28,29] The authors are aware of 2 reports of herpetic whitlow occurring in health care providers from accidental needle sticks during T-VEC administration.[15,27,30] T-VEC should not be prepared or administered by immunocompromised or pregnant individuals.[13,15] Some investigators have suggested the use of Luer-Lock needles to prevent needle detachment as the syringe develops high pressure when injecting fibrotic lesions.[15] Should an infection in a patient or health care provider occur, T-VEC has been designed to retain susceptibility to thymidine kinase inhibitors.[29,30] Of note, avoidance of thymidine kinase inhibitors in patients receiving T-VEC is recommended because of the potential to decrease oncolytic effect.[13]

Talimogene Laherparepvec Systemic Immune Effects and Pseudoprogression

The systemic immune effects of T-VEC are theorized to be caused by release of local tumor-derived antigens and virally encoded GM-CSF on destruction of injected tumor cells. Biopsies of regressing lesions, both injected and uninjected, from 11 T-VEC–treated patients were associated with the presence of MART-1 (melanoma antigen recognized by T cells 1)–specific cluster of differentiation (CD) [+]8 T cells and a reduction in CD4[+] regulatory T cells, providing evidence for systemic immune effects.[16,17] Benefits of systemic immune effects of T-VEC are noticed clinically (see **Table 3**).

A well-reported phenomenon related to the immunotherapies, including T-VEC, is pseudoprogression.[31,32] Pseudoprogression has been defined as a greater than 25% increase in total baseline tumor area or tumor burden or the appearance of a new lesion before clinical improvement.[17] Forty-eight percent of the T-VEC–treated OPTiM subjects who had a durable response experienced pseudoprogression before response (PPR). Importantly, PPR led to a delay in achieving durable response by approximately 3 months compared with those who did not experience PPR; however, there was no difference in duration of response or survival for those experiencing PPR.[17]

Pseudoprogression can create challenging clinical assessments of worsening tumor burden in the face of forthcoming improvement. There is not enough evidence to stratify T-VEC patients at greatest risk of pseudoprogression.[17] Immune-related response criteria or immune-related Response Evaluation Criteria in Solid Tumors (RECIST) can account for pseudoprogression and are more clinically appropriate for monitoring response to immunotherapies compared with the World Health Organization (WHO) criteria or RECIST.[15,32,33] Investigators have recommended maintaining T-VEC treatment for at least 6 months, as clinically appropriate, in anticipation of improvement of lesions.[13,15,19] This recommendation is consistent with OPTiM methodology of continuing treatment for at least 6 months regardless of occurrence of progressive disease (unless clinically appropriate alternative therapies are indicated).[18]

Table 6
Noteworthy ongoing clinical trials of injectables in melanoma

Study Agent	Description	Interventions	Phase	Clinical Trial
Nonviral Agents				
PV-10	Rose Bengal (inflammatory dye)	PV-10 vs systemic dacarbazine, temozolomide, or intralesional T-VEC	Phase III	NCT02288897
		PV-10 + pembrolizumab vs pembrolizumab	Phase Ib/II	NCT02257321
Tilsotolimod (IMO-2125)	TLR9 agonist	Intratumoral tilsotolimod + ipilimumab vs ipilimumab	Phase III	NCT03445533
CMP-001	TLR9 agonist	CMP-001 + nivolumab	Phase II	NCT03618641
		CMP-001 + pembrolizumab	Phase IB	NCT02680184
IL-2 and BCG	Inflammatory cytokine and attenuated *M bovis*	IL-2 + BCG vs IL-2	Phase II/III	NCT03928275
Viral Agents				
T-VEC	Herpesvirus	T-VEC + pembrolizumab vs placebo + pembrolizumab	Phase Ib/III	NCT02263508
		T-VEC neoadjuvant + surgery vs immediate surgery	Phase II	NCT02211131
		T-VEC + pembrolizumab	Phase II	NCT02965716
		Autologous CD1c (BDCA-1)+ myeloid dendritic cells + T-VEC	Phase II	NCT03747744
		T-VEC + hypofractionated radiotherapy vs T-VEC	Phase I	NCT02819843
		T-VEC + nivolumab	Phase II	NCT04330430
		T-VEC + pembrolizumab	Phase II	NCT03842943
		T-VEC + dabrafenib + trametinib	Phase Ib	NCT03088176
HF10	Herpesvirus	HF10 + nivolumab	Phase II	NCT03259425
ONCOS-102	Adenovirus	ONCOS-102 + pembrolizumab	Phase I	NCT03003676
OBP-301	Adenovirus	OBP-301	Phase 2	NCT03190824
CVA21	Coxsackievirus	CVA21 + pembrolizumab	Phase I	NCT02565992
		CVA21 + ipilimumab	Phase I	NCT02307149
PVSRIPO	Poliovirus/rhinovirus	PVSRIPO	Phase I	NCT03712358

Abbreviations: BCG, bacillus Calmette-Guérin; TLR, toll-like receptor.

Postmarket Studies

Although a large portion of OPTiM study subjects (45%) had advanced-stage disease (IV1b/IV1c), postmarketing case series of T-VEC monotherapy have shown better efficacy data than the OPTiM study owing to these primarily evaluating melanoma stage IIIB to IVM1a disease.[34–37] A case series, COSMUS-1 (Clinical Observational Study of talimogene laherparepvec use among Melanoma patients in routine clinical practice in the United States), included 76 patients, of whom 39% had stage IVM1b/c disease (compared with 45% in OPTiM). Patients received T-VEC as monotherapy (22%) or any combination of immunotherapy, targeted therapy, radiation, or chemotherapy occurring before, concurrent with, or after T-VEC therapy. Of patients completing T-VEC therapy, 19.7% achieved CR or no remaining injectable lesions, findings comparable with OPTiM (16.9% CR).[38]

Advancing the Clinical Utility of Talimogene Laherparepvec

T-VEC has the potential to advance melanoma treatment in a variety of situations. It can be considered for salvage therapy in patients having failed systemic chemotherapy and immunotherapy.[37,39,40] Given the lack of approved neoadjuvant treatment of resectable stage IIIB to IVM1a melanoma, an ongoing randomized controlled trial is assessing the utility of T-VEC as a neoadjuvant therapy (ClinicalTrials.gov identifier: NCT02211131).[41] One-year analysis of 150 patients with stage IIIB to IVM1a melanoma allocated in a 1:1 ratio for T-VEC neoadjuvant plus surgical resection versus surgical resection alone revealed recurrence-free rates of 33.5% versus 21.9% (HR, 0.73; $P = .048$) in favor of T-VEC neoadjuvant therapy.[41]

Other Available Injectables

Intralesional IL-2 is characterized as having a strong local response rate, minimal systemic response, and tolerable side effect profile. A phase II study evaluating IL-2 in 51 patients with metastatic melanoma found CR rates for 6 months or longer in 70% of injected metastases. However, there was no response in distant, uninjected metastases, which is a major limitation.[42] A 2014 systematic review analyzed 49 studies of IL-2 use for in-transit melanoma and found 78% CR rate per lesion and 50% CR rate per subject.[43] In contrast with the severe side effects seen with systemic IL-2, intralesional IL-2 is well tolerated from an AE perspective.[42,43] IL-2 is expensive, and each lesion requires multiple injections per week, which limits its clinical utility.

Rose Bengal is a photosensitizing dye selectively taken up by tumor-cell lysosomes. PV-10, a 10% Rose Bengal solution, has preliminary results suggesting efficacy in injected and uninjected metastatic melanoma lesions. PV-10 is only available in the clinical trial setting. The phase II study revealed an ORR of 51% in injected lesions and an ORR of 33% in uninjected lesions.[44] In addition, a phase Ib/II study comparing PV-10 plus pembrolizumab versus pembrolizumab alone is currently recruiting [NCT02557321].

Ongoing Clinical Trials

Table 6 summarizes ongoing investigations into intralesional treatments for melanoma.

SUMMARY

Head and neck cutaneous melanomas are challenging to treat, often because of the limited potential for surgical resection. Intratumoral injectables offer the benefit of local and potentially systemic responses, which are of particular value in unresectable lesions. T-VEC, an attenuated oncolytic HSV-1, is currently the most clinically relevant injectable for cutaneous melanoma. T-VEC has been shown to improve DRR, with suggested OS advantages compared with systemic GM-CSF therapy in patients with stage IIIB to IVM1a unresectable melanoma. These benefits are also most noticed in treatment-naive patients. The efficacy of T-VEC is maintained in patients with head and neck melanoma. The benefits of T-VEC are supported by real-world-use postmarketing studies. T-VEC plus systemic immunotherapies are being studied with promising preliminary data; however, the clinical utility of combination therapy is limited until more data are available. There are numerous ongoing clinical trials investigating other viral and nonviral injectables.

CLINICS CARE POINTS

- Ultrasound guidance can make injection of deeper tumors easier and more accurate.
- T-VEC is generally well tolerated with manageable flu-like reactions.
- Viral shedding risk is low but pregnant and immunocompromised individuals should be guarded against handing post injection drainage or contaminated bandages.
- T-VEC has been designed to retain susceptibility to thymidine kinase inhibitors.

DISCLOSURE

The authors have no commercial or financial conflicts of interest and did not receive funding for this article.

REFERENCES

1. Fadaki N, Li R, Parrett B, et al. Is head and neck melanoma different from trunk and extremity melanomas with respect to sentinel lymph node status and clinical outcome? Ann Surg Oncol 2013;20(9):3089–97.
2. Ellis MC, Weerasinghe R, Corless CL, et al. Sentinel lymph node staging of cutaneous melanoma: predictors and outcomes. Am J Surg 2010;199(5):663–8.
3. Golger A, Young DS, Ghazarian D, et al. Epidemiological features and prognostic factors of cutaneous head and neck melanoma: a population-based study. Arch Otolaryngol Head Neck Surg 2007;133(5):442–7.
4. Lachiewicz AM, Berwick M, Wiggins CL, et al. Survival differences between patients with scalp or neck melanoma and those with melanoma of other sites in the Surveillance, Epidemiology, and End Results (SEER) program. Arch Dermatol 2008;144(4):515–21.
5. Klop WMC, Elshot YS, Beck ACC, et al. Oncodermatology of the Head and Neck. Facial Plast Surg 2019;35(4):368–76.
6. Raja J, Ludwig JM, Gettinger SN, et al. Oncolytic virus immunotherapy: future prospects for oncology. J Immunother Cancer 2018;6(1):140.
7. Dock G. The influence of complicating diseases upon leukaemia. Am J Med Sci 1904;127:563–92.
8. Mastrangelo MJ, Bellet RE, Berkelhammer J, et al. Regression of pulmonary metastatic disease associated with intralesional BCG therapy of intracutaneous melanoma metastases. Cancer 1975;36(4):1305–8.
9. Bommareddy PK, Silk AW, Kaufman HL. Intratumoral approaches for the treatment of melanoma. Cancer J 2017;23(1):40–7.

10. Hamid O, Ismail R, Puzanov I. Intratumoral immunotherapy-update 2019. Oncologist 2020;25(3):e423–38.

11. Zheng M, Huang J, Tong A, et al. Oncolytic viruses for cancer therapy: barriers and recent advances. Mol Ther Oncolytics 2019;15:234–47.

12. Liang M. Oncorine, the world first oncolytic virus medicine and its update in China. Curr Cancer Drug Targets 2018;18(2):171–6.

13. Imlygic (talimogene laherparepvec) [prescribing information]. Thousand Oaks (CA): Amgen Inc; 2019.

14. Liu BL, Robinson M, Han ZQ, et al. ICP34.5 deleted herpes simplex virus with enhanced oncolytic, immune stimulating, and anti-tumour properties. Gene Ther 2003;10(4):292–303.

15. Harrington KJ, Michielin O, Malvehy J, et al. A practical guide to the handling and administration of talimogene laherparepvec in Europe. Onco Targets Ther 2017; 10:3867–80.

16. Kaufman HL, Kim DW, DeRaffele G, et al. Local and distant immunity induced by intralesional vaccination with an oncolytic herpes virus encoding GM-CSF in patients with stage IIIc and IV melanoma. Ann Surg Oncol 2010;17(3):718–30.

17. Andtbacka RH, Ross M, Puzanov I, et al. Patterns of clinical response with talimogene laherparepvec (T-VEC) in patients with melanoma treated in the OPTiM Phase III clinical trial. Ann Surg Oncol 2016;23(13):4169–77.

18. Andtbacka RH, Kaufman HL, Collichio F, et al. Talimogene laherparepvec improves durable response rate in patients with advanced melanoma. J Clin Oncol 2015;33(25):2780–8.

19. Andtbacka RHI, Collichio F, Harrington KJ, et al. Final analyses of OPTiM: a randomized phase III trial of talimogene laherparepvec versus granulocyte-macrophage colony-stimulating factor in unresectable stage III-IV melanoma. J Immunother Cancer 2019;7(1):145.

20. Andtbacka RH, Agarwala SS, Ollila DW, et al. Cutaneous head and neck melanoma in OPTiM, a randomized phase 3 trial of talimogene laherparepvec versus granulocyte-macrophage colony-stimulating factor for the treatment of unresected stage IIIB/IIIC/IV melanoma. Head Neck 2016;38(12):1752–8.

21. Robert C, Ribas A, Schachter J, et al. Pembrolizumab versus ipilimumab in advanced melanoma (KEYNOTE-006): post-hoc 5-year results from an open-label, multicentre, randomised, controlled, phase 3 study. Lancet Oncol 2019; 20(9):1239–51.

22. Chesney J, Puzanov I, Collichio F, et al. Randomized, Open-Label Phase II Study Evaluating the Efficacy and Safety of Talimogene Laherparepvec in Combination With Ipilimumab Versus Ipilimumab Alone in Patients With Advanced, Unresectable Melanoma. J Clin Oncol 2018;36(17):1658–67.

23. Long GVDR, Ribas A, Puzanov I, et al. Efficacy analysis of MASTERKEY-265 phase 1b study of talimogene laherparepvec (T-VEC) and pembrolizumab (pembro) for unresectable stage IIIB-IV melanoma. J Clin Oncol 2016;34(15_suppl): 9568.

24. Hodi FS, O'Day SJ, McDermott DF, et al. Improved survival with ipilimumab in patients with metastatic melanoma. N Engl J Med 2010;363(8):711–23.

25. Naidoo J, Page DB, Li BT, et al. Toxicities of the anti-PD-1 and anti-PD-L1 immune checkpoint antibodies. Ann Oncol 2015;26(12):2375–91.

26. Hu JC, Coffin RS, Davis CJ, et al. A phase I study of OncoVEXGM-CSF, a second-generation oncolytic herpes simplex virus expressing granulocyte macrophage colony-stimulating factor. Clin Cancer Res 2006;12(22):6737–47.

27. Administration UFaD. BLA 125518 talimogene laherparepvec (Amgen), in: Cellular, Tissue, and Gene Therapies Advisory Committee and Oncologic Drugs Advisory Committee Meeting. 2015.

28. Gangi A, Zager JS. The safety of talimogene laherparepvec for the treatment of advanced melanoma. Expert Opin Drug Saf 2017;16(2):265–9.

29. Senzer NN, Kaufman HL, Amatruda T, et al. Phase II clinical trial of a granulocyte-macrophage colony-stimulating factor-encoding, second-generation oncolytic herpesvirus in patients with unresectable metastatic melanoma. J Clin Oncol 2009;27(34):5763–71.

30. Soh JM, Galka E, Mercurio MG. Herpetic Whitlow-A case of inadvertent inoculation with melanoma viral therapy. JAMA Dermatol 2018;154(12):1487–8.

31. Hodi FS, Hwu WJ, Kefford R, et al. Evaluation of immune-related response criteria and RECIST v1.1 in patients with advanced melanoma treated with pembrolizumab. J Clin Oncol 2016;34(13):1510–7.

32. Wolchok JD, Hoos A, O'Day S, et al. Guidelines for the evaluation of immune therapy activity in solid tumors: immune-related response criteria. Clin Cancer Res 2009;15(23):7412–20.

33. Eisenhauer EA, Therasse P, Bogaerts J, et al. New response evaluation criteria in solid tumours: revised RECIST guideline (version 1.1). Eur J Cancer 2009;45(2): 228–47.

34. Perez MC, Miura JT, Naqvi SMH, et al. Talimogene Laherparepvec (TVEC) for the treatment of advanced melanoma: a single-institution experience. Ann Surg Oncol 2018;25(13):3960–5.

35. Franke V, Berger DMS, Klop WMC, et al. High response rates for T-VEC in early metastatic melanoma (stage IIIB/C-IVM1a). Int J Cancer 2019;145(4):974–8.

36. Louie RJ, Perez MC, Jajja MR, et al. Real-world outcomes of talimogene laherparepvec therapy: a multi-institutional experience. J Am Coll Surg 2019;228(4): 644–9.

37. Fröhlich A, Niebel D, Fietz S, et al. Talimogene laherparepvec treatment to overcome loco-regional acquired resistance to immune checkpoint blockade in tumor stage IIIB-IV M1c melanoma patients. Cancer Immunol Immunother 2020;69(5): 759–69.

38. Perez MC, Zager JS, Amatruda T, et al. Observational study of talimogene laherparepvec use for melanoma in clinical practice in the United States (COSMUS-1). Melanoma Manag 2019;6(2):Mmt19.

39. Seremet T, Planken S, Schwarze JK, et al. Successful treatment with intralesional talimogene laherparepvec in two patients with immune checkpoint inhibitor-refractory, advanced-stage melanoma. Melanoma Res 2019;29(1):85–8.

40. Chesney J, Imbert-Fernandez Y, Telang S, et al. Potential clinical and immuno-therapeutic utility of talimogene laherparepvec for patients with melanoma after disease progression on immune checkpoint inhibitors and BRAF inhibitors. Melanoma Res 2018;28(3):250–5.

41. Dummer R, Gyorki DE, Hyngstrom JR, et al. One-year (yr) recurrence-free survival (RFS) from a randomized, open label phase II study of neoadjuvant (neo) talimogene laherparepvec (T-VEC) plus surgery (surgx) versus surgx for resectable stage IIIB-IVM1a melanoma (MEL). J Clin Oncol 2019;37(15_suppl):9520.

42. Weide B, Derhovanessian E, Pflugfelder A, et al. High response rate after intratumoral treatment with interleukin-2: results from a phase 2 study in 51 patients with metastasized melanoma. Cancer 2010;116(17):4139–46.

43. Byers BA, Temple-Oberle CF, Hurdle V, et al. Treatment of in-transit melanoma with intra-lesional interleukin-2: a systematic review. J Surg Oncol 2014;110(6): 770–5.

44. Thompson JF, Agarwala SS, Smithers BM, et al. Phase 2 Study of Intralesional PV-10 in Refractory Metastatic Melanoma. Ann Surg Oncol 2015;22(7): 2135–42.

The Role of Mohs Surgery in Cutaneous Head and Neck Cancer

Gina D. Jefferson, MD, MPH

KEYWORDS

- Mohs micrographic surgery • Cutaneous cancer • Head and neck
- Basal cell carcinoma • Squamous cell carcinoma • Melanoma
- Merkel cell carcinoma

KEY POINTS

- MMS is most comonly used in treating basal cell and squamous cell cutaneous cancers.
- MMS allows the dermatologic surgeon to analyze 100% of the peripheral and deep margins by horizontal saucering technique.
- Certain, high-risk cSCC, and melanomas require consideration of alternative surgical interventions from MMS and additional therapies.

INTRODUCTION

In the 1930s, Frederic E. Mohs, while studying the effect of various substances injected into different neoplasms, encountered a 20% solution of zinc chloride that resulted in tissue necrosis without altering the microscopic structure of the tissue. Mohs conceptualized surgical excision of neoplasms after in situ fixation with zinc chloride to serially excise the neoplasm in total under the microscope. Furthermore, he developed a horizontal frozen section technique to evaluate 100% of the specimen margins, both deep and peripheral, in contrast to the traditional vertical section technique.[1,2] Mohs microsurgery has become the gold standard for treating a variety of cutaneous tumors.[3]

Evolution of Mohs Micrographic Surgery

The technique of Mohs micrographic surgery (MMS) was initially described as chemosurgery by Mohs. Chemosurgery references the application of dichloroacetic acid as a keratolytic followed by application of a zinc chloride paste combination with stibnite and bloodroot to a desired thickness in order to produce a predictable and

Head and Neck Oncologic and Microvascular Surgery, Department of Otolaryngology–Head & Neck Surgery, University of Mississippi Medical Center, 2500 North State Street, Jackson, MS 39216, USA
E-mail address: gjefferson@umc.edu

Otolaryngol Clin N Am 54 (2021) 439–447
https://doi.org/10.1016/j.otc.2020.11.015
0030-6665/21/© 2020 Elsevier Inc. All rights reserved.

oto.theclinics.com

controllable depth of penetration. These chemicals permitted in situ tissue fixation while preserving microscopic features necessary for evaluation of residual cancer cells. After tissue application, the patient's wound was dressed, and the patient returned the next day for surgical excision of the fixed tissue followed by excision of the first Mohs micrographic layer. The first micrographic layer is accomplished by incising around the tumor with a 1 mm to 5 mm margin with a scalpel beveled at a 30° to 45° angle to the desired depth. This permits excision of a saucer-shaped specimen that once flattened lends itself to deep and peripheral margin assessment. A surgeon may opt to perform debulking of the visible tumor first to submit for vertical histopathologic sections if warranted clinically. Both the resected tumor and the first micrographic layer were analyzed histologically with hematoxylin and eosin. The micrographic layer was inked, mapped, and examined under the microscope encompassing the entire peripheral and deep surface margins. If a tumor was seen, more fixative was applied to the resection site, and the process was repeated the following day until the cancer was completely resected.[1,3,4]

There were disadvantages to the originally described chemosurgery. Each stage of chemosurgery lasted an entire day, necessitating numerous consecutive days of treatment for patients requiring multiple stages for complete excision. The paste itself was painful, and some patients reportedly required hospitalization for pain management. Residual surgical defects required delayed reconstruction, given the additional 7 to 10 days typically required for the fixed tissue site to slough off, leaving the healthy bed of granulation tissue.[3]

In 1953, Mohs wanted to speed the procedure time for a patient with pigmented basal cell carcinoma (BCC) of the lower eyelid. He removed 2 additional layers after the excision of the tumor using local anesthetic without any fixation. Dr. Mohs published the technique in 1956 and presented the technique at a national meeting in 1969. Tromovitch and Stegman reported in 1974 a series of 102 head and neck BCCs treated by the fresh-tissue technique, demonstrating equivalent outcomes to the chemosurgery technique and thereby launching this fresh-tissue technique as the method utilized today.[1,3,5] In 1976, Mohs reported impressive results for patients he treated with either the fixed-tissue technique or the fresh-tissue technique. For a total of 9351 treated cancers, Mohs reported a 99.3% cure rate using the zinc chloride fixed tissue method, and 97% cure rate for the 127 patients treated by the fresh-tissue technique.[2,6]

The procedure was officially renamed Mohs micrographic surgery in 1985 to emphasize the microscopic evaluation and tumor mapping characteristic while permitting same-day resection and reconstruction. The MMS technique advantages include high rates of cure given the complete evaluation of the deep and peripheral tumor margin in contrast to the traditional vertical sectioning of tissue (**Fig. 1**). The vertical section method of pathologic assessment of margins permits sampling error while only evaluating 1% of the surface area for residual tumor. Another advantage is the conservation of normal, uninvolved tissue, resulting in the smallest possible defect. Because the dermatologic surgeon serves also as the pathologist, room for errors by tissue handoffs is minimized. Reconstruction is undertaken only after 100% margin evaluation confirms a completely free margin status.[1,3]

APPLICATION OF MOHS MICROGRAPHIC SURGERY IN THE HEAD AND NECK

Nonmelanoma skin cancer (NMSC) is the most common malignancy in the United States. Cutaneous BCC and squamous cell carcinoma (cSCC) are the most commonly diagnosed NMSCs, comprising over 1 million new cancer diagnoses annually. BCCs constitute 70% to 80% of all skin cancers, and 15% are cSCC. Melanoma makes up

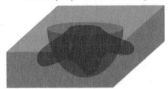

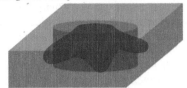

Cutaneous tumors frequently extend beyond the clinically evident borders. The tumor (red) is first excised (black) with a margin of visibly unaffected skin.

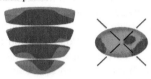

a. The Mohs excision is removed with a beveled angle, therefore allowing the deep and peripheral margin to be processed in the same plane.

a. The breadloafed section is excised with the edges at 90 degrees. The tissue is then sliced vertically in intervals along the specimen and these sections are examined.

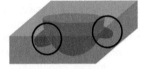

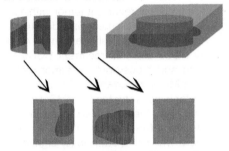

b. The Mohs section is processed horizontally, allowing for identification of 100% of the surgical margin. The positive margins are readily identified in the Mohs sections as shown above.

True positive   True positive   False negative

b. Examples of sampling errors from breadloafing tissue.

c. For Mohs tissue, additional layers are then taken from the mapped areas to ensure complete removal of the tumor, allowing for high cure rates. This technique allows for optimal tissue sparing of normal, uninvolved skin for smaller scars and more reconstructive options.

c. The breadloading technique sections the tissue in a vertical orientation. Typically, less than 1% of the specimen margin is evaluated. This may result in a higher rate of sampling error.

Fig. 1. Comparison of Mohs micrographic pathology technique compared with traditional vertical pathology sectioning. *From* Tolkachjov SN, Brodland DG, Coldiron BM, et al. Understanding Mohs Micrographic Surgery: A Review and Practical Guide for the Nondermatologist, Mayo Clin Proc 2017; 92(8):1261-71; with permission

most of the remaining cutaneous malignancies. BCC is locally aggressive but exhibits low likelihood for development of metastasis, while cSCC is biologically more aggressive, demonstrating perineural invasion (PNI) and regional cervical metastasis.[7] Surgical resection is the mainstay of treatment for these malignancies. Both wide local excision and MMS play a role in the management of these NMSCs.

Basal Cell Carcinoma

For primary BCC, MMS achieves high cure rates on the order of 98% to 99% compared with 91% to 95% for non-MMS treatment modalities.[8,9] Although the gold standard for primary treatment of BCC of the face is surgical excision, MMS is regarded as the treatment of choice for high-risk BCC. High-risk BCC is described as tumor location around the eyes, nose, lips and ears, also known as the H-zone; aggressive histopathologic types of morpheaform, infiltrative, micronodular and basosquamous; recurrent or incompletely excised lesions; lesions demonstrating perineural or perivascular involvement; and lesions excised with ill-defined margins.[8,10]

A randomized trial of 599 BCCs prospectively compared standard surgical excision to MMS for primary (n = 397) and recurrent (n = 202) BCC of the face where the primary outcome measure was clinical and biopsy-proven tumor recurrence after 5 years. The 5-year Kaplan-Meier estimated recurrence rate for primary BCCs treated by surgical excision was 4.1%, and for MMS, it was 2.5%, a nonsignificant difference (P=.397); all recurrences occurred in the H-zone. The authors surmised that the seemingly high recurrence rate after MMS was because all BCCs included in this study exhibited high-risk features. Regarding recurrent BCCs, the estimated Kaplan-Meier recurrence rate for tumors treated by surgical excision was 12.1% versus 2.4% for MMS, a difference in recurrence rate that was significant (P=.015).[8] This advantage in recurrence rate for recurrent BCCs treated by MMS may derive from the often infiltrative nature of recurrent tumor within scar tissue, whereby complete peripheral and deep margin assessment provides 100% excision capability.

Another prospectively performed randomized controlled trial inclusive of 408 primary BCCs and 202 recurrent BCCs assessed over a 10-year period for clinically evident and biopsy-proven tumor recurrence. The authors observed an estimated Kaplan-Meier recurrence rate of 12.2% for primary BCCs surgically excised and 4.4% for lesions treated by MMS, P=.10. For recurrent BCC lesions treated by surgical excision, the estimated recurrence rate was 13.5% and 3.9% for those lesions treated by MMS, significant with P=.023.[11]

There was not a statistically significant difference in recurrence between surgical excision and MMS for primary BCCs in either study. Surgical excision of most BCCs remains an efficacious and efficient means of management. MMS may provide added benefit for high-risk BCCs given this method's ability to assess 100% of the resection margin, particularly when the primary site occurs near vital structures in the head and neck.[8,11,12] Evidence that further supports this conclusion includes several studies demonstrating low recurrence rates of head and neck BCC after treatment via MMS of 1.4% to 4%.[9–11]

There is an apparent advantage when technically feasible to treat recurrent BCCs with MMS based on these 2 prospective studies. High-risk features such as perineural invasion or deep subcutaneous tumor extension that render BCC more likely to recur are features that MMS may more readily identify intraoperatively.[13] By virtue of MMS comprehensive intraoperative assessment of 100% of the peripheral and deep margins, another Mohs resection layer is possible in real time, thereby increasing the likelihood of margin clearance.

Head and neck surgeons may encounter patients who have recently undergone an attempt at surgical resection or MMS, where final pathologic evaluation reveals incomplete resection. A retrospective study of 1021 MMS performed on primary, residual, and recurrent BCCs showed a 2.6% 5-year recurrence rate for primary, 5.4% recurrence rate for residual, and 2.9% recurrence rate for recurrent BCCs. The higher rate of recurrence for residual tumors is likely because of repeat resection of a scar rather than the gross tumor itself. Gross tumor when present provides a visible periphery to guide margins. The authors also noted that there was a higher incidence of residual BCCs located in high-risk locations.[10] This study is demonstrative of the importance of a multidisciplinary tumor board for high-risk cutaneous cancer, where head and neck and Mohs micrographic surgeons, neuroradiologists, pathologists, and radiation and medical oncologists participate to provide the best treatment recommendations aimed at local disease control. High-risk regions, depth of tumor assessment with respect to underlying bone/cartilage, and surgical planning improve outcomes for complex head and neck cancer resection that is facilitated by tumor conference. Multidisciplinary discussion of complex head and neck tumors may result in almost 33% modification of the original treatment plan.[14]

Squamous Cell Carcinoma

Similar to BCC, MMS is regarded as the gold standard method of care for cSCC. For cSCC of the head and neck, there is a reported local recurrence rate of 3% to 5.2% for standard wide local excision compared with 1.2% to 3.9% for cSCCs treated by MMS.[15] However, there is a subset of high-risk cSCCs that warrant even greater attention when making treatment recommendations given greater risk for poor outcomes of local recurrence, metastasis, and even death.[16] The rate of nodal metastasis of cSCC ranges from 1.5% to 4%, and the disease-specific death rate is between 1.5% and 2.8%.[17]

High-risk cSCC is inconsistently defined in the literature.[16,18] An early study by Rowe and colleagues identified treatment modality, prior treatment history, location of tumor, size and depth of tumor, histologic differentiation, PNI, and immunosuppressed state as high-risk features for disease recurrence and metastasis. Other studies define high risk for recurrence and metastasis as location on the ear or lip, poor differentiation, desmoplastic or acantholytic histologic grades, and presence of lymphovascular involvement (LVI). There is also variability among studies with respect to the definition of tumor depth, with some using anatomic depth and others using Breslow thickness, differing definitions of PNI, and lack of control for confounding variables that commonly occur together such as tumor depth and PNI.[16]

A 5-year prospective, multicenter analysis of 745 cSCCs treated with MMS showed a local recurrence-free survival rate of 99.3%, nodal metastasis-free survival rate of 99.2%, and disease-specific survival rate of 99.4%. The authors identified Breslow depth as the only factor with associated increased hazard for local recurrence. For each 1 mm increase in Breslow depth, the hazard of nodal metastasis increased by almost 30%. Furthermore, no patient with incidental PNI received adjuvant treatment, and these tumors demonstrated no increased association with local recurrence, nodal metastasis, or disease-specific death when other variables were controlled. However, a separate analysis of tumors exhibiting perineural invasion showed a significant correlation of PNI greater than 0.1 mm with Breslow thickness, tumor invasion beyond subcutaneous fat, and poorly differentiated histology.[15]

Another retrospective study of 531 tumors demonstrated a 2.9% local recurrence rate, 4.8% nodal metastasis rate, 1.1% distant metastasis rate, and 1.1% disease-specific death rate after at least 1 year follow-up of MMS for cSCC. On multivariate analysis, poor tumor differentiation and tumor invasion beyond the subcutaneous fat were significantly associated with local recurrence and nodal metastasis.[18]

These 2 studies highlight the low incidence of poor outcomes for cSCC treated with MMS. In addition, a meta-analysis that compared standard wide local excision with MMS showed lower recurrence rates with MMS of 3.1% versus 8.1% for primary tumors. The improved cure rates were significant for higher-risk tumors with PNI. Local recurrence after MMS was 0% for tumors with PNI in comparison to 47.2% for those with PNI treated by standard wide local excision.[19] This is likely attributed to the enhanced examination of 100% of the tumor margins provided by MMS.

These studies also demonstrate that poor outcomes extend beyond local recurrence to include nodal and distant metastasis, and even death. The Brigham and

Women's Hospital (BWH) staging system for cSCC and eighth edition of the American Joint Committee on Cancer (AJCC) Staging both attempt to account for higher-risk tumors. These staging systems rely upon reporting of various pathologic and clinical features that are inconsistently reported. Regular reporting of tumor location, size, treatment history, rapid growth, neurologic symptoms, immune status of the patient, histologic differentiation, depth of invasion, presence of LVI or PNI would aid in identifying high-risk cSCC in need of further evaluation and aggressive treatment.[16] Reporting of these high-risk features would prompt appropriate imaging studies to evaluate for nodal metastasis. Imaging could change treatment 33% of the time through early detection and management of regional disease, thereby improving disease-free survival.[20] Discussion of high-risk cSCC patients with a multidisciplinary cutaneous malignancy tumor board is also recommended for discussion of adjuvant treatment modalities.

Melanoma

Cutaneous melanoma accounts for less than 5% of all skin cancers but contributes up to 60% of all skin cancer-related mortality. There is a well-documented role for MMS in the management of BCC and cSCC cancers, but as of yet there is no clearly defined role for MMS in the management of cutaneous melanoma.[21]

A prospective multicenter study evaluated 562 melanomas (377 noninvasive in situ and 185 invasive melanomas) treated with MMS. Melanoma antigen recognized by T cells-1 (MART-1) antigen immunostain was utilized on frozen section processing. The study objective was to recommend excision margins and to compare actual costs of tumor removal with MMS versus standard surgical excision. Recognizing that outlier melanomas characterized by wide subclinical extensions would create an unreasonable recommendation for margin guidelines to accomplish 100% complete excision rates, the authors chose a predetermined goal for 97% complete excision rate. They derived this 97% complete excision rate based on a historically known recurrence rate of 3% for standard wide local excision of melanoma. This resulted in recommendation for 12 mm margins for invasive and noninvasive melanoma of the head and neck region. With respect to cost, the authors found the use of MMS with MART-1 staining and immediate reconstruction resulted in a median cost of $1336.60 per tumor in a cohort inclusive of the head and neck (n = 345), hands/feet/genitalia (n = 13), extremities (n = 90), and trunk (n = 114). Tumors located on the head and neck average cost was $1459.22. Although the authors of this study mentioned other single institution retrospective reports of improved disease-specific survival rates and low marginal recurrence rates in treating melanoma with MMS, their own study did not report on disease-related outcomes. The authors did argue that the tendency of melanoma to extend beyond clinically visible tumor margin with amelanotic and subclinical invasion "reinforces the benefit of comprehensive margin evaluation."[22]

A summary of histopathologic pitfalls associated with MMS was recently reported, however, in which the authors highlighted the limitations of MMS assessment for melanoma. The accuracy of MMS for melanoma may improve by the use of IHC staining such as MART-1. Standard wide local excision is typically a 2-stage procedure because of the difficulty in interpretation of frozen sections with typical H&E stains. It is difficult to distinguish freeze artifact and actinic keratoses from junctional melanocytic proliferations on routine frozen sections stained with H&E.[23] Melanocytes are more readily identified in specimens that are formalin-fixed paraffin-embedded due to production of a clear halo artifact that differentiates the melanocyte from keratinocytes.[24]

To address concern regarding frozen section identification of melanocytes, and in particular subclinical extensions of disease, several Mohs surgeons have reported success of using immunostains for each Mohs layer including S100, HMB-45 and MART-1. One study directly compared the 3 aforementioned immunostains and noted that S100 failed in all cases because of inability to establish adequate controls for each case. HMB-45 was noted to fail at demonstrating the melanocyte proliferation at tumor edge that was visible with MART-1.

MART-1 was successful in all cases in this study, where only 10 cases were assessed by all 3 immunostains.[23] Sensitivity for MART-1 is reportedly 75% to 100%, with most reports in the 85% to 100% range, while sensitivity reported for HMB-45 ranges also from 75% to 100%, with most in the 70% to 80% range.[23] There is also potential difficulty with the MART-1 stain resulting in larger margins than typical for MMS of 5 mm. MART-1 staining of melanocytic hyperplasia due to solar damage may extend tumor margins artificially. MART-1 may also create false-positive interpretation with overstaining of certain inflammatory conditions, pigmented solar keratosis, and solar lentigo.[25] Furthermore, the horizontal sectioning by MMS technique does not permit assessment of maximal Breslow depth or evaluation of the melanoma growth characteristics. Breslow depth in particular is critical to the staging and prognostication of melanoma.[24]

A recent study derived from the National Cancer Database (NCDB) for head and neck melanoma inclusive of 50,397 cases reports a survival advantage for patients treated with MMS in comparison to WLE after controlling for potentially confounding variables. Patients treated with MMS were more likely than patients treated by standard WLE to survive 5 years (hazard ratio 1.181, 95% confidence interval 1.083–1.288, P<.001).[26] This overall conclusion requires cautious interpretation. On multivariate analysis, the survival benefit was only significant for melanomas less than 0.74 mm. Lentigo maligna was the only subtype on multivariate analysis to demonstrate survival advantage. Furthermore, there was a significantly disproportionate representation of melanomas treated by wide local excision (93% vs 7%), and most treated by MMS were thinner (mean Breslow depth of 0.8 mm) than those treated with wide local excision (mean Breslow depth of 1.7 mm).[26] The potential survival advantage of MMS may disappear with additional melanomas treated by MMS for comparison. Finally, a limitation of the NCDB database analysis is the lack of description of histologic examination of the MMS specimens. This is important in order to replicate outcomes because of the variety of methods described in the literature regarding histologic assessment.

Adoption of MMS for the treatment of cutaneous melanoma requires further investigation regarding margin assessment and outcomes compared with the standard technique of wide local excision. Furthermore, cutaneous melanoma requires evaluation of lymph node basins as per the National Comprehensive Cancer Network (NCCN) guidelines.[27] For this reason, wide local excision at the same time as sentinel node biopsy is often preferred over separate MMS.

Other Cutaneous Diseases

Merkel cell carcinoma (MCC), dermatofibrosarcoma protuberans (DFSP), and sebaceous and other adnexal carcinomas are rare and have propensity to recur locally. The technique of MMS has shown equal efficacy in the treatment of MCC and perhaps improved local control for DFSP and adnexal tumors all in retrospective reviews.[28,29] Although MMS appears efficacious in treating some rare cutaneous neoplasms, it is imperative to assess potential for regional disease with certain pathologies and to carefully surveil all patients undergoing either standard excision or MMS for treatment of these rare conditions.

SUMMARY

MMS represents an excellent means to address BCC and some cSCCs of the head and neck region, achieving excellent outcomes with respect to local recurrence rates and disease-specific survival. MMS by virtue of its technique maximally preserves uninvolved tissues of the head and neck, thereby maintaining form, cosmesis, and function to the greatest extent as dictated by the disease. However, the application of MMS for managing high-risk cSCC and melanoma requires additional investigation, and patients harboring these diseases should have case discussion with a cutaneous malignancy tumor board. MMS may also prove beneficial in treating rare cutaneous diseases such as MCC and DFSP while remembering to assess for regional spread of disease where applicable.

CLINICS CARE POINTS

- It is efficacious to utilize MMS for most head and neck BCCs and many cSCCs.
- There is not adequate evidence to suggest MMS allows for adequate margin assessment when treating melanoma.
- The use of MMS for melanoma does not permit appropriate staging of the cancer.

REFERENCES

1. Trost L, Bailin PL. History of Mohs surgery. Dermatol Clin 2011;29:135–9.
2. De Paola C. Frederic E. Mohs, MD, and the history of zinc chloride. Clin Dermatol 2018;36:568–75.
3. Wong E, Axibal E, Brown M. Mohs micrographipc surgery. Facial Plast Surg Clin North Am 2019;27:15–34.
4. Mohs FE. Mohs Micrographic Surgery. Stephen N, Snow, Mikhail GR, editors. In: Origin and progress of Mohs micrographic surgery. 2nd edition. Madison (WI): University of Wisconsin Press; 2004.
5. Tromovitch T, Stegman SJ. Microscopically controlled excision of skin tumors. Arch Dermatol 1974;110(2):231–2.
6. Mohs F. Chemosurgery for skin cancer: fixed tissue and fresh tissue techniques. Arch Dermatol 1976;1:37–41.
7. Mydiarz W, Weber RS, Kupferman ME. Cutaneous malignancy of the head and neck. Surg Oncol Clin N Am 2015;24:593–613.
8. Mosterd K, Krekels GAM, Nieman FHM, et al. Surgical excision versus Mohs' micrographic surgery for primary and recurrent basal-cell carcinoma of the face: a prospective randomised controlled trial with 5-years' follow-up. Lancet Oncol 2008;9(12):1149–56.
9. Leibovitch I, Huilgol SC, Franzco DS, et al. Basal cell carcinoma treated with Mohs surgery in Australia II. Outcome at 5-year follow-up. J Am Acad Dermatol 2005;53:452–7.
10. Kuiper E, VanDenBerge BA, Spoo JR, et al. Low recurrence rate of head and neck basal cell carcinoma treated with Mohs micrographic surgery: a retrospective study of 1021 cases. Clin Otolaryngol 2018;43:1321–7.
11. VanLoo E, Mosterd K, Krekels GAM, et al. Surgical excision versus Mohs' micrographic surgery for basal cell carcinoma of the face: a randomised clinical trial with 10 year follow-up. Eur J Cancer 2014;50:3011–20.
12. Clark C, Furnniss M, Mackay-Wiggan JM. Basal cell carcinoma: an evidence-based treatment update. Am J Clin Dermatol 2014;15:197–216.

13. Bichakjian C, Armstrong A, Baum C, et al. J Am Acad Dermatol 2018;78:540–59.
14. Wheless SAMK, Zanation AM. A prospective study of the clinical impact of a multidisciplinary head and neck tumor board. Otolaryngol Head Neck Surg 2010;143(5):650–4.
15. Tschetter A, Campoli MR, Zitelli JA, et al. Long-term clinical outcomes of patients with invasive cutaneous squamous cell carcinoma treated with Mohs micrographic surgery: a 5-year, multicenter, prospective cohort study. J Am Acad Dermatol 2020;82:139–48.
16. Bander T, Nehal KS, Lee EH. Cutaneous squamous cell carcinoma: updates in staging and management. Dermatol Clin 2019;37:241–51.
17. Karia P, Han J, Schmults CD. Cutaneous squamous cell carcinoma: estimated incidence of disease, nodal metastasis, and deaths from disease in the United States, 2012. J Am Acad Dermatol 2013;63(6):957–66.
18. Marrazzo G, Zitelli JA, Brodland D. Clinical outcomes in high-risk squamous cell carcinoma patients treated with Mohs micrographic surgery alone. J Am Acad Dermatol 2019;80:633–8.
19. Rowe D, Carroll RJ, Day CL. Prognostic factors for local recurrence, metastasis, and survival rates in squamous cell carcinoma of the skin, ear, and lip. Implications for treatment modality selection. J Am Acad Dermatol 1992;26(6):976–90.
20. Ruiz E, Karia PS, Morgan FC, et al. The positive impact of radiologic imaging on high-stage cutaneous squamous cell carcinoma management. J Am Acad Dermatol 2017;76(2):217–25.
21. Yan F, Knochelmann HM, Morgan PF, et al. The evolution of care of cancers of the head and neck region: state of the science in 2020. Cancers (Basel) 2020;12: 1543–66.
22. Ellison P, Zitelli JA, Brodland DG. Mohs micrographic surgery for melanoma: a prospective multicenter study. J Am Acad Dermatol 2019;81:767–74.
23. Albertini JGED, Libow LF, Smith SB, et al. Mohs micrographic surgery for melanoma: a case series, a comparative study of immunostains, an informative case report, and a unique mapping technique. Dermatol Surg 2002;28:656–65.
24. Franca K, Alqubaisy Y, Hassanein A, et al. Histopathologic pitfalls of Mohs micrographic surgery and a review of tumor histology. Wien Med Wochenschr 2018; 168:218.
25. Phan K, Onggo J, Loya A. Mohs micrographic surgery versus wide local excision for head and neck melanoma-in-situ. J Dermatolog Treat 2019;31:1–4.
26. Hanson J, Demer A, Liszewski W, et al. Improved overall survival of melanom of the head and neck treated with Mohs micrographic surgery versus wide local excision. J Am Acad Dermatol 2020;82:149–55.
27. Shaikh W, Sobanko JF, Etzkorn JR, et al. Utilization patterns and survival outcomes after wide local excision or Mohs micrographic surgery for Merkel cell carcinoma in the United States, 2004-2009. J Am Acad Dermatol 2018;78:175–7.
28. Lowe G, Onajin O, Baum CL, et al. A comparison of Mohs micrographic surgery and wide local excision for treatment of dermatofibrosarcoma protuberans with long-term follow-up. Dermatol Surg 2017;43:98–106.
29. Brady K, Hurst EA. Sebaceous carcinoma treated with Mohs micrographic surgery. Dermatol Surg 2017;43:281–6.

Special Article Series: Intentionally Shaping the Future of Otolaryngology

Editor

JENNIFER A. VILLWOCK

OTOLARYNGOLOGIC CLINICS OF NORTH AMERICA

www.oto.theclinics.com

Consulting Editor
SUJANA S. CHANDRASEKHAR

April 2021 • Volume 54 • Number 2

Special Foreword

Offering a Helping Hand to Future Colleagues

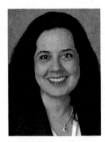

Sujana S. Chandrasekhar, MD, FACS, FAAOHNS
Consulting Editor

The great actress and humanitarian Audrey Hepburn famously said, "Remember, if you ever need a helping hand, it's at the end of your arm; as you get older, remember you have another hand. The first is to help yourself, the second is to help others." I first read this 4 years ago, when I was President of the American Academy of Otolaryngology–Head and Neck Surgery and writing a piece on mentorship and sponsorship. The 2 articles in the Special Article Series: Intentionally Shaping the Future of Otolaryngology in this issue speak to this concept.

Dr Jennifer Villwock spearheaded this series of articles, which will appear two at a time in *Otolaryngologic Clinics of North America*. The first articles were on Leadership and the dearth of diversity therein and appeared in the August 2020 issue. The next articles, in the October 2020 issue, covered the current state of the Otolaryngology workforce and defined diversity among our peers and why it is important. The subsequent articles, in the February 2021 issue, discussed the history of women and minorities in surgery and looked at leadership competencies in medicine. This issue's articles are on Mentorship and Sponsorship in a Diverse Population and on Otolaryngologic Training and Diversity.

These articles could not come at a more appropriate time. Our field has the doubtful distinction of being the lowest of all surgical specialties in percentage of African American residents and faculty, and we are near the bottom for all underrepresented in medicine (URIM), including blacks, Latinos, Native Americans, and Native Hawaiians. This disturbing, statistically significant data were presented based on a snapshot across medical school to residency to faculty representation in 2016.[1] We have more women in our residency programs than most surgical specialties, but less than general surgery and integrated plastic surgery. Women are 50% of medical school graduates but are underrepresented among otolaryngology residency applicants. However, they are equally represented between applicants and residents.

Otolaryngol Clin N Am 54 (2021) xvii–xix
https://doi.org/10.1016/j.otc.2021.01.004
0030-6665/21/© 2021 Published by Elsevier Inc.

African Americans apply to ENT programs in the same percentage as they exist in medical school; however, they are significantly not matching into programs. In terms of faculty, Asian Americans and Hispanics are underrepresented compared with their representation as residents.

Currently, Otolaryngology in the United States does not look like the populations we serve. Not only do diverse teams perform better across fields but also the presence of faculty and mentors who are racially concordant with potential applicants and/or trainees is vital to diversifying departments. A survey[2] of US Otolaryngology Program Directors showed the following: Over one-third of programs had matriculated 1 or fewer URIM residents. There was a significant association between the number of URIM faculty and the number of URIM residents matriculated. This highlights the importance of URIM faculty mentorship.

But just getting into an ENT program is not the end of the support. Ongoing mentorship and sponsorship are vitally important. Across specialties, URIM residents are dismissed at disproportionately high numbers. The ACGME (Accreditation Council on Graduate Medical Education) data from 2015 to 2016[3] show that black residents are dismissed at an alarming 6.1 to 1 rate compared with white residents in General Surgery. For other pipeline training programs, the rates are likewise bad: Anesthesiology fires 10.3 black residents to 1 white resident; Family Medicine has a rate of 3.3 to 1; Internal Medicine's rate is 12.3 to 1; Obstetrics and Gynecology has a rate of 3 to 1 for black residents and 4.8 to 1 for Latinx residents compared with non-Hispanic white residents; Pediatrics fires 6.7 black residents to 1 white resident; and Psychiatry has a rate of 4.2 to 1. Orthopedic Surgery is the worst, firing 14.75 Latinx and 31.25 black residents per white resident. Although Otolaryngology is not particularly evaluated because it is not defined as a pipeline program, the story is clear. These bright, high-achieving physicians who excelled through high school, college, and medical school and entered their chosen fields are confronting obstacles in training that we, as leaders and educators, need to identify and remove.

Otolaryngology lags behind other surgical specialties in representation of minorities and women. By deliberately focusing, we can correct this and enhance ENT health care for our population. I commend the authors of these 2 articles on clearly showing us what is and what can be, and what each of us can do to use our second hand to help others. I hope you read them and bring the message home to your own institution.

Sujana S. Chandrasekhar, MD, FACS, FAAOHNS
Consulting Editor
Otolaryngologic Clinics of North America
Past President
American Academy of Otolaryngology–
Head and Neck Surgery
Secretary-Treasurer
American Otological Society
Partner, ENT & Allergy Associates LLP
18 East 48th Street, 2nd Floor
New York, NY 10017, USA

Clinical Professor
Department of Otolaryngology–
Head and Neck Surgery
Zucker School of Medicine at Hofstra-Northwell
Hempstead, NY, USA

Clinical Associate Professor
Department of Otolaryngology–
Head and Neck Surgery
Icahn School of Medicine at Mount Sinai
New York, NY, USA

E-mail address:
ssc@nyotology.com

Website:
http://www.ears.nyc

REFERENCES

1. Ukatu CC, Welby Berra L, Wu Q, et al. The state of diversity based on race, ethnicity, and sex in otolaryngology in 2016. Laryngoscope 2020;130:E795–800.
2. Newsome H, Faucett EA, Chelius T, et al. Diversity in otolaryngology residency programs: a survey of otolaryngology program directors. PMID: 29664699 DOI: 10.1177/0194599818770614.
3. Available at: https://www.acgme.org/About-Us/Publications-and-Resources/Graduate-Medical-Education-Data-Resource-Book. Accessed January 4, 2021.

Special Preface

Meaningfully Moving Forward Through Intentional Training, Mentorship, and Sponsorship

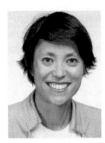

Jennifer A. Villwock, MD, FAAOA
Editor

The acquisition of effective strategies to successfully navigate both professional and personal realms, as well as the intersections between them, has never been more important. Medicine has always been a rapidly evolving field. However, these changes are amplified by factors like the increased availability of information, managing nontraditional spheres of influence like social media, emerging infectious disease concerns like the COVID-19 pandemic, and understanding how the social determinants of health and our own biases impact not only the care we provide but also the outcomes of our patients and communities.

Dr Cabrera-Muffly, creator, producer, and host of the podcast OtoMentor, discusses mentorship and sponsorship, with an emphasis on special considerations for the diverse population we are actively seeking to recruit to otolaryngology in her article, "Mentorship and Sponsorship in a Diverse Population." Mentorship and sponsorship are critical for success in general, but particularly for women and those who are underrepresented in medicine. The balance of the two are also important as "Mentors give you perspective. Sponsors give you opportunities." Said differently, "while a mentor is someone who has knowledge and will share it with you, a sponsor is a person who has power and will use it for you."[1] For example, women are likely to be overmentored but undersponsored.[2] This has long been known in the business world and is also seen in medicine. As noted in the *Harvard Business Review*, regardless of intentions, people tend to gravitate toward those who are like them on salient dimensions such as gender.[3] As such, in fields dominated by individuals with particular demographics, people sharing those characteristics are most likely to be proposed for new positions or opportunities. This can have longitudinal career implications.[1,2]

Otolaryngol Clin N Am 54 (2021) xxi–xxii
https://doi.org/10.1016/j.otc.2021.01.003
0030-6665/21/© 2021 Published by Elsevier Inc.

oto.theclinics.com

We cannot mentor and sponsor diverse otolaryngologists if we fail to recruit and effectively train them. Drs O'Brien and colleagues discuss historic and current trends in otolaryngology training, bringing special attention to the lack of diversity in our specialty, implications, and considerations moving forward in their article, "Otolaryngic Training and Diversity." As her team notes, Otolaryngology has one of the lowest percentages of Black physicians of any surgical specialty at 0.8%. Active steps are needed to recruit, retain, and effectively train a more diversified otolaryngology workforce. At a minimum, this includes early outreach, mentoring, and funded opportunities. As Corinne Pittman noted in her remarkable piece, "A Black medical student's plea for diversity, inclusion in otolaryngology residency," and points out that, given the shockingly low percentage of Blacks and women in Otolaryngology, there is a high likelihood that she will be the only Black person in her future residency training program. Ms Pittman also notes that exceptional candidates are often overlooked or unintentionally denied consideration for reasons that have nothing to do with the merit of their applications.[4]

I hope the information and insights presented in these special articles lay a foundation upon which further introspection regarding otolaryngology's past is done and provides a strong evidence base for how to intentionally pursue the goals of equity and justice in our field, its future, and the increasingly diverse communities we serve.

Jennifer A. Villwock, MD, FAAOA
Department of Otolaryngology, Head
and Neck Surgery
University of Kansas Medical Center
3901 Rainbow Boulevard, MS 3010
Kansas City, KS 66160, USA

E-mail address:
jvillwock@kumc.edu

REFERENCES

1. Ibarra H, Carter NM, Silva C. Why men still get more promotions than women. Harv Bus Rev 2010;88(9):80–5, 126.
2. Ayyala MS, Skarupski K, Bodurtha JN, et al. Mentorship is not enough: exploring sponsorship and its role in career advancement in academic medicine. Acad Med 2019;94(1):94–100.
3. Ibarra H. A lack of sponsorship is keeping women from advancing into leadership. Harv Bus Rev; 2019. Available at: https://hbr.org/2019/08/a-lack-of-sponsorship-is-keeping-women-from-advancing-into-leadership. Accessed November 16, 2020.
4. Pittman C. A Black medical student's plea for diversity, inclusion in otolaryngology residency. ENT Today; 2020. Available at: https://www.enttoday.org/article/a-black-medical-students-plea-for-diversity-inclusion-in-otolaryngology-residency/. Accessed November 16, 2020.

Mentorship and Sponsorship in a Diverse Population

Cristina Cabrera-Muffly, MD

KEYWORDS

- Mentorship • Sponsorship • Diversity and inclusion

KEY POINTS

- Mentorship and sponsorship are critical to the success of every otolaryngologist.
- Successful mentors and mentees demonstrate specific characteristics.
- Women and underrepresented minorities have additional mentorship needs that should be addressed.

INTRODUCTION

Imagine two residents (let us call them A and B) entering their chosen specialty of otolaryngology at the same time. They are the same gender and ethnicity, have the same board scores and class rank, have published the same number of peer reviewed research papers, and both have excellent letters of recommendation. Resident A matches into a department where every new resident is assigned a faculty mentor on arrival and expected to meet with them several times per year. On every rotation, resident A is asked to participate in research projects, and is coaxed into pursuing each rotations' subspecialty by faculty who give reasons why their field is the best. Resident B matches into a department where there is a more "hands off" approach to mentorship. Mentoring relationships are expected to evolve organically, and faculty expect residents to approach them with their interests in research and career planning. Unless Resident B is clear about their career path and goals, who do you think will publish more, develop better relationships with faculty, and be more comfortable pursuing their desired fellowship? Now imagine that in addition to these different training environments, Residents A and B are different genders, ethnicities, or both. Or perhaps Resident B is the first person in their family to graduate from college, let alone medical school, and has little idea of how to navigate the hierarchical world of surgery and academia. How will the careers of these two residents differ over a lifetime?

Department of Otolaryngology Head and Neck Surgery, University of Colorado School of Medicine, 12631 East 17th Avenue, Room 3110, Aurora, CO 80045, USA
E-mail address: cristina.cabrera-muffly@cuanschutz.edu

Otolaryngol Clin N Am 54 (2021) 449–456
https://doi.org/10.1016/j.otc.2020.11.016
0030-6665/21/© 2020 Elsevier Inc. All rights reserved.
oto.theclinics.com

MENTORSHIP AND SPONSORSHIP DEFINED

Mentorship occurs when a respected, experienced person within a field gives advice to a less experienced person to promote their success. Mentorship is typically developed in the context of a long-term professional relationship. The best mentors are more than just role models or teachers, serving as a coach, advisor, support person, and giver of (sometimes difficult) feedback. Sponsorship, in contrast, occurs when an experienced colleague recommends a less experienced protégé for career advancement opportunities. Mentors and sponsors can be the same person, but this is not always the case. In fact, sponsorship can occur in the absence of a personal relationship. Although mentorship is important, sponsorship is frequently necessary for career advancement (**Table 1**).[1]

Mentorship and sponsorship are important for medical students pursuing otolaryngology, residents in otolaryngology training programs, and otolaryngology faculty throughout their careers. Mentored individuals have been shown to be "promoted earlier, more likely to publish, more likely to follow initial career goals, and enjoy greater career satisfaction."[2] A systematic review of mentoring in academic medicine reported that "mentorship has an important influence on personal development, career guidance, career choice, and research productivity, including publication and grant success."[3]

Mentorship is categorized in a few different ways. One of the main divisions is between formal and informal relationships. In formal mentorship relationships, pairings are usually assigned, and there are often recommendations for the frequency and goals of each meeting. Informal mentoring is more flexible, with self-selected pairings and more fluid goal setting (**Table 2**).[4] The benefits of formal mentorship include an increase in the overall amount of mentorship with facilitated assignments.[5] This is especially important among women and underrepresented minority (URM) populations, who are less likely to have mentors.[4] There is no evidence that choosing a mentor leads to significantly better mentoring than an assigned pairing.[6] At the same time, informal mentors often serve as a role model, and mentees with informal mentors "demonstrate superior career development, higher income, and more promotions than those with only formal mentors."[2] Formal mentorship programs put the onus of support and training on the institution, whereas informal mentorship relies completely on the mentor and mentee's commitment to the relationship.

In addition to formal versus informal mentorship relationships, there are also various models of mentorship.[4] The most traditional of these is the apprenticeship model, where the mentee observes and emulates the skills of the mentor.[4] This is the model most training programs have relied on since the inception of residency. Team mentoring relies on a group of mentors with different skill sets to provide support to the

Table 1 Differences between mentorship and sponsorship	
Mentorship	**Sponsorship**
Longitudinal relationship	Episodic
Helpful for career development	Helpful for career advancement
More effective if personalities mesh well	More effective if sponsor is well-connected
More important early in career	More important later in career

Adapted from Ayyala MS, Skarupski K, Bodurtha JN, et al. Mentorship Is Not Enough: Exploring Sponsorship and Its Role in Career Advancement in Academic Medicine. Acad Med. 2019;94(1):94-100.

Table 2
Differences between formal and informal mentorship

Formal Mentorship	Informal Mentorship
Assigned pairings	Flexible, self-identified pairings
Focused goals	Self-directed goals
Specific timeline for meetings	Flexible meeting schedule
Benefit from mentor and mentee training	No training
Allows for inclusion of underrepresented groups	Relies on established social connections
Typically takes longer to achieve trust	Trust usually present from beginning

From Patel VM, Warren O, Ahmed K, et al. How can we build mentorship in surgeons of the future? ANZ J Surg. 2011;81(6):418-424.

mentee.[4] As training programs have expanded into large departments, team mentoring has become much more common. Competency mentoring is when specific goals are set by the mentor, who then helps the mentee achieve them.[4] The development and use of the otolaryngology milestones has introduced this type of mentorship into training programs.

CURRENT STATE OF MENTORSHIP IN OTOLARYNGOLOGY

What is the current state of mentorship in otolaryngology? Unfortunately, there is a paucity of data around mentorship at the medical student or faculty level. However, there are a few studies exploring mentorship in otolaryngology training programs. One study surveyed residents and program directors nationally, and found that 44% of otolaryngology programs had a formal mentorship program.[7] It was recommended by the authors that formal mentorship be included in all otolaryngology residencies.[7] The most important mentor characteristics for trainees included approachability, genuine caring, and supportiveness.[7] Residents rated senior faculty status and amount of influence in the field to be the least important.[7] Residents sought mentors with a compatible personality match and who were a good clinical role model.[7] A study examining 10 years of experience with mentorship at one training program found similar results, with honesty/integrity, being supportive, and being a good clinical role model rated as the most important mentor traits.[8] Mentors helped mentees the most with surgical skills, clinical decision making, and resident education, which supports the statement by the authors that "while all surgeons have role models, not every resident has a true mentor."[8] A common theme was the difficulty of finding time to provide mentorship, for the mentee, but even more so for the mentor. In another study, only 46% of mentors believed they had enough time and only 65% thought themselves effective mentors, whereas mentees demonstrated a much higher perception of accessibility and satisfaction rate with the process.[6] This suggests that mentors may be too hard on themselves, and that formal mentorship programs can fulfill trainees' needs for mentorship. A possible antidote to these feelings is formal training for mentors, especially in the areas of "career planning, providing feedback, and emotional wellbeing," which mentors self-identified as important.[6]

The formation of mentorship and sponsorship relationships is especially important for students, residents, and faculty who do not share the same gender identity, race, ethnicity, or sexual orientation as most of their peers in otolaryngology. People in these groups may have more difficulty identifying and connecting with mentors who they believe are similar to them in otolaryngology. Although women make up 50.8% of the US population and 47.4% of medical school graduates, only 34.7% of otolaryngology residents and 31.5% of otolaryngology academic faculty are female.[9] In general, women are more likely to perceive a lack of mentors as a barrier to their success.[2] Also, women may benefit more from mentors of the same gender for advice on issues relating to family and work-life balance.

The numbers of URM within otolaryngology are much lower, with African Americans and Blacks making up 12.6% of the US population, but only 2.1% and 2.4% of otolaryngology residents and faculty, respectively. Hispanic and Latinxs make up 17.3% of the US population, but only 5.5% and 2.9% of residents and faculty are Hispanic in otolaryngology.[9] "Black, Hispanic, and female residents have described value in identifying mentors with similar demographics and a shared sense of history."[10] Interviews with URM faculty at five academic medical institutions revealed a "lack of mentoring and role models."[11] Sponsorship becomes critical in these groups, because "mentorship may not be sufficient for career advancement, particularly for women and URM faculty."[1] Existing mentorship barriers include URM sense of isolation, lower rates of tenure and promotion, lack of role models, financial constraints, lack of social support, and racial bias.[12]

STRATEGIES FOR MENTORS AND SPONSORS

The most effective mentors share several characteristics. They are altruistic and care about their mentee's success, are available to their mentee, and are a positive role model. The Accreditation Council for Graduate Medical Education's Council of Review Committee Residents developed a group of resident mentorship milestones in 2016.[13] Although these milestones were meant to evaluate trainee development as a mentor, they are used for mentors at all levels of their career. Similar to specialty-specific Accreditation Council for Graduate Medical Education milestones, each mentorship milestone (availability, competence, and altruism) is accompanied by a progressive, four-level description of expertise.[13] For example, a novice mentor is just expected to demonstrate a willingness to participate in a mentoring program, whereas the expert mentor is able to transition their mentorship abilities beyond training.[13] Personal fit between mentor and mentee is also important, because a difference in values can undermine the relationship.[2] Effective mentors function in different roles at different times. Although they frequently provide career guidance, they are often also called on to provide emotional support and advice on work/life balance.[14]

Whether the mentorship relationship is established formally or informally, success is more likely if mentors discuss goals, priorities, and clear expectations with their mentee early on. Although these may change over time, early discussions set the tone for the relationship (**Box 1**).

Common pitfalls that accompany failed mentoring relationships include a lack of time committed to the relationship, breakdown in communication, and conflicts of interest. A mentor who is rarely available sends the message that their time is more valuable than the mentee's time, which can erode the relationship. Communication is influenced by many factors, including perceptions around hierarchy and status, introversion versus extraversion, culture of origin, level of trust, and perception of intent. Mentors may need to address these factors with their mentee. Mentors who are in a position to evaluate their mentee need to disassociate from this role when providing mentorship. Other conflicts of interest can arise around intellectual property, credit for work, or perceived competition.

Box 1
Strategies for mentors

1. Be available. Responding in a timely fashion to emails and telephone calls shows your mentee that you value their time.

2. Be prepared. For example, if you are meeting to discuss a research project, have your ideas and thoughts about the project readily accessible.

3. Actively listen. Do not interrupt your mentee when they are speaking. If you do not understand something, ask for clarification.

4. Be supportive and encouraging. Maintain a positive attitude about what your mentee has accomplished, while also encouraging them to progress in their goals. When mentees experience a setback, be empathic and listen to their concerns.

5. Recognize potential. If you are on a committee in which your mentee would flourish, encourage them to become part of this committee. Sponsor your mentee for projects and experiences that will help them grow.

6. Articulate expectations of your mentee. Do this early in the mentoring relationship. Set goals and high standards for their achievement.

7. Be a role model. Your mentee will look to you as an example for professional and personal behavior.

8. Build trust. Get to know your mentee as a person. Maintain confidentiality and provide candid feedback.

STRATEGIES FOR MENTEES

Characteristics of mentees who get more out of their mentoring relationship are similar to those of successful mentors. Availability, with the ability to be flexible in this regard, preparation for meetings, and open, honest communication allow for the relationship to flourish.[2] Humility in accepting feedback and gratitude for the mentor's reinforce trust within the relationship, and foster a deeper connection (**Box 2**).

Occasionally, a mentorship relationship becomes unhelpful, contentious, or even toxic. It is difficult to end a long-standing mentoring relationship, and an impartial third party may be needed to mediate. Keep in mind that confidentiality should be safeguarded even after the relationship is terminated (**Box 3**).

SPECIFIC MENTORSHIP AND SPONSORSHIP NEEDS AMONG DIVERSE POPULATIONS

In addition to the needs and strategies described previously, women, URM, and other populations have specific mentorship needs. "Structural disadvantage from racism, gender bias, social class, and other factors can compromise mentoring relationships."[15] Because URM and female faculty are unequally distributed among otolaryngology training programs, same race and same gender mentorship relationships may not be easy to establish within the same department. Mentees can establish relationships with mentors from different departments in the same institution or within otolaryngology at other institutions. This can help with retention of talent by limiting feelings of isolation and invisibility. Although "minority residents described a sense of responsibility for addressing the gaps in minority mentorship for future generations of physicians,"[10] leaders should think about the tax on women and URM to provide the bulk of diversity-related mentorship. Gender and racially discordant mentors should be encouraged to provide mentorship. The Association of Women Surgeons #HeForShe Task Force suggests that deliberate creation of mentoring partnerships helps to eliminate bias by facilitating interpersonal bonds.[16] Instead of purposefully assigning

---

Box 2
Strategies for mentees

1. Do not limit yourself to one mentor. Although one mentor may be having the type of career you want to pursue, they may not have similar hobbies or the same perspective on family life as you. It is okay and often necessary to be mentored in different realms by different people.

2. Have a set of goals in mind. Think about these questions: (1) What do you need to know or do to pursue your career path? (2) How can your mentor help you accomplish your goals? Try to be honest and open with your mentor about what you would like to get out of the relationship.

3. Respect your mentor's time. Set expectations about how often you will meet and for how long. Be prepared and punctual for these meetings.

4. Be open to feedback. Remember that failure is part of development. Your mentor will have high expectations of you and will push you. They are trying to make you the best you can be. Do not stop investing in a relationship because of a single failure or poor communication.

5. Remain confidential. This is a two-way street. You do not want your mentor to divulge information about you, but you also do not want to compromise your mentor's trust by divulging their comments to others.

6. Express gratitude for help. A simple "thank you for your time" goes a long way. Remember that your mentor is taking time away from their career development, family, and time off to help your development.

---

women or URM mentees with in-group mentors, leaders can decrease bias by assigning mentees with mentors outside of their demographic.[16] This allows for people to get to know others on an individual level instead of as a stereotype.[16] To be most effective, mentors should learn about perceived differences in mentoring by mentees of a different gender or race. It is "less important to have a coach identify as underrepresented than to have a coach who understands the importance of culture and how it might affect the coaching relationship."[17]

Specific issues to consider for women mentees can stem from the societal expectation that women be collaborative and agreeable. Women may not feel comfortable asking for a specific sponsorship opportunity or highlighting their own accomplishments.[18] Women with families can also experience "mommy track" bias, where mentors or sponsors assume they will not be interested in opportunities that require travel or evening meetings. Mentors can also have an impact overcoming the phenomenon in which women only apply for positions when they meet 100% of the qualifications, whereas men will apply if they meet 60% of the criteria. This is often ascribed to a lack of confidence but may also relate to women being socialized to follow the rules when it comes to meeting requirements.

Box 3
When to change mentors

1. Neglect: Your mentor does not respond to emails, fails to show up for meetings, and demonstrates a lack of interest.

2. Manipulation: Your mentor takes credit for your work, or threatens to cut off your relationship if you do not do projects he or she wants you to do.

3. Lack of experience: You want to learn to write a National Institutes of Health grant, but your mentor has not done this before. It is often useful to discuss these situations with another trusted mentor.

Table 3
Resources for racial- and gender-discordant mentorship relationships

Organization	Web Site
Alliance for Academic Internal Medicine	https://www.im.org/resources/diversity-inclusion
Association of American Medical Colleges	https://www.aamc.org/what-we-do/mission-areas/diversity-inclusion/unconscious-bias-training
Association of Program Directors in Radiology	https://www.apdr.org/program-directors/DEI-Curriculum
Association of Program Directors in Surgery	https://apds.org/program-directors/apds-diversity-and-inclusion-toolkit/

Specific issues to consider for URM mentees also frequently stem from societal expectations. Persons of color can suffer from the double-edged sword of being invisible and attracting attention. Because of societal expectations, the ideas, opinions, and needs of people of color may be ignored or given less weight. At the same time, people of color may be unfairly expected to speak for everyone in their ethnic group, be confused with the few other people of color in their organization, and expected to bear the burden of always being involved in any diversity-related initiatives.

Strategies for increasing women and URM within the field often overlap with mentoring. Such initiatives as creating a culture of inclusion, deliberate recruitment of diverse candidates, pay equity, funding for scholarly activities, and focusing on retention have a greater effect when mentorship relationships are also prioritized. Diversity programs with "greater intensity, defined as present for more than 5 years and with more components, are more effective."[12] It has been demonstrated within otolaryngology that the number of URM faculty within a department correlates with the number of URM residents matriculated to that program.[19] In addition, including diverse candidates in recruitment efforts increases the chance of hiring a minority only after there are two or more minority candidates.[19] It is therefore important to pursue recruitment and retention strategies deliberately at every career level.

Several excellent resources are available to strengthen mentorship initiatives among gender- or race-discordant relationships. An excellent resource is Osman and Gottlieb's MedEdPortal publication, Mentoring Across Differences, which provides interactive sessions for faculty training in mentoring.[15] Additional World Wide Web–based resources are found in **Table 3**.

SUMMARY

Mentorship and sponsorship are critically important for otolaryngologists at all levels of their career, from medical students first identifying an interest in the specialty, to mid and late career practicing otolaryngologists. Mentorship is typically found within a long-term professional relationship and provides career advice and support. Sponsorship is a more transactional relationship that promotes the mentee for specific career advancement opportunities. Both help mentees achieve more in their careers and have higher career satisfaction. Increasing the number of women and URM in otolaryngology is dependent on meeting the specific mentorship and sponsorship needs of these populations.

DISCLOSURE

The author has nothing to disclose.

REFERENCES

1. Ayyala MS, Skarupski K, Bodurtha JN, et al. Mentorship is not enough: exploring sponsorship and its role in career advancement in academic medicine. Acad Med 2019;94(1):94–100.
2. Sanfey H, Hollands C, Gantt NL. Strategies for building an effective mentoring relationship. Am J Surg 2013;206(5):714–8.
3. Sambunjak D, Straus SE, Marušić A. Mentoring in academic medicine: a systematic review. JAMA 2006;296(9):1103–15.
4. Patel VM, Warren O, Ahmed K, et al. How can we build mentorship in surgeons of the future? ANZ J Surg 2011;81(6):418–24.
5. Cohee BM, Koplin SA, Shimeall WT, et al. Results of a formal mentorship program for internal medicine residents: can we facilitate genuine mentorship? J Grad Med Educ 2015;7(1):105–8.
6. Lin SY, Laeeq K, Malik A, et al. Otolaryngology training programs: resident and faculty perception of the mentorship experience. Laryngoscope 2013;123(8):1876–83.
7. Gurgel RK, Schiff BA, Flint JH, et al. Mentoring in otolaryngology training programs. Otolaryngol Head Neck Surg 2010;142(4):487–92.
8. Geltzeiler MN, Lighthall JG, Wax MK. Mentorship in otolaryngology: 10 years of experience. Otolaryngol Head Neck Surg 2013;148(2):338–40.
9. Ukatu CC, Welby Berra L, Wu Q, et al. The state of diversity based on race, ethnicity, and sex in otolaryngology in 2016. Laryngoscope 2019. https://doi.org/10.1002/lary.28447.
10. Yehia BR, Cronholm PF, Wilson N, et al. Mentorship and pursuit of academic medicine careers: a mixed methods study of residents from diverse backgrounds. BMC Med Educ 2014;14:26.
11. Pololi L, Cooper LA, Carr P. Race, disadvantage and faculty experiences in academic medicine. J Gen Intern Med 2010;25(12):1363–9.
12. Lin SY, Francis HW, Minor LB, et al. Faculty diversity and inclusion program outcomes at an academic otolaryngology department. Laryngoscope 2016;126(2):352–6.
13. Khan NR, Rialon KL, Buretta KJ, et al. Residents as mentors: the development of resident mentorship milestones. J Grad Med Educ 2017;9(4):551–4.
14. Straus SE, Johnson MO, Marquez C, et al. Characteristics of successful and failed mentoring relationships: a qualitative study across two academic health centers. Acad Med 2013;88(1):82–9.
15. Osman NY, Gottlieb B. Mentoring across differences. MedEdPORTAL 2018;14:10743.
16. DiBrito SR, Lopez CM, Jones C, et al. Reducing implicit bias: Association of Women Surgeons #HeForShe task force best practice recommendations. J Am Coll Surg 2019;228(3):303–9.
17. Najibi S, Carney PA, Thayer EK, et al. Differences in coaching needs among underrepresented minority medical students. Fam Med 2019;51(6):516–22.
18. Levine RB, Ayyala MS, Skarupski KA, et al. "It's a little different for men"-sponsorship and gender in academic medicine: a qualitative study. J Gen Intern Med 2020. https://doi.org/10.1007/s11606-020-05956-2.
19. Newsome H, Faucett EA, Chelius T, et al. Diversity in otolaryngology residency programs: a survey of otolaryngology program directors. Otolaryngol Head Neck Surg 2018;158(6):995–1001.

Increasing the Number of Black Otolaryngologists

Erin K. O'Brien, MD*, Dontre' M. Douse, MD, Semirra L. Bayan, MD,
Janalee K. Stokken, MD, Kathryn M. Van Abel, MD

KEYWORDS

• Black • Bias • Diversity • Medical student • Residency

KEY POINTS

- Otolaryngology has one of the lowest percentages of Black physicians of any surgical specialty at 0.8%. The number of Black residents in otolaryngology has not increased in recent years, despite an emphasis on the need for increased diversity in the field.
- Metrics used for selection for otolaryngology residency positions, such as step 1 scores, clerkship grades, Alpha Omega Alpha membership, and number of publications, show evidence of racial bias and inequality and do not reliably predict successful residents. Overreliance on these criteria for interviews and rankings may disproportionately exclude Black medical students from matching into otolaryngology.
- In order to intentionally increase the number of Black physicians in the specialty, one must take active steps to recruit and mentor Black medical students through outreach in the first and second year of medical school, mentoring, and funded research and clinical opportunities.
- The number of Black trainees in otolaryngology has not increased in the last 13 years since the creation of the diversity committee of the American Academy of Otolaryngology–Head and Neck Surgery and the 5 years since the creation of the Society of University Otolaryngologists diversity committee.
- Residency interview selection should include a more holistic review of medical students' applications, implicit bias training for residency selection committee members, and intentional reviews of Black medical students' applications to identify candidates with qualifications that align with the department's goals, including the goal of increased diversity.

INTRODUCTION

Black Americans make up 13% of the population but only 5% of practicing physicians in the United States. The percentage of Black otolaryngologists is even lower, one of the lowest of any surgical specialty at 0.8%.[1] Although the percentage of Black matriculants into US medical schools has been slowly increasing (7.1% of all medical students in 2019), the percentage of Black trainees in the field has remained low and stagnant at

Department of Otolaryngology-Head and Neck Surgery, Mayo Clinic, 200 First Street, Rochester, MN 55905, USA
* Corresponding author.
E-mail address: obrien.erin@mayo.edu

Otolaryngol Clin N Am 54 (2021) 457–470
https://doi.org/10.1016/j.otc.2020.11.017
0030-6665/21/© 2020 Elsevier Inc. All rights reserved.

2.3% of residents in 2017.[2,3] This underrepresentation of the Black community is not only unethical, but has significant impact on quality patient care. Minority patients frequently report being more satisfied with the care they receive from racially concordant physicians, and having a diverse faculty results in improved training outcomes, promotes research that addresses disparity, and is associated with improved recruitment of diverse study populations into clinical trials.[4–9] In order to intentionally shape the future of otolaryngology to include more Black otolaryngologists, active steps must be taken now to improve recruitment, training, retention, and promotion of Black medical students to become otolaryngologists. In this article, the authors review the data on inequities in the grading and promotion of Black medical students that may negatively impact their opportunities to apply for and be accepted into otolaryngology residencies. The authors describe active measures to intentionally increase the number of Black and other underrepresented minority (URM) physicians into otolaryngology.

HISTORY

Racism and the active exclusion of Black Americans from medicine, surgical training, and otolaryngology grew out of the enslavement of African people more than 400 years ago. Despite the dissolution of slavery on June 19, 1865, systemic racism, race medicine, mass incarceration, poverty, education inequity, and both implicit and explicit bias, or racism, remain active barriers in 2020 to the education and upward mobility of Black Americans. Although this article focuses on access for Black medical students looking to become otolaryngologists, it is recognized that this is an incredibly small effort in what will truly be required to achieve racial parity within the field.

The history of medical training in the United States provides some background on inequities in the training of Black physicians. Born in 1762 and spending most of his life in slavery, James Durham was taught the practice of medicine by his owners and is considered the first African American physician in the United States.[10] In 1813, Dr James McCune Smith earned a medical degree in Glasgow, Scotland (because it was illegal for a Black man in the United States to earn an MD) and became the first practicing Black physician in the United States. Because of the "color line in medicine," it was not until 1847 that the first African American medical student graduated from a US institution.[11] From this momentous date, medical education of Black physicians, although still segregated, slowly but steadily grew until the publication of the Flexner Report.

Abraham Flexner was an education specialist who traveled to 155 medical schools in an effort to assess the state of medical education in the United States and Canada. He is credited with influencing the underlying structure of medical education in North America today and also with the disproportionately low numbers of Black physicians.[11,12] In his report in 1910 to the Carnegie Foundation, he cited a need for Black physicians, but stated that Black physicians should care only for Black patients. Flexner went on to say that Black physicians should be trained as "sanitarians" in "hygiene rather than surgery." He conceded that there would not be enough Black physicians to care for Black patients in the segregated system of health care that he described. Flexner's racist recommendations for improving medical education led to the closure of 5 of the 7 predominantly Black medical schools. The remaining 2 schools were subsequently responsible for training up to three-quarters of Black students until the 1960s when all medical schools were integrated.[12,13] This report had astonishing and lasting effects. The percentage of Black physicians in 1910 was 2.5%.[12] This number decreased, despite population growth, to 2.2% in the 1950s and 1960s.[14] Recent efforts to improve racial parity have result in growth to 5% of the workforce currently, but this lags far behind the US Black population.[12,14]

The lack of diversity in medicine has been associated with racial disparities in health outcomes. Minority patients are more likely to receive lower-quality care and have lower access to health care.[15] Because Black and URM physicians are more likely to care for minority patients in underserved areas with better patient satisfaction and communication, increasing the diversity of medical trainees may help address health disparities in medicine.[8,16,17] In addition, diversity in health care can improve cultural competency of the workforce, improve medical research, and influence health care policy.[18] Although race, as opposed to ancestry, is a social and not a genetic construct, it is associated with health disparities and survival differences for both pediatric and adult patients with otolaryngologic conditions.[19–22] Increasing the number of Black physicians in otolaryngology by increasing the number of Black residents in training programs could lead to a significant improvement in outcomes for Black and other minority patients.

Dr William Harry Barnes became the first practicing Black otolaryngologist after graduating from the University of Pennsylvania Medical School in 1913. Despite his legacy, the percentage of Black physicians in otolaryngology remains one of the lowest of any surgical specialty.[23,24] In a 2015 survey of members by the American Academy of Otolaryngology–Head and Neck Surgery (AAO-HNS), only 0.8% of the approximately 12,000 members identified as Black or African American.[1] Investigators of a study involving a survey of Black otolaryngologists identified only 124 Black physicians in the specialty.[1] As compared with increases in the population in the United States, the representation of Black otolaryngologists in the United States has decreased from 1990 to 2016 with underrepresentation of Black academic otolaryngologists at the assistant, associate, and full-professor level.[25] This low number of practicing and academic Black otolaryngologists is mirrored in the unacceptably low number of Black otolaryngology trainees.

The already low number of Black residents in otolaryngology decreased from 43 or 3.6% of otolaryngology residents in 1996 to 25 or 2.3% Black otolaryngology residents in 2004.[26] A more recent analysis of the number of women and minority applicants and residents in otolaryngology found that both the number of Black applicants and the number of Black residents decreased between 2008 and 2017; in 2017, there were just 37 Black residents, making up 2.3% of the trainee body, despite the growth of otolaryngology trainee positions.[3] A 2013 study found that unlike family medicine, internal medicine, and general surgery, from 1975 to 2010, otolaryngology did not have an increase in the number of Black residents.[27] This finding is in contrast to both women and other URM residents in otolaryngology, which, although still underrepresented, did increase.[27] A survey of program directors in otolaryngology reported in 2018 that more than one-third of respondents had matriculated one or fewer URM physicians into their program in the past 15 years. In this same study, more than half of the programs had one or fewer URM faculty member.[28] Despite increased recognition of the need to address diversity in otolaryngology, as outlined by Dr Steven Sims in an editorial in 2010[29] and in the responses by Academy leaders describing the efforts to address the lack of diversity,[30,31] these sentiments have not been reflected in the number of Black otolaryngology residents. The reasons for this lack of progress are not well delineated and may be related to both the historic disparity in the training of Black medical students and the modern selection process for residency positions in otolaryngology.

Otolaryngology has become incredibly competitive. A survey of medical students found that 80% considered matching into otolaryngology to be "near impossible" or "impossible."[32] In 2016, applicants to otolaryngology residency had an average United States Medical Licensing Examination (USMLE) step 1 score of 248, with

44.7% in the Alpha Omega Alpha (AOA) Honor Society with an average of 8.4 publications, abstracts, or presentations.[33] This number is significantly higher than most other specialties. The survey of medical students reported that students felt discouraged from applying to otolaryngology if they had a step 1 score less than the average for those applicants who matched from the previous year.[32] These metrics are used frequently as an initial screening filter by programs in an attempt to make the overwhelming number of applicants to their program more reasonable to review.

Traditionally, high emphasis has been placed on these metrics for matching into otolaryngology residency positions; however, there are no strong findings associating step 1 scores, AOA membership, or the number of publications with residency performance. A review by Daly and colleagues[34] found that USMLE scores did not correlate with faculty ranking of otolaryngology resident success and correlated with in-service scores only for the second year of residency. Although AOA membership was associated with faculty assessment in the top one-third of an otolaryngology residency class, in another study, AOA membership was not associated with a multisource assessment of professionalism of internal medicine residents at Mayo Clinic.[34,35] An applicant's number of publications was found to be associated with matching into otolaryngology but not with performance during residency.[36] Furthermore, an examination of publications cited on otolaryngology residency applications found between 9.8% and 23% of applicants misrepresented their contributions or number of publications.[37,38] Finally, up to 90% of program directors reported having at least 1 resident on active probation, despite these incredibly high scores and honors.[39]

Beyond being poor predictive metrics for performance in residency, there is evidence that step 1 and clerkship scores, AOA membership, the expectation of having a high number of publications, and summative Medical Student Performance Evaluations (MSPE) show bias against Black medical students. An examination of USMLE scores in 1994 identified both gender and racial differences in step 1 scores with lower scores for women and lower pass rates for Black students.[40] Further examination of step 1 scores in a 2019 paper found that Black students scored on average 16 points lower on all step examinations compared with white students, although when factoring in other covariates, such as undergraduate grades and MCAT scores, the difference was reduced to 4 to 5 points.[41] An examination of applicants to internal medicine residency found that step 1 cutoff scores would disproportionly exclude Black medical students from interview offers.[42]

Medical school clerkship grades, often based on some combination of subjective assessments and examinations, also demonstrate racial disparities. In the study of medical student residency applications from 2014 to 2016, the investigators found lower clerkship scores for Black students, findings similar to a 2007 study that also reported lower clerkship scores for Black students in all clinical rotations.[43,44] In another review of clerkship grades, URM medical students received lower clerkship director ratings than non-underrepresented students; although the difference was relatively small, the lower ratings resulted in minority students receiving half as many honors grades and being 3 times less likely to be inducted into an honors society.[45] The subjective nature of this grading system raises concerns about implicit bias or racism.

The AOA Honor Medical Society uses students' formal academic records to identify the upper quartile of a medical school class for eligibility for AOA. The weight of the metrics of criteria for selection into AOA, such as academics and leadership, is decided by each medical school's chapter, and nominees are voted on by active chapter members each year, with a majority vote required for selection.[46] In a study reviewing medical student applications to residency from 2014 to 2016, only 2.2% of AOA members identified as Black.[44] White students were found to be 6 times more likely to be selected for AOA membership than Black students, which could affect not only residency applications but also future career opportunities in academic medicine.[47] The evidence of bias in AOA selection has resulted in several medical schools, including Icahn School of Medicine at Mount Sinai in New York, abandoning AOA altogether.[48]

Recently, the number of presentations, abstracts, or publications has increased to an average of 8.4 per successful otolaryngology applicant.[33] In fact, it is increasingly becoming the norm that medical students striving toward an otolaryngology residency position take a year or more to accomplish research in the hopes of improving their competitiveness.[33] There is little evidence that research productivity as a medical student is associated with success as a resident, and much evidence to the contrary.[36,49–51] In addition, most of the 1-year research positions offered at academic centers do not offer funding to trainees seeking to engage in research for the year. The lack of funding to cover living expenses for students discriminates against applicants who are unable financially to support themselves in an unpaid position for that period of time. Although there are some scholarships available, these are few and far between, leaving Black applicants with yet another barrier between themselves and a successful application to otolaryngology.

Finally, an examination of words to describe medical students in the summative MSPE found significant differences by race, with white students described more often by "standout" or "ability" keywords and Black students more often described as "competent"; the competency adjectives however only had a positive connotation 37% of the time for Black students but 57% of the time for white students.[52] The racial differences in step 1 scores, AOA selection, clerkship grades, and even dean's letter (MSPE) descriptors lead to what these investigators describe as small differences in medical school adding up to an "amplification cascade" of large consequences in the careers of URM physicians (**Table 1**).[45]

Although these barriers to improving diversity within otolaryngology and access for Black residents in the field are daunting, they are not insurmountable. It must first be acknowledged that despite recent efforts to improve diversity, there remains an unacceptable lack of improvement in recruiting and maintaining Black and URM otolaryngology residents.[30] We must then engage in honest and humble discussion, dedicate ourselves as a specialty to educating ourselves about these issues, and commit as a community to making a change. We must identify and implement strategies that actively address recruitment and retention into otolaryngology, no longer relying on Black and URM medical students to break through the nearly impossible barriers set before them to be the change we all need. We propose several intentional steps to actively recruit Black medical students and address biased metrics used in residency interview selection and rankings with the goal of training and retaining Black otolaryngologists.

DISCUSSION

The "leaky pipeline" involves a loss of URM students and physicians in each step of training and promotion.[53,54] Intentional interventions can increase retention of underrepresented undergraduate and medical students, who may then ultimately go on to a successful career in otolaryngology. Programs to increase the number of Black and URM students in medicine should begin as early as primary and secondary school with access to STEM curriculum, mentorship, and identification of financial opportunities. Current Black otolaryngology residents have cited undergraduate and post-baccalaureate programs focused on URM students as having made a significant impact in their opportunity to attend medical school (personal communication Shannon Fayson, MD, 2020). A program created by surgeons to increase the number of

Table 1
Traditionally used metrics that contribute to the "amplification cascade" of barriers for Black and underrepresented minority students to successfully match into otolaryngology–head and neck surgery residency

Metric	Unfavorable Impact
High mean USMLE step 1 score	Black and URM students disproportionally excluded from interview offers at residency programs with high step 1 cutoffs typically used for otolaryngology–head and neck surgery (oto-HNS)
AOA membership	AOA not offered by all medical schools, and AOA membership significantly skewed based on race, with a disproportionately low number of Black students
Mean number of publications, presentations, and/or abstracts (>8.4)	Disproportionate exclusion of Black and URM students who may not have as many research opportunities at their home institution or may not be have the financial resources to support themselves during an unpaid research internship
Clerkship grade/MSPE	Black students are less likely to receive honors in clinical clerkships Possible exclusion of potential Black or URM residents who may be described as "competent" instead of "standout" secondary to implicit bias associated with word choice

women and URM students applying to procedure-based residencies provides a roadmap for increasing the number of Black trainees in otolaryngology.[55] The authors review the successive steps in the pipeline beginning with medical students. Focusing on educational opportunities at earlier time points, although critical, is outside the scope of this publication.

Medical School

Increasing the number of Black physicians in otolaryngology residencies begins with increasing interest in the field early in medical school and providing both mentorship and research opportunities. The goal is to foster curiosity and interest in otolaryngology while helping each student create a competitive application through meaningful experiences, the creation of a relationship with a mentor, and an increased number of publications. The Nth Dimensions Pipeline Initiatives Curriculum was created by a non-for-profit organization of general surgeons to increase the number of women and URM medical students applying for surgery and other procedure-based residencies.[55] The program focused on 3 steps: (1) increasing initial exposure and hands-on experience such as bioskills and surgical technique workshops; (2) clinical and research experience with shadowing physicians and completing a research project with poster presentation; and (3) mentoring and professional development for second through fourth year of medical school. Initial results from the Nth Dimensions program found increased retention of women and URM students applying for and matching into surgical and procedural residencies (72.3%).[55] Studies in our own specialty have cited the benefit of similar interventions in the choice and success in matching into otolaryngology.

Early exposure may be critical to a Black medical student's decision to pursue a career in otolaryngology. Black otolaryngologists surveyed about their specialty choice reported that early exposure to otolaryngology and enjoyment of their otolaryngology rotation were significant factors in applying for residency in the specialty.[1] Otolaryngology faculty and current residents should offer more opportunities for interactions with medical students early in their medical school careers, with hands-on procedural skills workshops and shadowing opportunities. Additional exposure through active engagement by otolaryngology faculty in anatomy courses during the first 2 years of the students' preclinical training should be encouraged. These opportunities should be intentionally offered and encouraged for URM and Black medical students through medical school diversity programs and minority organizations, such as the Student National Medical Association (SNMA) medical school chapter.

Clinical and research experience for URM students has been shown to be effective for matriculation into otolaryngology training programs. To increase the pipeline of URM students applying for otolaryngology residency, Johns Hopkins Department of Otolaryngology–Head and Neck Surgery created the Clerkship Program for Underrepresented Minority Medical Students.[56] Fifteen URM students from 10 medical schools completed a 1-month clinical rotation or a 3-month research clerkship. The students averaged 1.7 publications after completing the program. Six students matched into otolaryngology and 6 students matched into other surgical specialties. Three of the students matched at Johns Hopkins, increasing the number of URM residents in their program.[56] This early evidence-based approach suggests that the creation of a structured program designed to support exposure, mentorship, and research efforts resulted in successful application to surgical specialties, including otolaryngology. Additional resources for both programs and students can be found on the Web site Headmirror.com, which includes a diversity and inclusion page with a list of resources for URM students, including grants for summer clinical and research programs from the American Head and Neck Society and individual otolaryngology departments, grants to support travel for clinical rotations from the Society of University Otolaryngologists (SUO), the American Society of Pediatric Otolaryngologists, and the AAO-HNS, and the Harry Barnes, MD Endowment Leadership Grant to support otolaryngology residents of African descent from the United States, Canada, or the Caribbean to attend the AAO-HNS annual meeting.[57] Research and travel opportunities must be funded so that opportunities are not preferentially available for students with economic means. Programs emulating the goals set forth by the Johns Hopkins clerkship program should be considered at institutions across the country.

Mentorship is a critical component to successful career advancement, regardless of the field. However, likely because of the highly competitive nature of matching into otolaryngology, Black otolaryngologists in practice cited mentorship as *less* impactful than exposure and rotations in otolaryngology when choosing their specialty.[1] Despite the low number of Black and URM faculty at academic institutions, which makes identifying race-concordant mentors challenging, an association was seen between being mentored as a student and currently mentoring students and faculty, including mentoring at other institutions.[1] In addition, because faculty mentors may be less visible and ultimately spend less time with medical student trainees, residents may have a stronger influence as role models than faculty.[58,59] Although race-discordant mentorships should not be discredited, programs offering mentorship from faculty with diverse backgrounds are critical to the comfort, feelings of belonging, and support for URM students and residents.[28,60] In fact, it appears that both female and nonwhite applicants may actually cancel interviews at institutions because of a lack of women and diverse residents and faculty.[58]

Mentorship does not always require face-to-face interaction, which may allow for dedicated mentors to reach students that have few other mentorship opportunities.

For medical schools without otolaryngology programs and institutions with a high number of minority students such as medical schools affiliated with historically Black colleges and universities (HBCU), otolaryngologists can provide virtual or distance mentoring. The SUO Web site provides a list of diversity champions in academic programs for URM students interested in research opportunities, mentorship, and clinical rotations. Regardless of the race, gender, role, or physical location of a mentor, a successful mentorship requires that the mentor be invested in the mentee. Mentors should be prepared to meet regularly with their mentee to map out a strategy for successful application to otolaryngology, read and revise personal statements, host mock interviews for students, write strong letters of recommendation, and make personal telephone calls on behalf of their mentee.

Efforts to address racial inequity require active steps to address past racism and exclusion with nonblinded programs for Black and URM students. These efforts need to be funded so that mentors and preceptors are financially supported for their academic time and students receive financial resources for travel, work, and housing. In addition, mentorship should not fall primarily onto the shoulders of URM faculty; this role should be shared by all academic otolaryngologists and even by nonacademic otolaryngologists in practice. Because the number of Black trainees in otolaryngology has not increased in the last 13 years since the creation of the diversity committee of the AAO-HNS and the 5 years since the creation of the SUO diversity committee, more must be done to increase the number of Black medical students applying for and being accepted into otolaryngology residencies.

Application to Residency

In addition to increasing the number of Black medical students with an interest in otolaryngology and support for their applications with mentorship, clinical rotations, and research opportunities, we must examine how student applications are reviewed and how interviews are conducted to increase the number of accepted Black residents. Given the racial differences in clerkship scores, the MSPE or dean's letter, AOA membership and step 1 scores, the criteria for review of applications must be evaluated to decrease racial biases. Although Bowe and colleagues[61] found that, on average, medical students who matched into otolaryngology programs had above average board scores, publications, and AOA membership, these very selective metrics were not found to be associated with higher success in residency. The investigators proposed that qualifying criteria, such as minimum step 1 scores of 220 to 230, 3 publications, and top one-third of their class, be used to screen applicants for otolaryngology residency with more focus on holistic qualities in ranking applicants for interview offers. Recently, the USMLE announced that the step 1 score will be reported as pass/fail rather than a numeric 3-digit score, a change that some feel may help increase diversity, especially in the "the most competitive, and simultaneously least diverse, medical specialties."[62]

Individual programs may identify specific areas of scholarship or skills that align best with the goals of their department, such as basic science or clinical research, education, or innovation; identifying students with similar interests or experiences may identify appropriate candidates for interviews more than specific scholarship metrics like grades or scores. For departments looking to increase their own minority recruitment, the knowledge and experiences of their own residents can help improve their institutional efforts. In addition, the leadership and volunteer efforts of minority medical students often through diversity council or admissions committee positions, leadership positions in SNMA, community service, and minority student mentoring and recruitment, which require significant time commitments beyond medical school course work and rotations, speak to their ability to balance their time, efforts, and energy beyond school. Residency application review committees should discuss the value they place on extracurricular and leadership experience as they review medical students. Committees should consider the ability to overcome adversity, crisis management, and demonstration of grit and professional will, all of which have been identified as clear differentiators of success for Black medical students and physicians.[1] In addition, committees should consider "unblinded" application reviews of URM applicants in order to provide additional or secondary reviews of candidates who might not meet the most stringent academic criteria for interview selection or may have been given lower ranking for interview selections because of unconscious biases.

The review committees should participate in training on an unconscious bias as well as learning the history of racial inequity in medical education and racial differences in traditional metrics for assessing scholarship. The selection and interview committee itself should be diverse, allowing a variety of inputs and viewpoints and backgrounds. When reviewing applications, program directors and administrators can "turn off" the photographs on the Electronic Residency Application Service applications by marking photographs as nonviewable while committee members review the applications to try to decrease the potential for bias. A study on the role of physical attributes and race or ethnicity in application photographs in addition to academic metrics in selection for radiology resident interviews found that facial attractiveness more strongly predicted reviewer ratings than AOA membership or clerkship grades; race or ethnicity was less influential but still a significant predictor of reviewer ratings.[63] A follow-up study found that reviewers with more self-awareness of the potential for implicit bias were able to mitigate this risk as they reviewed applications and could compensate for potential biases, supporting the role of implicit bias testing and training.[64] Implicit bias testing and education were associated with 1 medical school's admission committee members reporting more consciousness of their own potential biases as they interviewed candidates; in the year following the implicit bias exercise, that medical school matriculated the most diverse class in the school's history, further supporting the value of this training.[65]

Interviews

Once applicants are selected for interviews, the program schedule and interviews should be structured in a way to reduce potential biases, highlight support for both past and current Black and URM trainees and faculty, and emphasize the value of diversity in the program's selection process and training program. Programs can provide access for URM candidates to meet with minority residents and faculty and provide information on the academic achievements and careers, such as publications, grants, fellowships, and leadership roles of past URM trainees. Similar strategies for improving recruitment of URM residents have been outlined by other specialties, such as work groups for increasing diversity in emergency medicine.[66]

Interviews should be structured to reduce the potential for biases and identify qualities sought by the program in their trainees. A review of literature on the value of in-person interviews to predict future performance in residency failed to establish a relationship between interview performance and success or problems for trainees during residency. The investigators did recommend that programs avoid traditional, unstructured interviews and offer standardized questions to improve interrater reliability and decrease potential biases by interviewers.[67] A surgical skills assessment during the otolaryngology residency interview was predictive of performance in residency as determined by faculty evaluations.[68] Behavioral questions regarding professionalism, leadership, trainability/suitability for the specialty, and fit for the program were found

Table 2
Proposed efforts to increase diversity in otolaryngology resident selection

Medical School Efforts	Application Review	Interview Strategies
• Hands-on bioskills oto-HNS workshops for first- and second-year medical students • Mentoring by oto-HNS faculty and residents locally and remotely, especially at HBCUs and schools without oto-HNS programs • Funded research internships • Funded clinical clerkships for visiting students	• Minimum criteria for scholastic metrics for application review • Holistic application review, including weighting leadership, mentoring, and service experience • Faculty training on racial inequities in medical school training and evaluations • Implicit bias training for faculty and residents	• Highlight support for Black and URM trainees and faculty • Provide opportunities to speak with current and past Black and URM trainees • Structured interview questions with MMI format to reduce potential for bias • Funded "second-look" weekends for Black and URM candidates

to provide information on leadership and attrition in obstetrics and gynecology residency interviews.[69] Multiple mini interviews (MMI) include stations with a behavioral descriptor or situational judgment-type question addressing a specific core competency; these MMI style interviews have been found to have correlation with future clinical examination testing and may correlate with specialty success.[67] In addition, the use of the MMI format during medical school interviews was found to result in a higher acceptance of diverse racial and ethnic candidates, whereas reliance on numbers and letters about the candidates had the potential to decrease URM applicants' acceptance.[70]

To indicate their commitment to recruiting and supporting Black trainees, some programs have used second-look weekends with opportunities for candidates to meet additional department members, trainees in other departments, Black faculty, and community members. Financial support for these second-look weekends further signals a commitment to increasing diversity and supporting trainees. Although there is no literature to show a significant correlation between participation in second-look trips and successful a match, candidates have indicated that they find these opportunities helpful in making decisions regarding their rankings of programs. Developing relationships between the department and institutional or community organizations that support diversity and minority citizens can also provide valuable connections in the recruitment of candidates who are considering moving themselves and potentially their families to these communities where they will be training.

SUMMARY

Given the lack of improvement in the disparity between the percentage of Black citizens in the United States, Black physicians in the United States, and Black physicians within otolaryngology, intentional steps must be taken to address factors that affect the opportunity to train in otolaryngology for Black medical students (**Table 2**). By understanding the disparities in the grading and promotion of Black medical students, historically, and more recently, including board scores, grades, honors, and publications, and how the overemphasis on these metrics in the selection of otolaryngology residents disproportionately excludes Black applicants, medical schools and otolaryngology training programs can be more intentional in recruiting, mentoring, interviewing, and matching Black otolaryngology residents, ultimately addressing many of the leaks in the pipeline from medical school to becoming a practicing otolaryngologist. These same measures of inclusion may extend to all underrepresented minorities, therefore improving the diversity within the specialty as part of the goal of improving care for all patients.

ACKNOWLEDGMENTS

The authors thank Shannon Fayson, MD for sharing her perspectives on the role of post–baccalaureate programs in supporting Black students in matriculating to medical school.

DISCLOSURE

The authors have nothing to disclose.

REFERENCES

1. Faucett EA, Newsome H, Chelius T, et al. African American otolaryngologists: current trends and factors influencing career choice. Laryngoscope 2020;130(10): 2336–42.
2. Percentage of matriculants to U.S. medical schools by race/ethnicity (alone), academic year 2018-2019. Available at: https://www.aamc.org/data-reports/workforce/interactive-data/figure-8-percentage-matriculants-us-medical-schools-race/ethnicity-alone-academic-year-2018-2019. Accessed August 6, 2020.
3. Lopez EM, Farzal Z, Ebert CS Jr, et al. Recent trends in female and racial/ethnic minority groups in U.S. Otolaryngology Residency Programs. Laryngoscope 2020. https://doi.org/10.1002/lary.28603.
4. Saha S, Komaromy M, Koepsell TD, et al. Patient-physician racial concordance and the perceived quality and use of health care. Arch Intern Med 1999; 159(9):997–1004.
5. Komaromy M, Grumbach K, Drake M, et al. The role of black and Hispanic physicians in providing health care for underserved populations. N Engl J Med 1996; 334(20):1305–10.
6. Moy E, Bartman BA. Physician race and care of minority and medically indigent patients. JAMA 1995;273(19):1515–20.
7. Cohen JJ. The consequences of premature abandonment of affirmative action in medical school admissions. JAMA 2003;289(9):1143–9.
8. Marrast LM, Zallman L, Woolhandler S, et al. Minority physicians' role in the care of underserved patients: diversifying the physician workforce may be key in addressing health disparities. JAMA Intern Med 2014;174(2):289–91.
9. Branson RD, Davis K, Butler KL. African Americans' participation in clinical research: importance, barriers, and solutions. Am J Surg 2007;193(1):32–9.
10. 10 History-Making Black Physicians. Available at: https://www.mdlinx.com/physiciansense/10-history-making-black-physicians/. Accessed August 6, 2020.
11. Black History Month: A Medical Perspective: Education. Available at: https://guides.mclibrary.duke.edu/blackhistorymonth/education. Accessed August 6, 2020.
12. Hlavinka E. Racial Bias in Flexner Report Permeates Medical Education Today. 06/18/2020, 2020.
13. Sullivan LW, Suez Mittman I. The state of diversity in the health professions a century after Flexner. Acad Med 2010;85(2):246–53.

14. Petersdorf RG. Not a choice, an obligation. Acad Med 1992;67(2):73–9.
15. Institute of Medicine Committee on I. Policy-level strategies for increasing the diversity of the USHW. In: Smedley BD, Butler AS, Bristow LR, editors. The nation's compelling interest: ensuring diversity in the health-care workforce. Washington, DC: National Academies Press (US) Copyright; 2004. p. 32, by the National Academy of Sciences. All rights reserved; 2004.
16. Shen MJ, Peterson EB, Costas-Muniz R, et al. The effects of race and racial concordance on patient-physician communication: a systematic review of the literature. J Racial Ethn Health Disparities 2018;5(1):117–40.
17. Laveist TA, Nuru-Jeter A. Is doctor-patient race concordance associated with greater satisfaction with care? J Health Soc Behav 2002;43(3):296–306.
18. Cohen JJ, Gabriel BA, Terrell C. The case for diversity in the health care workforce. Health Aff (Millwood) 2002;21(5):90–102.
19. Stein E, Lenze NR, Yarbrough WG, et al. Systematic review and meta-analysis of racial survival disparities among oropharyngeal cancer cases by HPV status. Head Neck 2020;42(10):2985–3001.
20. Ruthberg JS, Khan HA, Knusel KD, et al. Health disparities in the access and cost of health care for otolaryngologic conditions. Otolaryngol Head Neck Surg 2020; 162(4):479–88.
21. Jabbour J, Robey T, Cunningham MJ. Healthcare disparities in pediatric otolaryngology: a systematic review. Laryngoscope 2018;128(7):1699–713.
22. Chou V. How science and genetics are reshaping the race debate of the 21st century. Available at: http://sitn.hms.harvard.edu/flash/2017/science-genetics-reshaping-race-debate-21st-century/. Accessed August 6, 2020.
23. Francis CL, Villwock J. Diversity and inclusion-why does it matter. Otolaryngol Clin North Am 2020;53(5):927–34.
24. Ukatu CC, Welby Berra L, Wu Q, et al. The state of diversity based on race, ethnicity, and sex in otolaryngology in 2016. Laryngoscope 2020;130(12): E795–800.
25. Lett LA, Orji WU, Sebro R. Declining racial and ethnic representation in clinical academic medicine: a longitudinal study of 16 US medical specialties. Plos One 2018;13(11):e0207274.
26. Andriole DA, Jeffe DB, Schechtman KB. Is surgical workforce diversity increasing? J Am Coll Surg 2007;204(3):469–77.
27. Schwartz JS, Young M, Velly AM, et al. The evolution of racial, ethnic, and gender diversity in US otolaryngology residency programs. Otolaryngol Head Neck Surg 2013;149(1):71–6.
28. Newsome H, Faucett EA, Chelius T, et al. Diversity in otolaryngology residency programs: a survey of otolaryngology program directors. Otolaryngol Head Neck Surg 2018;158(6):995–1001.
29. Sims HS. More of the same: why isn't otolaryngology becoming more diverse? ENTtoday 2010.
30. Kuppersmith RBAT, Regan J. Change is already here. ENTtoday 2010.
31. Miller RH. Resonpse from the editor. ENTtoday 2010.
32. Kaplan AB, Riedy KN, Grundfast KM. Increasing competitiveness for an otolaryngology residency: where we are and concerns about the future. Otolaryngol Head Neck Surg 2015;153(5):699–701.
33. Bowe SN, Schmalbach CE, Laury AM. The state of the otolaryngology match: a review of applicant trends, "impossible" qualifications, and implications. Otolaryngol Head Neck Surg 2017;156(6):985–90.

34. Daly KA, Levine SC, Adams GL. Predictors for resident success in otolaryngology. J Am Coll Surg 2006;202(4):649–54.
35. Cullen MW, Reed DA, Halvorsen AJ, et al. Selection criteria for internal medicine residency applicants and professionalism ratings during internship. Mayo Clin Proc 2011;86(3):197–202.
36. Calhoun KH, Hokanson JA, Bailey BJ. Predictors of residency performance: a follow-up study. Otolaryngol Head Neck Surg 1997;116(6):647–51.
37. Beswick DM, Man LX, Johnston BA, et al. Publication misrepresentation among otolaryngology residency applicants. Otolaryngol Head Neck 2010;143(6):815–9.
38. Sater L, Schwartz JS, Coupland S, et al. Nationwide study of publication misrepresentation in applicants to residency. Med Educ 2015;49(6):601–11.
39. Bhatti NI, Ahmed A, Stewart MG, et al. Remediation of problematic residents—a national survey. Laryngoscope 2016;126(4):834–8.
40. Case SM, Swanson DB, Ripkey DR, et al. Performance of the class of 1994 in the new era of USMLE. Acad Med 1996;71(10 Suppl):S91–3.
41. Rubright JD, Jodoin M, Barone MA. Examining demographics, prior academic performance, and United States Medical Licensing Examination scores. Acad Med 2019;94(3):364–70.
42. Edmond MB, Deschenes JL, Eckler M, et al. Racial bias in using USMLE step 1 scores to grant internal medicine residency interviews. Acad Med 2001;76(12):1253–6.
43. Lee KB, Vaishnavi SN, Lau SK, et al. Making the grade:" noncognitive predictors of medical students' clinical clerkship grades. J Natl Med Assoc 2007;99(10):1138–50.
44. Wijesekera TP, Kim M, Moore EZ, et al. All other things being equal: exploring racial and gender disparities in medical school honor society induction. Acad Med 2019;94(4):562–9.
45. Teherani A, Hauer KE, Fernandez A, et al. How small differences in assessed clinical performance amplify to large differences in grades and awards: a cascade with serious consequences for students underrepresented in medicine. Acad Med 2018;93(9):1286–92.
46. Alpha Omega Alpha How Members Are Chosen. Available at: https://alphaomegaalpha.org/how.html#gsc.tab=0. Accessed July 31, 2020.
47. Boatright D, Ross D, O'Connor P, et al. Racial disparities in medical student membership in the Alpha Omega Alpha Honor Society. JAMA Intern Med 2017;177(5):659–65.
48. Gordon M. A medical school tradition comes under fire for racism. Available at: https://www.npr.org/sections/health-shots/2018/09/05/643298219/a-medical-school-tradition-comes-under-fire-for-racism. Accessed July 31, 2020.
49. Bhat R, Takenaka K, Levine B, et al. Predictors of a top performer during emergency medicine residency. J Emerg Med 2015;49(4):505–12.
50. Tolan AM, Kaji AH, Quach C, et al. The Electronic Residency Application Service application can predict accreditation council for graduate medical education competency-based surgical resident performance. J Surg Educ 2010;67(6):444–8.
51. Grewal SG, Yeung LS, Brandes SB. Predictors of success in a urology residency program. J Surg Educ 2013;70(1):138–43.
52. Ross DA, Boatright D, Nunez-Smith M, et al. Differences in words used to describe racial and gender groups in Medical Student Performance Evaluations. Plos One 2017;12(8):e0181659.

53. Barr DA, Gonzalez ME, Wanat SF. The leaky pipeline: factors associated with early decline in interest in premedical studies among underrepresented minority undergraduate students. Acad Med 2008;83(5):503–11.

54. Freeman BK, Landry A, Trevino R, et al. Understanding the leaky pipeline: perceived barriers to pursuing a career in medicine or dentistry among underrepresented-in-medicine undergraduate students. Acad Med 2016;91(7): 987–93.

55. Mason BS, Ross W, Chambers MC, et al. Pipeline program recruits and retains women and underrepresented minorities in procedure based specialties: a brief report. Am J Surg 2017;213(4):662–5.

56. Nellis JC, Eisele DW, Francis HW, et al. Impact of a mentored student clerkship on underrepresented minority diversity in otolaryngology-head and neck surgery. Laryngoscope 2016;126(12):2684–8.

57. Diversity and Inclusion. Available at: https://www.headmirror.com/diversity-and-inclusion. Accessed August 6, 2020.

58. Fairmont I, Farrell N, Johnson AP, et al. Influence of gender and racial diversity on the otolaryngology residency match. Otolaryngol Head Neck Surg 2020;162(3): 290–5.

59. Jagsi R, Griffith KA, DeCastro RA, et al. Sex, role models, and specialty choices among graduates of US medical schools in 2006–2008. J Am Coll Surgeons 2014;218(3):345–52.

60. Deas D, Pisano ED, Mainous AG 3rd, et al. Improving diversity through strategic planning: a 10-year (2002-2012) experience at the Medical University of South Carolina. Acad Med 2012;87(11):1548–55.

61. Bowe SN, Laury AM, Gray ST. Associations between otolaryngology applicant characteristics and future performance in residency or practice: a systematic review. Otolaryngol Head Neck Surg 2017;156(6):1011–7.

62. Youmans QR, Essien UR, Capers Qt. A test of diversity - what USMLE pass/fail scoring means for medicine. N Engl J Med 2020;382(25):2393–5.

63. Maxfield CM, Thorpe MP, Desser TS, et al. Bias in radiology resident selection: do we discriminate against the obese and unattractive? Acad Med 2019;94(11): 1774–80.

64. Maxfield CM, Thorpe MP, Desser TS, et al. Awareness of implicit bias mitigates discrimination in radiology resident selection. Med Educ 2020;54(7):637–42.

65. Capers Qt, Clinchot D, McDougle L, et al. Implicit racial bias in medical school admissions. Acad Med 2017;92(3):365–9.

66. Boatright D, Branzetti J, Duong D, et al. Racial and ethnic diversity in academic emergency medicine: how far have we come? Next steps for the future. AEM Educ Train 2018;2(Suppl Suppl 1):S31–9.

67. Stephenson-Famy A, Houmard BS, Oberoi S, et al. Use of the interview in resident candidate selection: a review of the literature. J Grad Med Educ 2015;7(4): 539–48.

68. Moore EJ, Price DL, Van Abel KM, et al. Still under the microscope: can a surgical aptitude test predict otolaryngology resident performance? Laryngoscope 2015; 125(2):E57–61.

69. Strand EA, Moore E, Laube DW. Can a structured, behavior-based interview predict future resident success? Am J Obstet Gynecol 2011;204(5):446.e1-3.

70. Terregino CA, McConnell M, Reiter HI. The effect of differential weighting of academics, experiences, and competencies measured by multiple mini interview (MMI) on race and ethnicity of cohorts accepted to one medical school. Acad Med 2015;90(12):1651–7.